Preventing Eating-Related and
Weight-Related Disorders

Contents

Acknowledgements

This edited volume is the outcome of an international conference hosted in May 2008 by the Department of Community Health Systems Resource Group at The Hospital for Sick Children in Toronto, Ontario, entitled *Improving the prevention of eating-related disorders: Linking collaborative research, advocacy, and policy change*. The purpose of the meeting was to bring together researchers, practitioners, and decision-makers from the fields of eating disorders and obesity to continue our dialogue about ways to seek common ground to promote health. The partnerships that have evolved as a result of these cross-discipline and cross-sector talks and collaborations provide a strong foundation for team building in prevention.

We would like to thank our co-authors for their insights shared during the conference and throughout this volume and for their continued collaborations. The topics covered in each of the book chapters are cutting-edge and pivotal for the success of future prevention work in our field. We appreciate the authors' generous sharing of their knowledge to help advance the field of prevention. Their individual and collective contributions provide a refreshing and much-needed perspective on the type of innovative intervention research and rigorous methodology required to move the field forward. We are grateful to Karima Kinlock and Sarah Bovaird for their extensive involvement in coordinating and organizing the international conference and the editing of this volume. We would like to thank Sarah Collier, Katie Walker, and Heather Harrison for their assistance with the organizing of the conference and the editing of the book.

First and foremost, I would like to acknowledge the support of my co-editors Dr. Michael Levine, Dr. Niva Piran, and Dr. Bruce Ferguson, without whom this book would not have been made possible. Their individual and collective scholarly contributions led to the success of both the edited volume and the international conference that preceded these writings. Both Niva and Michael spent countless hours planning and organizing the details of the conference and the content of the book, as well as sharing their wealth of editorial experience and expertise. I am grateful for their intellectual input. With role models like Michael and Niva, it is only a matter of time before our field reaches heightened awareness and credibility. Thank you to Michael for travelling to Toronto to jump-start the planning phase of these two important initiatives.

In addition to my personal passion for prevention research, what motivates me the most in my professional life is the unwavering support I receive daily from my mentor and co-editor Dr. Bruce Ferguson. Bruce's vision for a better world includes a steadfast commitment to improving the lives of children and youth. His loyalty and devotion to this lifelong ambition are modelled in the way he interacts with children and youth and his drive to create a supportive environment for learning, growth, well-being, and fun. Bruce's mentoring and leadership skills have touched the lives of countless students, trainees, educators, health professionals, and decision-makers, all of whom now share and embody his passion for finding ways to create a brighter future for our children and youth.

I am grateful for the support I am afforded on the home front. A huge thank-you goes to Anna and Bernie for their inspiration and ongoing support of my prevention work.

Finally, I would like to dedicate this book to my close colleagues and friends from public health—a circle of health promotion specialists who have been my collaborators and support system during my seventeen-year program of community-based prevention research. Collaborative working relationships paired with the pooling of interdisciplinary expertise and resources have created the perfect landscape for translating prevention research findings into practice and policy. In particular I would like to acknowledge Joanne Beyers, as well as Sari Simkins, Lora Stratton, Mary Turfryer, Diana Wardrope, Nancy Voorberg, Lucy Valleau, Lesley Andrade, Elaine Murkin, Cindy Scythes, Ella Manowiec, Carol MacDougall, and Jennifer Cowie-Bonne, for their expert contributions and unwavering support.

— *Gail L. McVey, PhD*

I want to thank my wife (Dr. Mary Suydam) and my co-editors—who will always be colleagues and friends. I also want to acknowledge the support and guidance I've received from so many women who have shown me (sometimes none too delicately) the important and exciting connections between the personal, the professional, and the political. My sincere thanks to (in alphabetical order): Amy, Ann, Beth, Brenda, Bryn, the Carolyns, Deb, Dianne, Eleanor, Jess, Laura, Lori, Margo, Mary, Judy, Linda, Paula, Ruth, Sarah, and Susan.

— *Michael P. Levine, PhD*

I want to thank my family, Andre, Adam, and Steven Garber for their support of my work, and for inspiring me in their generosity and insights. I am also thankful to the many participants in the Embodiment projects, to the research teams, and my colleagues, including the co-editors of this volume—Gail McVey, Michael Levine, and Bruce Ferguson—and the contributors to this volume, for shared processes and forums of knowledge construction.

— *Niva Piran, PhD*

I want to thank the authors of this volume for bringing breadth and intensity to this important area. I am grateful to my co-editors for creating a process that was always committed to excellence but also edifying and fun. Sarah Bovaird and Karima Kinlock worked hard to make it easy for me to contribute to the process. Finally, I would like to acknowledge the members of the Community Health Systems Resource Group at SickKids whose passion, focus, and knowledge keep me humble and curious and maintain my conviction that together we can and will make a difference in the lives of our children and youth.

— *H. Bruce Ferguson, PhD*

Introduction

Michael P. Levine, *Kenyon College*
Gail L. McVey, *The Hospital for Sick Children, University of Toronto*
Niva Piran, *Ontario Institute for Studies in Education, University of Toronto*
H. Bruce Ferguson, *The Hospital for Sick Children, University of Toronto*

Over the past decade, there has been an enormous amount of social and professional concern about an array of disorders related to weight, body shape, body image, and eating. On the one hand, there is research that documents that this spectrum of disordered eating and eating disorders is prevalent, serious, and often chronic (Hudson, Hiripi, Pope, & Kessler, 2007; Jones, Halford, & Dooley, 1993; Keski-Rahkonen et al., 2007; Sihvola et al., 2009). This spectrum ranges from body dissatisfaction or negative body image to restrictive dieting and disordered eating patterns (such as binge eating and compensatory behaviours that are used to counteract the ingestion of calories such as self-induced vomiting, laxative use, and excessive exercise). Furthermore, disordered eating patterns are associated with other health and mental health challenges, such as depression, anxiety disorders, and substance abuse (Gadalla & Piran, 2007; Piran & Gadalla, 2006; Seeley, Stice, & Rohde, 2009; Stice, Shaw, & Marti, 2007).

Obesity, in turn, has raised social concerns related to recent increases in its prevalence (Tremblay, Katzmarzyk, & Willms, 2002; World Health Organization, 2001), associated health challenges (Reilly et al., 2003), as well as the social stigma connected to individuals who are perceived to be obese (MacLean et al., 2009; Puhl & Heuer, 2009). Moreover, a number of risk factors for the development of clinical eating disorders, such as negative body image, restrictive dieting, binge eating, and purging behaviours, were found to be present among at least a segment of individuals who are obese (Haines & Neumark-Sztainer, 2006; Neumark-Sztainer et al., 2006;

1

Stice, Ng, & Shaw, 2010). This information has led researchers to suggest that the understanding and related health-promoting interventions of both disordered eating patterns and obesity could be enhanced through examining new, and possibly shared, theoretical lens and research programs (Neumark-Sztainer et al., 2007). The importance of addressing both disordered eating patterns and obesity relates to the prevalence of both phenomena in modern, industrialized countries across the world (Keel & Klump, 2003; Keski-Rahkonen et al., 2007).

In terms of eating disorders, across studies, the prevalence of full-blown (i.e., diagnosable) eating disorders appears to be in the range of 2-3% of the population and 5% of adolescent girls and young women. This number translates to 600,000 to 990,000 Canadians with symptoms sufficient for an eating disorder diagnosis at any one time. Moreover, two Canadian studies reveal that an even larger number of females aged 15 to 29—perhaps as many as 20-25% or another 675,000 to 850,000—while not meeting the criteria for an eating disorder, have significant subclinical symptoms that can be seriously debilitating (Jones, Bennett, Olmsted, Lawson, & Rodin, 2001; McVey, Pepler, Davis, Flett, & Abdolell, 2002).[1] There is also growing evidence that many males are troubled by their body size (i.e., being underweight or overweight) and that these concerns are correlated with body image dissatisfaction, disordered eating, and unhealthy attempts at muscle gain (Cohane & Pope, 2001; Croll, Neumark-Sztainer, Story, & Ireland, 2002; McCabe, Ricciardelli, & Finemore, 2002; McCreary & Sasse, 2002). Attention is being paid as well to the earlier ages of onset, with children as young as seven years presenting to eating disorder treatment programs.

With regard to obesity, the cause for concern worldwide is well documented (see, e.g., Kraak & Story, 2010). In Canada, the proportion of older children and adults that are either overweight or obese was twice as high in 1996 (26% in girls, 32% in boys) as it was in 1981 (13.1% in girls, 10.6% in boys) in nine of 10 provinces (Tremblay et al., 2002; Willms, Tremblay, & Katzmarzyk, 2003). In North America, the increase in percentage of obese and overweight children and youth is greater than the increase in any other disease or risk factor over the last century (Frank, Engelke, & Schmid, 2003).

Prevention is the only answer to the interlocking concerns of experts, parents, economists, and other citizens. For example, even though it is clear that the spectrum of disordered eating constitutes a significant public health problem, there will never be enough skilled clinicians across the many disciplines represented in this volume to effect a substantial reduction in using the traditional medical approach of "identify it–detect it–treat it." For example, the Institute for Health Information (2006) estimates the number of psychologists in Canada in 2004 at slightly less than 15,000.

The Canadian Psychiatric Association states that there are approximately 4,100 psychiatrists.[2] Thus, if there are approximately 19,000 psychologists and psychiatrists, and if we estimate very conservatively that the number of people suffering from an eating disorder or from significant symptoms of an eating disorder to be 1,000,000, then each professional would need to have the time, the skill, and the support to work with 52 or 53 people. Moreover, even if such a group of experts existed, and even if therapy were successful in nearly all instances—and, then, even if we were to eliminate the well-documented personal and socio-cultural barriers to treatment seeking or treatment provision (see, for example, Cachelin and Striegel-Moore, 2006)—therapeutic interventions would not have an impact on the incidence of new "cases." The implication is inescapable: we must devote considerable resources, skill, and sustained effort to prevention and we must think well beyond the paradigm of identify it–detect it–treat it/head it off.

Prevention programs seek to avoid or delay significantly the development of disordered eating and full-blown weight-related disorders. These programs intentionally and systematically intervene in ways that are designed to reduce risk factors, to increase the protective factors that provide resilience in the face of risk, and to promote health and hardiness in general. The categorization of prevention programs varies across reviews and can be confusing (see Levine and Smolak, 2006, 2008, 2009, for extended discussions). In the present book, we use the terminology championed by the National Research Council and the Institute of Medicine (NRC/IOM) (2009), branches of the National Academy of Sciences in the United States.

The NRC/IOM (2009, p. 67) proposes a continuous arc of "mental health intervention spectrum" from mental health promotion → universal prevention → selective prevention → targeted prevention → treatment → after-care, and maintenance of treatment gains. Universal prevention programs seek to change and reinforce government policies, social institutions, and common cultural practices in order to improve the "public health" of extremely large groups of citizens who have not been distinguished or segregated on the basis of individual risk. Selective prevention also has a public policy component, but the primary audience consists of people "whose risk of developing [the disorder in question] is significantly higher than average" (p. 66), as well as those who are not yet at high risk because they are non-symptomatic. The third major point on the IOM's continuum is indicated or targeted prevention. The potential participants "targeted" for this third category of programs have been identified, selected (versus selective), or screened as being "at high risk." Thus, screening "indicates" that certain people are at high risk for an eating disorder because they have high levels of negative body image, weight concerns, and/or unhealthy forms of weight management—all of which may well be "precursors" or even "warning signs" of an eating disorder.

Universal and selective forms of prevention constitute what many people still refer to as "primary prevention," whereas targeted or indicated prevention corresponds to "secondary prevention" (Levine & Smolak, 2006). Selective, as well as universal, programs are "primary" because, by definition, they have a closer connection to a fundamental goal of prevention: reducing the incidence of a disorder. According to meta-analysis reviews of outcome research, there are several promising trends in the area of targeted prevention (Stice, Shaw, & Marti, 2007). In particular, the most promising interventions for reducing symptoms of an eating disorder consist of multiple interactive sessions designed for females at late adolescence or early adulthood who show some level of weight and shape preoccupation. Quite a bit of attention has focused on several lines of research using cognitive dissonance-based interventions (Stice, Shaw, Becker, & Rohde, 2008). These methodologically rigorous research programs have made enormous contributions to establishing the prevention of disordered eating as a major part of efforts to integrate research and practice. Nevertheless, a significant shortcoming of targeted prevention is its limited reach to relatively small and select groups of individuals (mostly female) who are already adversely affected by a host of risk factors, which leaves untouched a very large portion of the population who could benefit from prevention (Austin, 2001).

Beginning in the late 1990s, studies of universal-selective prevention programs designed for non-clinical populations (individuals or groups not affected by symptoms) have emerged that have the advantage of trying to prevent risk factors and symptoms before they appear in larger samples of people. This research has been reviewed in detail by scholars in Canada (McVey, 2004; Piran, 2005, 2010), the United States (e.g., Levine & Smolak, 2006, 2008), Australia (O'Dea, 2005), and Spain (López-Guimerà & Sánchez-Carracedo, 2010). Outcome-based studies have revealed some promising trends (reviewed in Chapter 1); however, the effects sizes published to date have been small (Fingeret, Warren, Cepeda-Benito, & Gleaves, 2006; Stice & Shaw, 2004). Nevertheless, before conclusions are drawn about the efficacy of universal-selective (that is, primary) prevention programs, there is a need to improve upon the rigorousness of the research by adopting more stringent criteria such as grounding the intervention in theoretical models and extending the follow-up evaluation to assess outcome in a more meaningful way.

What else can be done to improve the effectiveness of prevention? Although this is one of the central questions we posed to each author in this volume, including ourselves, we offer some preliminary conclusions for comparison with each contributor's ideas. First, primary prevention programs need to expand beyond the individual risk factor approach and include interventions that target multiple levels (e.g., environmental factors, group norms, and social psychological processes). In the substance abuse literature, there is evidence that when we add environmental aspects of intervention (i.e., those that target multiples levels), there is a jump in effect sizes (Pentz, 2000). Second, we need to carefully select multi-level outcome indicators that are broad enough to be sensitive to the intended changes brought on by multi-level interventions (outcome and process indicators), all the while trying to shed light on the active ingredients (indirect indicators) that make an intervention sustainable over time (Green & Tones, 1999). Moreover, as noted, there is a need to address the broad spectrum of weight-related disorders in our prevention programming and provide broad, overlapping support for reducing harmful social norms and harmful but normative practices such as weight-and-shape-related teasing.

This task is particularly challenging since, on the one hand, what is considered the "norm-al," but not the normative, body in our environment is an "ideal" that is at a minimum extremely lean, contoured, and sculpted. On the other hand, our environment features innumerable activities and labour-saving devices and practices that facilitate a sedentary lifestyle while providing a clear majority of people with access to the consumption of a diet high in fat and calories and low in cost (Battle & Brownell, 1996). These adverse social factors are further enhanced through the association of low socio-economic status with heavier weight and the social stigma of obesity (Gortmaker, Must, Perrin, Sobol, & Dietz, 1993; MacLean et al., 2009). Health-promoting strategies related to both disordered eating and obesity are therefore inherently complex and require the shared creativity of researchers and professionals from varied health and mental health disciplines.

Between 2007 and 2008, two national knowledge exchange events were held in Canada: Obesity and Eating Disorders: Seeking Common Ground to Promote Health (McVey et al., 2008) and Preventing Eating-Related Disorders: Collaborative Research, Advocacy and Policy Change.[3] These two meetings were convened to enable clinical and community psychology, experimental psychology, public health, and education to (1) collectively brainstorm barriers and potential facilitators for integrating prevention research and work across the spectrum of weight-related disorders by bringing together stakeholders from the two fields of eating disorders and obesity; (2) explore theoretical frameworks drawn from the fields of public health, health promotion, prevention science, and feminist paradigms to broaden and deepen understanding about the complex issues in body weight and health; and (3) encourage dialogue among researchers, practitioners, advocates, and policy-makers involved in the prevention of weight-related disorders so as to build a foundation for collaborating on effective, multi-level approaches to promoting the health of children and youth. At a minimum, these knowledge exchange events were intended to explore ways to put into place strategies to optimize positive health outcomes by avoiding conflicting messages and by minimizing the risk of unintended harmful consequences inherent in some existing prevention strategies.

Aiming at interdisciplinary exchange, these meetings brought together stakeholders from the fields of prevention theory, public health, education (both practice and policy), program development, risk factor research, and prevention outcome research. This exchange provided unique opportunities for these individuals to share knowledge about current ideas, practices, and findings in the prevention of weight-related disorders, eating disorders, and disordered eating at a time when provincial mandates in education and public health were under review. A great deal is known about these individual disorders (see, e.g., Thompson, 2004). How they relate to each other and what this means for a broad, social systems perspective within prevention science and public health remains uncharted or poorly charted territory. Consequently, the symposia fostered communication and collaboration between internationally recognized researchers, whose expertise spanned the topics of risk, resilience, and prevention of weight-related disorders from the broader social systems perspective, and local practitioners and decision-makers from education and public health whose mandate was to promote healthy weights.

With respect to theory and knowledge that could have a significant, positive effect on public policy, there were suggested recommendations on two fronts. The first is a better integration of the prevention of weight-related disorders such as eating disorders and obesity with (1) efforts to prevent chronic diseases through more generalized processes related to healthy eating, active living, healthy weights, and smoking cessation; and (2) a focus on the promotion of mental health and other resources that foster resilience to both normative and unusual stressors. The second development is the expansion from more clinical approaches focusing directly on the individual to ecological models of prevention that target multiple contexts including individual, family, school/community, neighbourhoods, and different governmental agencies such as health and education.

The present book is one specific outcome of the symposium on collaborative research, advocacy, and policy change, although its goals and content are heavily influenced by the symposium addressing the common ground of obesity and eating disorders. The contributions to this book provide a framework for further developments in the field by shedding light on neglected and sometimes very complicated areas of theory and research and by examining the ways in which a public health approach to the universal prevention of the spectrum of weight-related disorders might help improve upon existing prevention models. The Public Health Model, as compared to a medical causal model that centres on individual responsibility, reflects the belief that psychological, health, and social problems result from the interaction between individuals and their larger environments, as shaped by familial, academic, social, cultural, economic, and political factors. This model offers a non-stigmatizing way to share the responsibility for developing, implementing, evaluating, disseminating, and sustaining healthy lifestyle strategies equally across all children, youth, and their families. Moreover, in promoting universal prevention (but integrating it with other levels of prevention and treatment), the focus is on the collaborative, community-based construction of optimal healthy environments for children and youth and their families rather than on individually targeting, for example, children and adolescents at a very high risk for eating disorders or working solely with larger children and focusing exclusively on their eating and/or activity levels.

We are excited and proud to have internationally recognized authors from Canada, the United States, and Australia contribute chapters that are current, innovative, and forward thinking. The prevention-related topics deviate from those typically presented during conferences on prevention, and we encouraged the authors and each other to highlight what is currently on or even beyond the horizon. For example, relatively little prevention outcome research has focused on addressing children and youth's needs in multiple contexts and on examining ways to link the various systems of care that wrap around our children and youth. Consequently, the first section of this book examines the need for, and status of, ecological-systemic approaches to prevention. These approaches are outlined and elaborated through the lens of theory and various types of applied research. A variety of perspectives are represented, including prevention science, feminist theory, developmental psychopathology, public health, and media literacy. In Chapter 1, after consideration of the basic concepts and terminology, Michael Levine and Gail McVey examine the field of prevention science, an important development for improving programming, research, dissemination, and advocacy. They consider central current trends in prevention theory and outcome research. Special attention is given to innovative socio-ecological models derived from feminist principles, which appear to have implications for the synchronous prevention of eating disorders, obesity, and other mental health disorders. The

Feminist-Ecological-Developmental-Ecological Model provides a road map to guide research and practice by adults related to the health needs of children and youth (Levine & Smolak, 2006; Piran, 1999, 2001). Child development and, to a very real degree, the personal and professional development of adults committed to prevention must be understood in the context of interrelated systems that determine, and are determined by, the developing child. This understanding necessitates collaborative and integrative approaches to prevention, to professional development, and to social change — of which the Ontario Project, also described in Chapter 1 — is highlighted.

The contributions by Lindsay McLaren and Niva Piran in Chapter 2 and by Susan Paxton in Chapter 3 provide an in-depth review of how to move prevention forward through population-based research. These chapters emphasize that a population health approach aims to improve the health of the entire population and to reduce health inequities among population groups. To achieve population-level impact, the direct target of change is the conditions in which behaviours occur rather than the behaviours themselves. McLaren and Piran introduce the population health framework (e.g., the public health intervention ladder) and identify how it applies to the prevention of weight-related disorders. They describe the Health-Promoting School Model of the European Network of Health-Promoting Schools as an example of a community-based intervention that provides a possible path to sustained, population-level prevention of disordered eating. Paxton's chapter describes innovative steps that have been taken at the public policy/government level in Victoria, Australia, to bring about changes that promote healthy social and physical environments. One such initiative is Body Image and Health Incorporated, which has as its goal to change the social environments that encourage the endorsement of an unhealthy body ideal and weight loss practices, with a focus on the fashion industry and media (e.g., collaboration with fashion companies to promote models with a wider range of body types and the marketing of designer clothes in all sizes).

The importance of improving the cultural environment though activism and advocacy in the field of the prevention of weight-related disorders is accentuated in Chapter 4 by Levine and Joe Kelly and in Chapter 5 by Manuela Ferrari. Levine and Kelly distinguish *activism* (responding negatively to unhealthy messages and positively to healthy messages) from *advocacy* (using principles and forms of mass media to promote and market positive social changes). They describe how the rapidly evolving "new media" pose ongoing challenges to the development of media literacy by both professionals and youth so that various constituencies can bring individual, group, and organizational strategies to bear on media activism and media advocacy. Definitions, applications, current controversies, and limits of media literacy are described in terms of their relevance to the prevention of weight-related disorders. Ferrari subsequently explores ways in which cyberactivism can extend the benefits of the more traditional methods of activism at the cultural level. Up-to-date Internet-based tools and communication strategies are proposed as potential and potent vehicles to optimize interactive social networking to bring about changes in social systems and policies.

Risk factor research remains a cornerstone of prevention science and public health. The second section of the book highlights theory and research in the areas of risk and resilience that have important implications for the prevention of the spectrum of weight-related disorders. In Chapter 6, Linda Smolak distinguishes between malleable and fixed-risk factors and delineates the requirements for establishing a risk factor as causal. Biological, socio-cultural, and psychological risk and protective factors (each of which varies with age, gender, ethnicity, social class, and other broad culturally defined factors) are described in terms of their roles in a feminist-ecological-developmental perspective regarding the etiology of body image concerns and disordered eating. Borrowing from the disciplines of philosophy, critical sociology, and psychology, Piran and Tanya Teall introduce in Chapter 7 an innovative developmental theory of embodiment and explain its important implications for understanding and preventing disordered eating and body weight preoccupation. They also discuss differences between the constructs of embodiment and body image. Piran's theory of embodiment proposes that interpersonal and other social experiences, related to the intersection of gender, weight, ethnicity, and other aspects of social location, activate three core pathways that shape an individual's experience of his or her body: (1) experiences in the physical domain; (2) experiences in the mental domain produced by exposure to dominant social labels and expectations; and (3) experiences related to social power. The authors describe a long-standing program of qualitative and quantitative risk factor and prevention research conducted by Piran in Ontario, Canada, which supports embodiment theory and its significance for prevention.

In Chapter 8, Smolak and Piran address the critically important topic of gender differences in the nature and etiology of body image, with an emphasis on how differences in the "lived" experience of boys and girls contribute to the gendering of positive and negative body image as well as disordered eating. Smolak and Piran demonstrate how objectification, sexism, and violence against females must be acknowledged and then integrated into a feminist-ecological-developmental approach to prevention. This chapter reinforces Piran's (2010, pp. 183-84) recent contention that

> the goal of feminist informed prevention programs is the transformation of social systems towards the goal of equity, with an emphasis on the body being a site of rights, agency, and freedom. Such a transformation, which counteracts the adverse influences of patriarchy and other systems of privilege, is the responsibility of all stakeholders in the community and is shaped by and empowers members of the community most adversely affected, in the case of eating disorder prevention most often girls and women of diverse social locations.

The chapters by Smolak and Piran leave no doubt that the concepts of risk and risk reduction are very important components of current and future prevention work. In Chapter 9, Leora Pinhas and Benjamin Taylor delve deeper into the matter of conceptualizing and communicating about risk for professional and lay audiences. Pinhas and Taylor outline the interplay between risk perception, risk communication, and health behaviour, illuminating how these apparently simple, yet ultimately slippery, ideas apply to obesity and eating disorders. Limitations of the body mass index (BMI) as a measure of individual risk are discussed, as are the potential negative health, psychological, and behavioural effects arising from risk classification of children at early stages of development. Although epidemiology continues to have an important place in prevention and public health, important changes in standards and definitions of obesity play a role in the reporting and prevalence figures for obesity. Pinhas and Taylor's chapter stresses, therefore, that numbers alone, without consideration of context or explanation, can be misleading and should never serve as the sole source for decision-making concerning prevention policy and/or funding allocation. The authors also point out that despite increases in the prevalence of weight bias, which parallel reported rates of age and race discrimination, there remain no legal or social sanctions against this form of discrimination. Yet, the negative emotional and physical health consequences associated with weight discrimination act as barriers to the acceptance and proliferation of the very same health promotion behaviours that are implicated in the prevention of weight-related disorders. Finally, Pinhas and Taylor point out that the risk perception surrounding the obesity "epidemic" has overshadowed the seriousness and prevalence of eating disorders, pushing aside efforts to develop public health models of prevention that could assist in the prevention of the full spectrum of weight-related disorders.

Chapter 10, authored by McLaren and colleagues, concludes the book's second section. As noted earlier, Piran's embodiment theory, supported by her previous investigations of prevention (see, e.g., Piran, 2001), indicts disparities in, and abuses of, social power as one pathway in the development of negative body image and disordered eating. Consequently, we asked McLaren and her colleagues to describe the association between socio-economic position, health status, and weight-related disorders and to address the need to take social inequalities into consideration when developing prevention efforts. Inequalities occur along multiple axes including race/ethnicity, gender, immigration, education, and employment. From a prevention perspective, it is important to adapt efforts to the particular socio-economic circumstances of the groups defined as being in need of intervention. For example, in the case of obesity prevention, one might consider group-based and income-related barriers to a diet of nutritious foods. Regardless, there is a need to gather population-based data on weight-related disorders in general and on disordered eating in particular so that trends can be monitored over time, and large-scale prevention initiatives can be developed that involve more upstream approaches (e.g., changes to food policy or private sector initiatives to promote a healthier ideal body size) with substantial community input, and these can be evaluated more effectively for their impact on individual and community well-being.

We hope this book will take an important place alongside other useful reviews of what we know about the prevention of negative body image, disordered eating, and eating disorders. However, beyond this goal, we have sought to develop a resource that enables a relatively atypical collection of professionals to consider what we ourselves do not know enough about. Thus, our intent is for this collection of chapters to showcase where the opportunities are to learn more and to collaborate more by doing more. How do we break down "silos" (i.e., large but ultimately narrow, vertical constraints) in order to gain a better understanding of the interrelationships among the relevant fields of study and the relevant risk factors that pertain to the spectrum of weight-related disorders? How can participants from different fields work together—and, more importantly, work with the very people whom they hope to empower as they empower themselves—over extended periods to develop shared conceptual and methodologic frameworks that integrate their respective disciplinary perspectives? And how can new discoveries and the resultant excitement and hope be disseminated effectively and then sustained within the context of disparate, individual communities? It is our hope that individually and collectively the chapters will contribute valuable knowledge about the ways to maximize reach across communities, foster mental health wellness and resiliency, and build healthier children and healthier communities.

Notes

1 Statistics Canada. Retrieved from http://www40.statcan.gc.ca/l01/cst01/demo10a-eng.htm.
2 Canadian Psychiatric Association. Retrieved from http://www.cpa-apc.org/browse/documents/19.
3 Preventing Eating-Related Disorders: Collaborative Research, Advocacy and Policy Change. Retrieved from http://www.chsrgevents.ca.

References

Austin, S. B. (2001). Population-based prevention of eating disorders: An application of the Rose prevention model. *Preventive Medicine, 32,* 268-283.

Battle, E. K., & Brownell, K. D. (1996). Confronting a rising tide of eating disorders and obesity: treatment versus prevention and policy. *Addictive Behaviors, 21*(6), 755-765.

Cachelin, F., & Striegel-Moore, R. H. (2006). Help seeking and barriers to treatment in a community sample of Mexican American and European American women with with eating disorders. *International Journal of Eating Disorders, 39,* 154-161.

Cohane, G. H. & Pope, H. G. (2001). Body image in boys: A review of the literature. *International Journal of Eating Disorders, 29,* 373-379.

Croll, J., Neumark-Sztainer, D., Story, M., & Ireland, M. (2002). Prevalence and risk and protective factors related to disordered eating behaviours among adolescents: Relationship to gender and ethnicity. *Journal of Adolescent Health, 31*(2), 166-175.

Fingeret, M. C., Warren, C. S., Cepeda-Benito, A., & Gleaves, D. H. (2006). Eating disorder prevention research: A meta-analysis. *Eating Disorders: Journal of Treatment and Prevention, 14,* 191-213.

Frank, L. D., Engelke, P. O., & Schmid, T. L (2003). *Health and community design: The impact of the built environment on physical activity.* Washington, DC: Island Press.

Gadalla, T. M., & Piran, N. (2007). Co-occurrence of Eating Disorders and Alcohol Use Disorders in Women: A Meta Analysis. *Archives of Women's Mental Health, 10*(4), 133-140.

Gortmaker, S. L., Must, A., Perrin, J. M., Sobol, A. M., & Dietz, W. H. (1993). Social and economic consequences of overweight in adolescence and young adulthood. *New England Journal of Medicine, 329,* 1008-1012.

Green, J., & Tones, K. (1999). For debate: Towards a secure evidence base for prevention. *Journal of Public Health, 21*(2), 133-139.

Haines, J., & Neumark-Sztainer, D. (2006). Prevention of obesity and eating disorders: A consideration of shared risk factors. *Health Education Research, 21,* 770-782.

Hudson, J. I., Hiripi, E., Pope, H. G., & Kessler, R. C. (2007). The prevalence and correlates of eating disorders in the NCS Replication. *Biological Psychiatry, 61*(3), 348-358.

Institute for Health Information (2006). *Psychologists.* Retrieved from http:// secure.cihi.ca/cihiweb/products/Psychologists.pdf

Jones, L. M., Bennett, S., Olmsted, M. P., Lawson, M. L., & Rodin, G. (2001). Disordered eating attitudes and behaviours in teenage girls: A school-based study. *Canadian Medical Association Journal, 165,* 547-552.

Jones, L. M., Halford, W. K., & Dooley, R. T. (1993). Long-term outcome of anorexia nervosa. *Behaviour Change, 10,* 93-102.

Keel, P. K., & Klump K. L. (2003). Are eating disorders culture-bound syndromes? Implications for conceptualizing their etiology. *Psychological Bulletin, 129,* 747-769.

Keski-Rahkonen, A., Hoek, H. W., Susser, E. S., Linna, M. S., Sihvola, E., Raevuori, A., Bulik, C. M., Kaprio, J., & Rissanen, A. (2007). Epidemiology and course of anorexia nervosa in the community. *American Journal of Psychiatry, 164,* 1259-1265.

Kraak, V. I., & Story, M. (2010). A public health perspective on healthy lifestyles and public private partnerships for global childhood obesity prevention. *Journal of the American Dietetic Association, 110,* 192-200.

Levine, M. P., & Smolak, L. (2006). *The prevention of eating problems and eating disorders: Theory, research, and practice.* Mahwah, NJ: Lawrence Erlbaum Associates.

Levine, M. P., & Smolak, L. (2008). "What exactly are we waiting for?" The case for universal-selective eating disorders prevention programs. *International Journal of Child and Adolescent Health, 1,* 295-304.

Levine, M. P., & Smolak, L. (2009) Prevention of negative body image and disordered eating in children and adolescents: Recent developments and promising directions. In L. Smolak & J. K. Thompson (Eds.), *Body image, eating disorders, and obesity in youth* (2nd edition, pp. 215-239). Washington, DC: American Psychological Association.

López-Guimerà, G., & Sánchez-Carracedo, D. (2010). Prevención de las alteraciones alimentarias: Fundamentos teóricos y recursos prácticos [Preventing eating disorders: Theoretical and practical resources]. Madrid: Pirámide.

MacLean, L., Edwards, N., Gerrard, M., Sims-Jones, N., Clinton, K., & Ashley, L. (2009). Obesity, stigma and public health planning. *Health Promotion International, 24*(1), 88-93.

McCabe, M. P., Ricciardelli, L. A., & Finemore, J. (2002). The role of puberty, media and popularity with peers on strategies to increase weight, decrease weight and increase muscle tone among adolescent boys and girls. *Journal of Psychosomatic Research, 52*(3), 145-153.

McCreary, D. R., & Sasse, D. K. (2002). Gender differences in high school students' dieting behavior and their correlates. *International Journal of Men's Health, 1,* 195-213.

McVey, G. (2004). Eating disorders. In L. Rapp-Paglicci, C. Dulmus, & J. Wodarski (Eds.), *Handbook of preventive interventions for children and adolescents* (pp. 275-300). New York: Wiley and Sons.

McVey, G., Adair, C., deGroot, J., McLaren, L., Plotnikoff, R., Gray-Donald, K., Collier, S. (2008). Obesity and eating disorders: Seeking common ground to promote health. A national meeting of researchers, practitioners and policy-makers, November 2007, final report. Retrieved from http://www.ocoped.ca/DNN/PDF/Obesity_eating_disorders_2007.pdf

McVey, G. L., Pepler, D., Davis, R., Flett, G., & Abdolell, M. (2002). Risk and protective factors associated with disordered eating during early adolescence. *Journal of Early Adolescence, 22*, 75-95.

National Research Council and Institute of Medicine of the National Academies (NRC/IOM). (2009). *Preventing mental, emotional, and behavioral disorders among young people: Progress and possibilities.* Committee on prevention of Mental Disorders and Substance Abuse among Children, Youth, and Young Adults: Research Advances and Promising Interventions (Mary Ellen O'Connell, Thomas Boat, and Kenneth E. Warner, Editors). Washington, DC: National Academies Press.

Neumark-Sztainer, D., Wall, M., Guo, J., Story, M., Haines, J., & Eisenberg, M. (2006). Obesity, disordered eating, and eating disorders in a longitudinal study of Adolescents: How do dieters fare 5 years later? *Journal of the American Dietietic Association, 106*, 559-568.

Neumark-Sztainer, D. R., Wall, M. M., Haines, J. I., Story, M. T., Sherwood, N. E., & van den Berg, P. A. (2007). Shared risk and protective factors for overweight and disordered eating in adolescents. *American Journal of Preventive Medicine, 33*, 359-369.

O'Dea, J. (2005). School-based health education strategies for the improvement of body image and prevention of eating problems: An overview of safe and effective interventions. *Health Education, 105*, 11-33.

Pentz, M. (2000). Institutionalizing community-based prevention through policy change. *Journal of Community Psychology, 28*(3), 257-270.

Piran, N. (1999). Eating disorders: A trial of prevention in a high risk school setting. *Journal of Primary Prevention, 20*(1), 75-90.

Piran, N. (2001). Re-inhabiting the body from the inside out: Girls transform their school environment. In D. L. Tolman & M. Brydon-Miller (Eds.), *From subjects to subjectivities: Handbook of interpretative and participatory methods* (pp. 218-38). New York: New York University Press.

Piran, N. (2005). Prevention of eating disorders: A review of outcome evaluation research. *Israel Journal of Psychiatry and Related Sciences, 42*(3), 172-77.

Piran, N. (2010). A feminist perspective on risk factor research and on the prevention of eating disorders. *Eating Disorders: Journal of Treatment and Prevention, 18*(3), 183-198.

Piran, N., & Gadalla, G. (2006). Eating disorders and substance abuse in Canadian women: A National Study. *Addiction, 102*, 105-113.

Puhl, R. M., & Heuer, C. A. (2009). The stigma of obesity: A review and update. *Obesity, 17*, 941-964.

Reilly, J. J., Methven, E., McDowell, Z. C., Hacking, B., Alexander, D., Stewart, L., & Kelnar, C. J. H. (2003). Health consequences of obesity. *Archives of Disease in Childhood, 88,* 748-752.

Seeley, J., Stice, E., & Rohde, P. (2009). Screening for depression prevention: Identifying adolescent girls at high risk for future depression. *Journal of Abnormal Psychology, 118*(1), 161-170.

Sihvola, E., Keski-Rahkonen, A., Dick, D. M., Hoek, H. W., Raevuori, A., & Rose, R. J. (2009). Prospective associations of early-onset Axis I disorders with developing eating disorders. *Comprehensive Psychiatry, 50,* 20-25.

Stice, E., Ng, J., & Shaw, H. (2010). Risk factors and prodromal eating pathology. *Journal of Child Psychology and Psychiatry, 51,* 518-525.

Stice, E., & Shaw, H. (2004). Eating disorder prevention programs: A meta-analytic review. *Psychological Bulletin, 130,* 206-227.

Stice, E., Shaw, H., Becker, C., & Rohde, P. (2008). Dissonance-based interventions for the prevention of eating disorders: Using persuasion principles to promote health. *Prevention Science, 9,* 114-128.

Stice, E., Shaw, H., & Marti, C. N. (2007). A meta-analytic review of eating-disorder prevention programs. *Annual Review of Clinical Psychology, 3,* 207-223.

Thompson, J. K. (Ed.). (2004). *Handbook of eating disorders and obesity.* Hoboken, NJ: Wiley.

Tremblay, M. S., Katzmarzyk, P. T., & Willms, J. D. (2002). Temporal trends in overweight and obesity in Canada, 1981-1996. *International Journal of Obesity, 26,* 538-543.

Willms, J. D., Tremblay, M. S., & Katzmarzyk, P. T. (2003). Geographic and demographic variation in the prevalence of overweight Canadian children. *Obesity Research, 11*(5), 668-673.

World Health Organization. (2001). *Obesity: Preventing and managing the global epidemic,* Report of WHO Consultation on Obesity, 3-5 June 1997, Geneva. Geneva, Switzerland: World Health Organization.

PART ONE

Working with Larger and Broader Systems

Prevention, Prevention Science, and an Ecological Perspective: A Framework for Programs, Research, and Advocacy

Michael P. Levine, *Kenyon College*
Gail L. McVey, *The Hospital for Sick Children, University of Toronto*

There are many detailed analyses of the current and increasingly complex state of affairs in the prevention of negative body image, disordered eating, and related conditions such as abuse of steroids and food supplements (Becker, Stice, Shaw, & Woda, 2009; Holt & Ricciardelli, 2008; Levine & Smolak, 2006, 2008, 2009; Piran, 2005, 2010; Sinton & Taylor, 2010; Wilksch & Wade, 2009; Yager & O'Dea, 2008). This chapter examines the field of prevention science, with an eye towards improving programming, research, dissemination, and advocacy in the prevention of eating disorders. Special attention is given to innovative socio-ecological models, derived from feminist principles that appear to have important implications for the synchronous prevention of eating disorders, obesity, and other mental health disorders. Challenges associated with the implementation of multi-level interventions for multiple, intersecting problems are discussed, as are directions for future research.

Moving towards Prevention Science

Eating disorders prevention began in earnest in the mid-1990s—that is, less than 20 years ago. In contrast, prevention theory and research have been a focus of public health, community psychology, and psychiatry, social work, cardiovascular health, and substance abuse for two to three times longer (Levine & Smolak, 2006, Chapters 1, 9, & 10). Indeed, there is a body of knowledge demonstrating that prevention can work. For example, school-based prevention programs that are interactive and engaging and that emphasize positive peer norms, resistance skills, media literacy, stress management, and other life skills have been shown to prevent initiation and escalation of the use of tobacco, alcohol, and other drugs by adolescents ages 11 through 13 (effect size = ~ .15; Botvin & Griffin, 2002; Tobler et al., 2000). Over the past twenty years, this and similar facts, theories, and methods have become the foundation of a broad and significant development in the general field of prevention called "prevention science" (Committee on the Prevention of Mental Disorders and Substance Abuse, 2009, Chapter 10; Reese, Wingfield, & Blumenthal, 2009; Weissberg, Kumpfer, & Seligman, 2003).

Technically, the prevention sciences (plural) are a set of disciplines that apply scientific methods to an understanding of the etiology, development, and prevention of physical and psychological disorders as well as of other social problems such as youth crime (see Table 1). Albee's (1983) non-specific vulnerability-stressor model of risk, resilience, and prevention contributes several important lessons in prevention science (see Levine & Smolak, 2006, Chapter 7). This ecological model emphasizes that psychological, health, and social problems result from the interaction between individuals and their larger environments, as shaped by familial, academic, social, cultural, economic, and political factors. The powerful role of socio-economic, socio-political, and other socio-cultural factors in the development of cumulative risks and in the maintenance of disorder, illness, and health has two immediate and significant implications. First, prevention work is necessarily an integra-

---

TABLE 1: PREVENTION SCIENCE'S SIX CORE PRINCIPLES OF EFFECTIVE PROGRAMMING

---

1. Uses a research-based risk and protective factor framework that involves families, peers, schools, and communities as partners to target multiple outcomes.
2. Is long-term, age-specific, and culturally appropriate.
3. Fosters development of individuals who are healthy and fully engaged through teaching them to apply social-emotional skills and ethical values in daily life.
4. Aims to establish policies, institutional practices, and environmental supports that nurture optimal development.
5. Selects, trains, and supports interpersonally skilled staff to implement programming effectively.
6. Incorporates and adapts evidence-based programming to meet local community needs through strategic planning, ongoing evaluation, and continuous improvement.

Source: All principles are direct quotations (italics removed) from different paragraph headings in Weissberg, Kumpfer, and Seligman (2003). Principle 1 is quoted from page 428; the remaining principles are quoted from page 429.

tion of science and social justice (see Kenny, Horne, Orpinas, & Reese, 2009; Levine & Maine, 2010; Piran, 2001). Second, all of the phases of the prevention cycle involve the planning, advocacy, interpersonal skills, and patience necessary for establishing multiple productive working relationships with granting agencies, key community stakeholders (e.g., leaders of cultural and ethnic communities and school district leaders), those who work in the setting in which the intervention will take place (e.g., health system and prison system staff), those who will participate (e.g., families and youth), and policy agencies (Piran, 1999a, 1999b, 2001, 2010; see also Levine & Smolak, 2006).

Prevention science strongly supports Piran's long-standing argument, based on the intensive case study (Piran, 1999b, 2001) and outcome (Piran, 1999a) of a whole school prevention program implemented in a residential ballet school, that programs designed to change the contexts within which body image problems and disordered eating develop are likely to be particularly valuable (see also O'Dea, 2005; Piran, 2005, 2010). In general, social ecological models highlight four concentric arenas of risk and resilience that each individual exists within: *individual* (biological and personal history factors, such as temperament, level of physical maturation, age, and history of abuse), *relationship* (peer, family, and intimate partner influences), *community* (the neighbourhood, school, athletic, or workplace influences), and *societal* (greater cultural and social norms). Thus, an ecological approach is entirely consistent with the fundamental definition of universal prevention as a health-promoting enterprise that works by improving public policies and institutions such as school systems (Cowen, 1973; see Levine & Smolak, 2006, Chapter 1).

School Environment

The school setting is ideal for primary prevention work (Levine, 1987; Levine & Smolak, 2006; Wilksch & Wade, 2009). It offers a unique opportunity to reach out to large groups of children and youth as well as to their teachers, parents, and other adult stakeholders who care for them. Different programs have tried to address the school environment to different degrees. The Very Important Kids (VIK) program developed by Haines and colleagues focused on changing the peer environment within the school (e.g., the establishment of peer group rules of no teasing or harassment). The VIK program also aimed to engage children, community members, and parents in a theater production related to body image and weight-related issues as well as to inform parents and teachers about ways to provide children with a healthy developmental context (Haines, Neumark-Sztainer, & Morris,

2008; Haines, Neumark-Sztainer, Perry, Hannan, & Levine, 2006). The Planet Health program sought to change the school culture regarding eating patterns by changing and integrating the school curriculum to create consistency in the body of knowledge transmitted to students and in the school's emphasis on increasing the children's physical activity (Austin, Field, Wiecha, Peterson, & Gortmaker, 2005). In their Healthy Schools–Healthy Kids program, McVey and colleagues provided all of the aforementioned components and also established all-girl peer groups that were facilitated in school by local public health practitioners whom McVey partnered with and trained for the purpose of the study (McVey, Lieberman, Voorberg, Wardrope, & Blackmore, 2003a; McVey, Tweed, & Blackmore, 2007). Of note, the graduates of these Girl Talk peer groups subsequently disseminated media literacy strategies to the rest of the student body. To summarize, examples of components included across these programs were education and training of teachers and other staff regarding healthy influences on body image, nutrition, and physical activity; classroom curricula embedded into all grade levels and across multiple topics; live theatre highlighting the negative influence of the media and/or appearance-based teasing; after-school programs; posters and public service announcements underscoring messaging about size acceptance, healthy eating, and active living; and inclusion to some extent of parents, teachers, or other school personnel in the intervention.

Randomized controlled trials conducted on these ecologically based interventions reveal stronger effect sizes compared to curriculum-based universal programs (Stice, Shaw, & Marti, 2007). Significant intervention effects were reported for disordered eating (McVey et al., 2007—effect sizes = 0.39 at eight-month follow-up and 0.27 at 14-month follow-up; Austin et al., 2005—effect size = 0.09 at 21-month follow-up) and also for decreases in established risk factors such as the internalization of media stereotypes (McVey et al., 2007—effect sizes = 0.02 at eight-month follow-up and 0.22 at 14-month follow-up) and weight-based teasing (Haines et al., 2006—effect size = 0.63).

Disordered eating, media influences, and weight-based teasing also play a role in the development of overweight/obesity, suggesting that these ecologically based interventions could simultaneously help prevent the spectrum of weight-related disorders (Bauer, Haines, & Neumark-Sztainer, 2009; Neumark-Sztainer et al., 2007). In fact, building individual and peer group resilience through the modification of peer norms and the involvement of teachers and parents has the potential to help prevent a multitude of risky behaviours (e.g., substance abuse, smoking, risky sexual behaviour) and problems (e.g., depression and anxiety). Such multi-topic prevention programs would help reduce numerous economic and other burdens on these schools—which, in fact, represent the majority of schools in general—which are genuinely concerned about, and committed to helping stem, the tide of emotional and behavioural problems in students.

The achievements of the ecologically based programs are noteworthy in the face of the challenges they have encountered. For example, some intervention schools in the Healthy Schools–Healthy Kids project developed by McVey and colleagues were unco-operative when carrying out the teacher-delivered curriculum, despite it being matched to the Ontario, Canada, Ministry of Education's expectations and despite the fact that teaching responsibilities were spread across various course topics. In addition, the time allotted to the researchers for teacher training was minimal. This reluctance highlights the importance of advocating for teacher training to be integrated into ministry guidelines (Gortmaker et al., 1999; McVey, Tweed, & Ferrari, 2005; Piran, 1999a, 1999b, 2001). Finally, as many researchers have painfully discovered (Neumark-Sztainer et al., 2006), parental participation in the programs discussed to this point has been very low (McVey et al., 2007).

Changing Social Norms

In addition to the Non-Specific Vulnerability-Stressor Model, another paradigm in the prevention of negative body image and weight-related disorders that emphasizes a contextual, ecological approach is the Feminist-Empowerment-Relational Model pioneered in Canada by Piran (1995, 1999c, 2001, 2010; see also Levine & Piran, 2004; Levine & Smolak, 2006, Chapter 8). The risk factors emphasized by feminist theories have been solidly supported by cross-sectional (correlational), experimental, and even some prospective data (Smolak & Murnen, 2007; see Chapters 6, 7, & 8 in this volume).

The Ballet School Studies

Although Steiner-Adair (1994) has long championed a feminist perspective in thinking about prevention, the first description of a comprehensive and programmatic feminist approach to the prevention of eating disorders was published in 1995 by Piran (concerning her 1985 program in implementation) and subsequently in a chapter three years later (Piran, 1998; see also Piran, 1999a, 1999b). This feminist perspective has affected trends in the field, such as the emphasis on dialogical-participatory interactions with various stakeholders and an ecological perspective in the form of multi-level interventions that focus on contextual factors. Given the pronounced gender differences across the spectrum of weight-related disorders, and given the empirical evidence for the effectiveness of the feminist approach, the argument that it makes good sense to explore further feminist theories and methodologies for preventing body image disturbance and weight-related problems is compelling (Levine & Smolak, 2006, Chapters 8 & 9; Piran, 2010).

The feminist approach and prevention science share an insistence on the necessity of assessing, understanding, and changing peer norms, the behaviour of adults, and the physical and social contexts that form the ecology of children and adolescents (see also Perry, 1999; Ranby et al., 2009; Smolak & Levine, 1996).[1] Piran (2001, p. 261) explains that in "social groups where body weight and shape preoccupation has become entrenched in the social life of the group, the establishment of constructive group norms regarding body weight and shape actually involves the creation of a shift in the peer group experience." Piran (1998, 1999c, 2001) was the first in the body image and eating disorder fields to focus her prevention work on peer group norms, conducting over 300 focus groups with students aged 10 to 18 years in a competitive, residential, and co-educational dance school. Using participatory action research, Piran worked collaboratively with the girls to (1) solicit their descriptions of events that affected how they felt about their bodies; (2) critically interpret those events; and (3) develop action plans to create system-wide changes.

Most programs since then have not made intervention at the peer group level a focus of their prevention work, which plausibly might account for the low-effect sizes reported across universal prevention studies (Stice et al., 2007). Notable exceptions are, for example, studies conducted by (in chronological order) O'Dea and Abraham (2000), Steiner-Adair and colleagues (2002), McVey and colleagues (2003a, 2003b, 2007), Elliot and colleagues (2006; reviewed later in this article), Haines and colleagues (2006), and Becker and colleagues (Becker, Bull, Schaumberg, Cauble, & Franco, 2008; Becker et al., 2009; Perez, Becker, & Ramirez, 2010). Peer group components in these programs ranged from (1) the development of creative strategies designed to reduce or eliminate "fat talk" and/or weight-related teasing (both of which sustain and extend normative but unhealthy concerns about weight and shape); (2) group-based training in various resilience skills to boost resistance against societal prejudices and norms; (3) interventions designed in part, and then led, by peers; (4) the activation of networks and social systems that collectively influence policy-concerning equity; and (5) the engagement of community partners in a manner that shares power and decision-making in order to increase and integrate knowledge about health problems, to improve problem solving, and to sustain the implementation and improvement of prevention programming.

One benefit of changing peer norms is that the program continues to have an impact once the circumscribed interventions are complete. The primary prevention program conducted by Piran (1999a, 1999b, 1999c) in a high-risk residential school setting (which was technically a selective intervention; see the introduction in this volume) led to system-wide changes that were sustained for over a decade. Moreover, Piran's 15 years of prevention work at the school produced sustained decreases in the incidence of disordered eating (see Levine & Smolak, 2006, Chapter 8).

Sorority Body Image Program

For over six years, Becker has worked closely with local and national members of the Delta Delta Delta (Tri-Delta) Sorority to develop, implement, evaluate, refine, sustain, and disseminate *Reflections*, the Sorority Body Image Program (SBIP).[2] Engagement of peers and changes in peer norms are an essential part of the specific program for sorority sisters that have been repeatedly shown to be effective in producing positive outcomes at follow-up with small to moderate effect sizes (Becker et al., 2008; Becker et al., 2009; Perez et al., 2010).

In the spring of 2007, the Office of Student Affairs at Trinity University officially noted that the SBIP had fundamentally and "historically" altered the entire sorority system by teaching the sororities to collaborate instead of compete and to find a common voice concerning an important issue (body image and health) of common interest (Becker, Ciao, & Smith, 2008). Further, local changes in peer norms have "trickled up" to the national and international levels to influence the ways in which Tri-Delta publicizes, funds, and otherwise supports this program and other prevention activities (Becker & Woda, 2010). Tri-Delta is committed to making SBIP available to all sorority members nationwide, not just its own members (Becker et al., 2009, p. 269). Consequently, Tri-Delta has plunged into advocacy work, using resources, marketing skills, and pre-established networks that prevention research invariably lacks in order to build interest in SBIP and other dissonance-based interventions.

From a feminist-empowerment-relational perspective, it is important to note also that one peer norm at the forefront of Becker's work is the assumption that sororities are an excellent foundation for prevention work because their commitment to sisterhood, community service, and leadership are the heart and lifeblood of an effective ecological approach to prevention and health promotion (Becker et al., 2009). That is, Becker and her colleagues in sororities vigorously reject the assumption that sororities should be a "target" of prevention efforts because they are a shallow drowning pool of values and people that breed negative body image and disordered eating.

Consistent with Piran's Feminist Model, the authentic, respectful collaborations and participatory research that produced *Reflections* have generated not only a strikingly successful prevention project but also a host of other positive phenomena in the prevention and advocacy fields. These include (1) Tri-Delta's infusion of hundreds of thousands of dollars and hundreds of thousands of woman hours into prevention, public education, and advocacy on a national and international scale; (2) the Body Image Academy, which uses a training manual that is ultimately intended for mass distribution to provide ongoing training of adult and peer leaders seeking to implement and evaluate *Reflections* on their campus (Becker & Stice, 2008; Becker et al., 2009);[3] and (3) the rapidly expanding and media-friendly Fat Talk Free Week.[4]

Girl-Talk Groups

Sustainability was also a goal of McVey and her colleagues' (2003a, 2003b, 2007) all-girl peer groups, and it was achieved by integrating it into routine public health service delivery in the province of Ontario, Canada, using the practitioners whom McVey had consulted and trained in her collaborative study. The nurse practitioners were involved in the development of, and ongoing consultation with, the researchers throughout the period of study. McVey and her colleagues' (2007) comprehensive school-based program was integrated into the Ontario Ministry of Education's curriculum and translated in a timely way to teachers and public health professionals through province-wide professional development training (McVey et al., 2005, 2010; McVey, Gusella, Tweed, & Ferrari, 2009). This Integrative Prevention Model, which has its roots in the Comprehensive School Health (CSH) Model, is advocated and otherwise supported by many organizations throughout Ontario and Canada (for example, the Canadian Association for School Health and the Ontario Society of Nutrition Professionals in Public Health) (O'Dea & Maloney, 2000; Piran, 1999c).[5] The CSH platform rests on four pillars intended to support the interdependence of health and education at the level of the entire school: social and physical environment; teaching and learning; healthy school living; and partnerships and services. This means that adopting the CSH Model to prevent weight-related disorders fits with various other initiatives being brought forward to the school setting and presented to educators, school support staff, students, and families—initiatives that are eliminating duplication and increasing the consistency of health promotion information (for example, actions concerning sexual harassment, bullying and teasing, nutrition, an active life style, and the ability to cope with stress). Arguably, this distillation of essential messaging towards multiple prevention purposes is critical, given the academic pressures that teachers already face in today's schools.

Finally, and in the same vein, there is a need to identify and publish information about indirect indicators—that is, factors that often go unreported but are essential to the success of a program. Such factors include the advocacy of the program to and with key stakeholders, the training of personnel delivering the programs, and the creative measurement of the buy-in from gatekeepers and its impact on future uptake. Knowledge derived from participatory approaches and intensive case studies such as the one reported by Piran (2001) provide enriching information that goes beyond the lessons learned from experimental designs.

Sports Settings

Competitive athletics offer many benefits for girls and boys. Indeed, they offer significant opportunities for embodiment, physical vigor, and mental health (Menzel & Levine, 2010). However, for females, at least, competitive sports become a high-risk setting for disordered eating when there are direct pressures to attain an ideal body size, shape, or weight in order to perform at a high, if not elite, level (Smolak, Murnen, & Ruble, 2000). Although competitive athletic programs come with a unique set of challenges, their structure and culture in general allow for team-centred education, positive social norm development, an intensity of contact, and other potential mechanisms for prevention that are absent in general school settings (Goldberg & Elliot, 2005; Thompson & Sherman, 2010). Two recent programs, one from the United States and the other from Canada, have been designed to facilitate selective prevention in young female athletes.

The ATHENA Program

In the United States, a program entitled Athletes Targeting Healthy Exercise and Nutrition Alternatives (ATHENA) is intended to prevent eating problems and unhealthy weight/shape management or performance-enhancing practices—including the use of diet pills, nicotine, "nutritional" supplements, and anabolic-androgenic steroids—among female athletes, cheerleaders, and members of the dance and drill teams (Elliot et al., 2006, 2008; Ranby et al., 2009).[6] ATHENA is based on the Adolescents Training and Learning to Avoid Steroids program (ATLAS), whose well-documented and award-winning ability to prevent use and abuse of anabolic steroids and food supplements (and drinking and driving) by young male football players has made it a "model" program championed by the United States Department of Education (Elliot et al., 2008; Goldberg & Elliot, 2005; Goldberg et al., 2000).[7] Both ATLAS and ATHENA integrate psycho-education, positive norm development, media literacy (see Chapter 4 in this volume), drug resistance skills, and competence building (life skills) with many well-established practices in the design and evaluation of drug prevention programs (see Levine & Smolak, 2006, Chapter 10). ATHENA's ecological elements include the use of face-to-face interactions within a team context, guided practice in meaningful work towards real team goals, program delivery by peer athletes, and carefully tailored manuals to train coaches and peers ("squad leaders" for groups of five) in order to administer the program within the framework of the team's usual practices during the competitive season (Goldberg & Elliot, 2005). Coaches and peers implementing the ATHENA program work closely with small groups of student athletes to establish and reinforce healthy norms within a cohesive group, clear expectations for healthy behaviour in support of self and others, and desired skills.

A large-scale randomized controlled evaluation of ATHENA by Elliot and colleagues (2006) revealed many of the predicted prevention effects (Ranby et al., 2009). Relative to girls on teams in the comparison schools, ATHENA participants aged 14 to 16 were significantly less likely to begin using diet pills, amphetamines, anabolic steroids, and muscle-building supplements. In addition to reporting healthier-eating behaviours and fewer injuries, participants also reduced their intentions to lose weight and to use self-induced vomiting and drugs for weight control. Just as important, ATHENA successfully increased four potentially significant mediators: media literacy, drug resistance skills, self-efficacy in controlling mood, and the perception that few peers endorse and use body-shaping drugs. Although many of the relative gains demonstrated in the short term were not maintained over the one-to-three-year follow-up period, this program is certainly deserving of further development and evaluation (Elliot et al., 2008).

BodySense

In Canada, working with a multi-disciplinary steering committee of community-based health professionals as well as with a national advisory group composed of experts in various fields and of relevant associations (e.g., the Canadian Association for the Advancement of Women and Sport and Physical Activity), Buchholz, Mack, McVey, and their colleagues (2008) designed and evaluated the effectiveness of a three-month selective prevention program entitled BodySense: A Positive Body Image Initiative for Female Athletes.[8] The foundation for this psycho-educational program is 10 integrated "BodySense basics" pertaining to, for example, body health ("the facts"), unique body size and shape ("respect for the individual"), physical activity for enjoyment ("natural and healthy bodies"), stress management ("coping in healthy ways"), and modelling healthy attitudes and behaviours ("role modelling"). The BodySense basics were presented in workshops at gymnastic clubs: one workshop for parents and coaches and one for the gymnasts.

Participants in the Bodysense program were competitive female gymnasts (ages 11 to 18 years), parents, and coaches from seven gymnastic clubs. Four clubs were randomly designated to receive the three-month BodySense program, whereas the remaining clubs formed a control group. As predicted, participation in the BodySense program resulted in athletes perceiving a reduction in pressure from their sports clubs to be thin. However, there was no significant between-group difference in the change in the female athletes' eating attitudes or behaviours. Low participation of coaches and parents in the follow-up evaluation precluded any cogent conclusions about its impact on the adult stakeholders. Lessons learned from Piran's and Becker's selective prevention work in a highly competitive dance school and in a well-known sorority, respectively—namely, the need to focus on system-wide change over an extended period of time—should inform future prevention work conducted with athletes.

Coalitions and Collaboration: The Example of the Ontario Project

Facilitating universal-selective prevention, by definition, requires changes in the people, institutions, beliefs, and practices that make up a community or intersecting communities (Albee, 1983; Cowen, 1973; Levine & Smolak, 2006; Perry, 1999; Piran, 2001, 2010). Since no one person could accomplish such social change, coalitions have been the cornerstones of universal-selective prevention. With its etymology in "to grow from," a coalition is a coming together of distinct, sometimes disparate, elements to form a "gestalt" that organizes for, and acts towards, at least one common purpose. In practice, coalitions represent an array of local organizations and individuals who construct a power base that works to publicize mutual concerns and to effect lasting social changes. A well-organized, broad-based coalition will be successful in creating policy change, increasing public knowledge, creating a network, and developing innovative solutions to complex problems.

The Ontario Project

Since 1996, McVey (2006) has been organizing multiple collaborative working groups and coalitions in the province of Ontario, Canada. Their mutual purpose has been the development, implementation, and refinement of a model of health promotion that integrates universal, selective, and targeted prevention. This prevention model and the participating coalitions have brought together and co-ordinated the following: research, policy and program development, coalition building and advocacy, knowledge dissemination, and multi-disciplinary professional development.

One significant element of the Ontario Project is McVey's series of studies of prevention programs aimed at specific age groups of children, youth, and young adults as well as at the adults who mentor them (McVey, 2005). These programs promote positive body image in an attempt to reduce or help prevent disordered eating, but McVey has recently expanded her prevention efforts and research to align with public health chronic disease prevention mandates to promote healthy weights (Ontario Ministry of Health Promotion, 2010). The project's diverse prevention studies have spanned efficacy trials (McVey & Davis, 2002; McVey et al., 2007); effectiveness trials to demonstrate success in real life settings (McVey et al., 2003a, 2003b); implementation research to break down common barriers and promote the sustainability of best practices (McVey et al., 2010); grounded theory for program development (Ferrari, Tweed, Rummens, Skinner, & McVey, 2009); and translational research to align with existing organizational structures that are responsible for policy development (McVey et al., 2005; McVey et al., 2009) in an effort to build capacity across various health and mental health systems in the province. The co-ordination of prevention research and knowledge translation activities has been made possible by McVey's active membership in various coalitions (e.g., the Ontario Healthy Schools Coalition, the Body Image Coalition of Peel, and the Canadian Association of School Health) and through her delivery of many face-to-face, community-based prevention workshops across the province of Ontario (McVey et al., 2005). These cross-disciplinary, academic/community, and inter-ministerial collaborations have led to the establishment of partnerships that have, in turn, increased the sustainability and the credibility of prevention research and earned McVey and other project members invitations to participate in various government "think tanks" geared towards curriculum development and/or policy development in the realm of education and public health.

Knowledge Translation and Dissemination

One potentially important function and advantage of coalitions is the development of, and then the translation of, research-based and other forms of practical knowledge into forms that can be disseminated to those who can use it in day-to-day prevention practices. In the Ontario Project, knowledge translation of best practices in prevention is occurring in many forms. These include advocacy at the government level to update and revise policies in schools; training workshops delivered in the community to various professionals who work with children, youth, and their families (McVey et al., 2005);[9] and accessible and free-of-cost online curriculum resources that are matched to Ministry of Education learning objectives to maximize uptake by teachers (McVey et al., 2009).[10]

Training local staff to facilitate interventions deepens the connection of programs to the ecology of implementation and helps sustain programs beyond the scope of the research. This has been the case for the ongoing involvement of public health nurses in the Girl Talk support groups for middle-school girls, which were originally established as part of programmatic prevention outcome research (McVey et al., 2003a, 2003b; McVey et al., 2007). At the university level, McVey and her colleagues (2010) partnered with university-based practitioners to build capacity for promoting positive body image among professionals who work with young adults. The research team arranged for a body image intervention to be integrated into their peer health educator-training program that is facilitated annually by health promotion staff across three universities in Ontario. As documented in the SBIP reviewed earlier, peer health educators as newly trained agents of change can affect the rest of the student population positively in how they model body satisfaction and in how they actively engage with the issues they believe in as well as in the knowledge and practices that they disseminate. Plans are under way to collaborate with additional universities across Ontario to conduct and evaluate an assessment of the level of readiness (both individually and at the organizational level) of university-based health personnel to carry out prevention, early identification, and early intervention services in the area of eating disorders. Finally, McVey and her collaborators from public health in Ontario are preparing to develop, implement, and evaluate a sensitivity training model for professionals to encourage their reflection on ways to avoid transmitting negative messages about food, weight, and shape to children and youth and to integrate mental health promotion into their daily practice.

An increasingly important form of knowledge translation—and one with the potential for further research, coalition building, and advocacy—is the Web-based training of teachers and public health practitioners. The online program *The Student Body: Promoting Health at Any Size* was designed to assist teachers and local public health practitioners in promoting positive body image in children before they reach early adolescence, a high-risk period for the development of negative body image, disordered eating, and depression in females (McVey et al., 2009; Smolak & Levine, 1996). The online format makes it accessible to facilitators (both during and outside of school hours), and the classroom activities, previously shown through research to improve body satisfaction and eating behaviour, were carefully matched to two provincial government's mandated objectives (McVey et al., 2004). A controlled randomized evaluation of the impact of the Web-based training program revealed that after 60 days in effect the program improved the teachers' knowledge concerning dieting, while increasing the public health practitioners' self-efficacy to fight weight bias. In general, participants reported an overall improvement in awareness of how weight bias can, even inadvertently, be present in their teaching practices, and how this bias can trigger body image concerns among their students. These findings support further investigations into the use of the Web to disseminate knowledge and practical ideas for engaging teachers—and possibly other influential professionals (e.g., pediatricians and coaches)—in the prevention of the spectrum of disordered eating among children and adolescents (see Chapter 5 in this volume).

Merging Prevention Research, Knowledge Translation, Coalition Building, and Advocacy

Government support of, and its direct involvement in, the prevention of eating disorders and the promotion of positive body image is not unique to Canada (see Chapter 3 in this volume). What is unique to Ontario, Canada, is the merging of prevention research and knowledge translation activities with established training and advocacy practices and with the building of a provincial network of specialized eating disorder treatment programs.[11] Through this network, workshops and consultations are carried out across the province in an effort to standardize best practices in the assessment, treatment, early identification, and multi-level prevention of eating disorders. And, all the while, local regions are encouraged and supported in their efforts to form their own respective body image or eating disorder coalitions. This effort enables the newly gained knowledge and resources to be tailored to fit the unique needs of this community, such as advocating for less fat talk; training local teachers to incorporate evidence-based curriculum into their daily teaching practices; helping school staff to understand how racism and prejudice that are built on social class feed negative body image and unhealthy weight management; and sensitizing preschool caregivers and after-school leaders about ways to be an effective role model (Piran, 2001, 2010). Research indicates that these training activities can significantly increase knowledge and the level of comfort of educators and practitioners to deliver body image curriculum and early intervention strategies, respectively (McVey et al., 2005; Piran, 2004). A bigger success is noted in the establishment of (1) a "community of practice" among eating disorder service providers who meet regularly to exchange knowledge and expertise related to their daily treatment practices and (2) a less formal yet equally thriving prevention hub that blends research, practice, and policy.

Thus, the metropolis of Toronto and the province of Ontario more broadly benefit from a geographical scaffolding or network of health, public health, mental health professionals, non-profit groups (e.g., the National Eating Disorder Information Centre and Sheena's Place), and other concerned citizens who are united in efforts to promote health and decrease disease related to the intersection of body image, obesity, and eating disorders.[12] This action lays the groundwork for many creative collaborative initiatives that seem to blossom within the formation and maintenance of these relationships. The resultant upsurge in professional morale and enthusiasm is very likely to improve practitioners' relationships with the children, families, and adults whom they serve. Scaffolding of this sort also serves as a model for other treatment and prevention topics.

Conclusions, Implications, and Key Issues

Conclusion 1: We must continue to improve our understanding of the ecology of children and youth so as to be able to challenge and change unhealthy elements while strengthening positive aspects
Work from other public health fields, such as drug abuse prevention, clearly demonstrates the value of changing the ecology in which children live (Levine & Smolak, 2006; Perry, 1999). Tobler and colleagues' (2000) meta-analysis of over 200 drug prevention studies found that programs facilitating "system-wide" changes had the highest weighted effect size (+ .27). The evidence currently available indicates that the ecological approach is also strongly recommended in the prevention of the spectrum of negative body image and disordered eating (Levine & Smolak, 2006; Piran, 2010).

With respect to the important setting of the school system, we need to continue developing and carefully evaluate universal-selective and selective-targeted programs that integrate multifaceted curricular interventions with the training of teachers, coaches, and other staff and with the involvement of parents and other key stakeholders in the community. Evaluations of such research should make use of sophisticated study designs that capture outcome indicators other than those associated with individual (or aggregate) attitudinal or behavioural changes, such as policy and/or organizational change, changes in weight-related group norms, and feelings of connectedness to, and engagement with, positive, health-promoting features of the social and physical environment (Levine & Smolak, 2006, Chapter 12). An ecological perspective in evaluation also points to the need to measure the processes involved in the implementation of multi-level, systemic interventions and their interaction with mediating variables, such as the critical thinking by key players that leads to modification and evolution of a program (see Green & Tones, 2010).

Framing this type of research is the fundamental issue of developing valid assessments of the risk and protective features (or potentials) of various environments. This process will advance efforts to identify exactly which elements of the ecology of children and youth are most amenable to change and to clarify how best to change them. The hard-won lessons of prevention science and the Feminist-Empowerment-Relational Model indicate that, whether the setting is a school system, an elite dance academy, an athletic team, or an organization such as the Girl Scouts, it is likely that the most effective ecological approaches will promote health, resilience, and prevention through the following methods: (1) lessons in a variety of subjects, (2) peer leadership, (3) education and training of adults in the position of mentors, and (4) attempts to change and integrate the norms of peer groups and the policies of organizations (Levine & Smolak, 2006; Perry, 1999; Piran, 1995, 2010). It is also very likely that conceptualizing and assessing ecological changes will require the exploration of ways to combine the standards of evidence operating within clinical psychology and prevention science with quantitative and qualitative methods from, at the very least, the more participatory fields of health promotion, anthropology, and public health (Society for Prevention Research, 2004).

Conclusion 2: We must incorporate elements of the Feminist-Empowerment-Relational Model into our ecological approaches to prevention

There is now a substantial body of theory, basic research, and prevention outcome research to support the effectiveness of feminist-ecological and participatory approaches to strengthening girls and women while changing the many environments that demean the value of females (and males) and that equate femininity with the thin body ideal and physical objectification (Becker, Piran, & Haines, 2007; Levine & Smolak, 2006; Piran, 1998, 1999b, 1999c, 2001, 2010; Smolak & Murnen, 2007; see also Chapters 7 & 8 in this volume). The development and co-ordination of efforts to convince schools and other organizations to institute and enforce policies for gender equity in the classroom or on the playing fields, and against teasing or harassment, will not be easy. We will constantly be reminded of both the clear role of advocacy in prevention and the feminist dictum that "the personal is the political." Nevertheless, promoting respect for females and males is entirely consistent with the mission statements of most institutions and, in particular, schools. A great many schools have an overt and abiding commitment to facilitating learning and to promoting youth development through fairness, safety, citizenship, and leadership. Further, people committed to prevention—and especially those seeking to enter the field via thesis and dissertation—work are reminded that, even after nearly 25 years of research and advocacy work by Neumark-Sztainer, McVey, Paxton, Piran, Steiner-Adair, Smolak, and others, there is still a great need for the development and/or systematic long-term evaluation of programs that embody and teach feminist attitudes (Levine & Smolak, 2006; Levine & Piran, 2004; Piran, 2010). Such programs would incorporate respect for women and their achievements, a critical analysis of media and other societal images of women, and the de-emphasis of appearance in favour of competence, values, positive personality characteristics, health, and vitality.

Conclusion 3: We must improve our ability to involve parents

Parents have a significant impact on their children's eating habits, body image, activity levels, and emotional functioning. They are also children's earliest models, and, arguably, children's beliefs and confidence in these critical areas of development are calibrated first on their parent's beliefs. Consequently, many experts have championed the need to involve parents in prevention efforts. In her doctoral dissertation, Trost (2007) randomly assigned parents to either a wait-list control or three weekly 90-minute workshops designed to help them understand and challenge the slender beauty ideal and then to communicate effectively with their middle-school daughters in ways that reduce the internalization of that ideal and improve body image. At the three-month follow-up, the program reduced significantly the parents' internalization of the thin ideal and the parents' body dissatisfaction and produced a non-significant trend towards similar reductions in the daughters' internalization, body dissatisfaction, and bulimic symptoms. Trost's (2007) preliminary study points to the potential value of further research to evaluate the effectiveness, for example, of methods to improve parents' indirect and direct influences on the body image development and eating behaviour of their daughters (or sons) (see also Russell-Mayhew, Arthur, & Ewashen, 2007).

As noted previously, engaging parents in programs for preventing eating disorders has proven to be very challenging (Haines et al., 2006; McVey et al., 2007). Nevertheless, it is possible to involve substantial numbers of parents in ways that matter, as documented in Shepard and Carlson's (2003) review of school-based programs that have successfully applied an ecological approach to health promotion and drug abuse prevention (see also Perry, 1999). Parents are optimally positioned as agents of change in these efforts. Parents are the adult role models who stay with children the longest, and prevention scientists should work with parents rather than being independent of them whenever possible.

Conclusion 4: We must continue to develop collaborative, integrative approaches

Projects in Canada (McVey, 2006), Australia (see Chapter 3 in this volume), Germany (Berger, Sowa, Bormann, Brix, & Strauss, 2008), Spain (D. Sanchez, personal communication, 12 February 2009), and the United States (Becker et al., 2009; Elliot et al., 2008) provide exciting examples of ways to address a continuum of weight-related disorders by developing community partnerships—and, in some instances, collaborations—between government, foundations, non-profit corporations, communities, and researchers. These dynamic working relationships are designed to integrate risk factor research, risk identification, a continuum of prevention, program dissemination, professional development, and, in an increasing number of instances, public policies in regard to health promotion.

A "participatory" approach to this type of collaboration acknowledges, engages, and, hopefully, empowers various stakeholders within the school and the community (for examples pertaining to prevention of negative body image and weight-related disorders, see Becker et al., 2007; MacLean et al., 2010; Piran, 1999, 2001, 2010). A variety of qualitative and quantitative methods, including patient, respectful dialogues with a variety of local interests, are employed to generate knowledge from—and for—both the researchers and the people being researched. The theory and practice of participatory research reinforces the tremendous need to involve teachers and students (i.e., peers) in the decision-making process concerning the development, implementation, and evaluation of programs for promoting positive body image in the school setting (see, for example, Rosskam, 2009).

Notes

1 Prevention science subsumes a broad array of theoretical perspectives, including problem behaviour theory (Perry, 1999), social cognitive theory (Goldberg and Elliot, 2005; Perry, 1999), the feminist ecological developmental perspective (Levine and Smolak, 2006, chapter 15; Smolak and Levine, 1996), and principles of team-centred education (Goldberg and Elliot, 2005, figure 1, p. 70).

2 Technically, Delta Delta Delta (Tri-Delta) was founded as, and remains, a "fraternity" (https://www.tridelta.org/AboutUs/). However, to avoid confusion and to emphasize its commitment to sisterhood, we refer to it as a "sorority." Note that Carolyn B. Becker, Ph.D., was not or is not a member of Tri-Delta or any other such "fraternal" organization (Becker and Woda, 2010).

3 Body Image Academy. Retrieved from http://thecenter.tridelta.org/our-programs/reflections-body-image-program/body-image-academy-faqs.

4 Fat Talk Free Week. Retrieved from http://endfattalk.org/; see also the Fat Talk Free Week sites on youtube.com.

5 Comprehensive school health model. Retrieved from http://www.safehealthyschools.org/csh.htm.

6 Athletes Targeting Healthy Exercise and Nutrition Alternatives (ATHENA). Retrieved from http://www.ohsu.edu/xd/education/schools/school-of-medicine/departments/clinical-departments/medicine/divisions/hpsm/research/athena.cfm.

7 Adolescents Training and Learning to Avoid Steroids program (ATLAS). Retrieved from http://www.ohsu.edu/xd/education/schools/school-of-medicine/depart ments/clinical-departments/medicine/divisions/hpsm/research/atlas.cfm.

8 BodySense: A Positive Body Image Initiative for Female Athletes. Retrieved from http://www.bodysense.ca.

9 Ontario Community Outreach Program for Eating Disorders. Retrieved from http://www.ocoped.ca [OCOPED].

10 The Student Body: Promoting Health at Any Size. Retrieved from http://research.aboutkidshealth.ca/thestudentbody/home.asp.

11 OCOPED, *supra* note 9. It is worth noting that the adjective "provincial" is short-hand for a political entity that covers over a million square kilometers (> than 400,000 square mi.) and more than 12 million people (i.e., greater than a third of Canada's total population. See Canada Online, http://canadaonline.about.com/cs/provinces/p/ontariofacts.htm.

12 National Eating Disorder Information Centre. Retrieved from http://www.nedic.ca. Sheena's Place. Retrieved from http://www.sheenasplace.org.

References

Albee, G. W. (1983). Psychopathology, prevention, and the just society. *Journal of Primary Prevention, 4,* 5 40.

Austin, S. B., Field, A. E., Wiecha, J., Peterson, K. E., & Gortmaker, S. L. (2005). The impact of a school-based obesity prevention trial on disordered weight-control behavior in early adolescent girls. *Archives of Pediatric and Adolescent Medicine, 159,* 225-230.

Bauer, K. W., Haines, J., & Neumark-Sztainer, J. (2009). Obesity prevention: Strategies to improve effectiveness and reduce harm. In L. Smolak & J. K. Thompson (Eds.), *Body image, eating disorders, and obesity in youth* (2nd ed., pp. 241-260). Washington, DC: American Psychological Association.

Becker, C. B., Bull, S., Schaumberg, K., Cauble, A., & Franco, A. (2008). Effectiveness of peer-led eating disorders prevention: A replication trial. *Journal of Consulting and Clinical Psychology, 76,* 347-354.

Becker, C. B., Ciao, A. C., & Smith, L. M. (2008). Moving from efficacy to effectiveness in eating disorders prevention: The Sorority Body Image Program. *Cognitive and Behavioral Practice, 15,* 18-27.

Becker, C. B., Piran, N., & Haines, J. (2007, May). *Sustainable eating disorder prevention programs: Using the participatory approach to facilitate both science and long-term implementation.* Workshop presented at the International Conference on Eating Disorders, Baltimore, MD.

Becker, C. B., & Stice, E. (2008). *The Sorority body image program: Group leader guide*. New York: Oxford University Press.

Becker, C. B., Stice, E., Shaw, H., & Woda, S. (2009). Use of empirically supported interventions for psychopathology: Can the participatory approach move us beyond the research-to-practice gap? *Behaviour Research and Therapy, 47,* 265-274.

Becker, C. B., & Woda, S. (2010). *Reflections Body Image Program: Partnering with sororities in eating disorders prevention and advocacy* (workshop presented at the Academy for Eating Disorder's International Conference on Eating Disorders, Salzburg, Austria).

Berger, U., Sowa, M., Bormann, B., Brix, C., & Strauss, B. (2008). Primary prevention of eating disorders: Characteristics of effective programs and how to bring them to broader dissemination. *European Eating Disorder Review, 16,* 173-183.

Botvin, G. J., & Griffin, K. W. (2002). Preventing substance use and abuse. In K. M. & G. G. Bear (Eds.), *Preventing school problems—promoting school success: Strategies and programs that work* (pp. 259-298). Bethesda, MD: National Association of School Psychologists.

Buchholz, A., Mack, H., McVey, G. L., Feder, S., & Barrowman, N. (2008). BodySense: An evaluation of positive body image intervention on sport climate for female athletes. *Eating Disorders: Journal of Treatment and Prevention, 16,* 308-321.

Committee on the Prevention of Mental Disorders and Substance Abuse among Children, Youth, and Young Adults [National Research Council and Institute of Medicine of the National Academies]. (2009). *Preventing mental, emotional, and behavioral disorders among young people: Progress and possibilities.* Washington, DC: National Academies Press.

Cowen, E. L. (1973). Social and community intervention. *Annual Review of Psychology, 24,* 423-472.

Elliot, D. L., Goldberg, L., Moe, E. L., DeFrancesco, C. A., Durham, M. B., McGinnis, W. J., & Lockwood, C. (2008). Long-term outcomes of the ATHENA (Athletes Targeting Healthy Exercise and Nutrition Alternatives) program for female high school athletes. *Journal of Alcohol and Drug Education, 52,* 73-92.

Elliot, D. L., Moe, E. E., Goldberg, L., DeFrancesco, C. A., Durham, M. B., & Hix- Small, H. (2006). Definition and outcome of a curriculum to prevent disordered eating and body-shaping drug use. *Journal of School Health, 76,* 67-73.

Ferrari, M., Tweed, S., Rummens, J. A., Skinner, H., & McVey, G. (2009). Health materials and strategies for the prevention of immigrants' weight-related problems. *Qualitative Health Research, 19,* 1259-1272.

Goldberg, L., & Elliot, D. L. (2005). Preventing substance use among high school athletes: The ATLAS and ATHENA programs. *Journal of Applied Social Psychology, 21,* 63-87.

Goldberg, L., MacKinnon, D. P., Elliot, D. L., Moe, E. L., Clarke, G., & Cheong, J. (2000). The Adolescents Training and Learning to Avoid Steroids Program: Preventing drug use and promoting healthy behaviors. *Archives of Pediatrics and Adolescent Medicine, 154*, 332-338.

Gortmaker, S. L., Peterson, K. E., Wiecha, J., Sobol, A. M., Dixit, S., Fox, M. K., & Laird, N. (1999). Reducing obesity via a school-based interdisciplinary intervention among youth: Planet Health. *Archives of Pediatric Adolescent Medicine, 153*, 409-418.

Green, J., & Tones, K. (2010). *Health promotion: Planning and strategies* (2nd ed.). London: Sage.

Haines, J., Neumark-Sztainer, D., & Morris, B. (2008). Theater as a behavior change strategy: Qualitative findings from a school-based intervention. *Eating Disorders: Journal of Treatment and Prevention, 16*, 241-254.

Haines, J., Neumark-Sztainer, D., Perry, C. L., Hannan, P. J., & Levine, M. P. (2006). V.I.K. (Very Important Kids): A school-based program designed to reduce teasing and unhealthy weight control behaviors. *Health Education Research, 21*, 884-895.

Holt, K. E., & Ricciardelli, L. A. (2008). Weight concerns among elementary school children: A review of prevention programs. *Body Image, 5*, 233-243.

Kenny, M. E., Horne, A. M., Orpinas, P., & Reese, L. E. (Eds.). (2009). *Realizing social justice: The challenge of preventive interventions.* Washington, DC: American Psychological Association.

Levine, M. P. (1987). *How schools can help combat eating disorders.* Washington, DC: National Education Association.

Levine, M. P., & Maine, M. (2010). Are media an important medium for clinicians? Mass media, eating disorders, and the Bolder Model of treatment, prevention, and advocacy. In M. Maine, B. H. McGilley, & D. W. Bunnell (Eds.), *Treatment of eating disorders: Bridging the research-practice gap* (pp. 53-67). New York: Elsevier.

Levine, M. P., & Piran, N. (2004). The role of body image in the prevention of eating disorders. *Body Image, 1*, 57-70.

Levine, M. P., & Smolak, L. (2006). *The prevention of eating problems and eating disorders: Theory, research, and practice.* Mahwah, NJ: Lawrence Erlbaum Associates.

Levine, M. P., & Smolak, L. (2008). "What exactly are we waiting for?" The case for universal-selective eating disorder prevention programs. *International Journal of Child and Adolescent Health, 1*, 295-304.

Levine, M. P., & Smolak, L. (2009). Prevention of negative body image and disordered eating in children and adolescents: Recent developments and promising directions. In L. Smolak & J. K. Thompson (Eds.), *Body image, eating disorders, and obesity in youth* (2nd ed., pp. 215-239). Washington, DC: American Psychological Association.

MacLean, L. M., Clinton, K., Edwards, N., Gerrard, M., Ashley, L., Hansen-Ketchum, P., & Walsh, A. (2010). Unpacking vertical and horizontal integration:

Childhood overweight/obesity programs and planning, a Canadian perspective. *Implementation Science, 5*, 36.

McVey, G. (2005). Preventing eating disorders by educating teachers, coaches, and counselors. In D.K. Katzman & L. Pinhas (Eds.), *Help for eating disorders: A parent's guide to symptoms, causes and treatments* (pp. 266-277). Kingston, ON: Robert Rose.

McVey, G. (2006, June). *A developmental and community-wide approach to the prevention of disordered eating: Findings from outcome-based research.* Oral presentation by the Prevention Special Interest Group during a panel discussion on Prevention Update: An International Perspective at the Academy for Eating Disorders International Conference on Eating Disorders, Barcelona, Spain.

McVey, G. L., & Davis, R. (2002). A program to promote positive body image: A one-year follow-up evaluation. *Journal of Early Adolescence, 22*, 96-108.

McVey, G. L., Davis, R., Kaplan, A. S., Katzman, D. K., Pinhas, L., Geist, R., Heinmaa, M., Forsyth, G. (2005). A community-based training program for eating disorders and its contribution to a provincial network of specialized services. [Supplemental material]. *International Journal of Eating Disorders, 373*, 5-40.

McVey, G. L., Davis, R., Tweed, S., & Shaw, B. P. (2004). Evaluation of a school-based program designed to improve body image satisfaction, global self-esteem, and eating attitudes and behaviors: A replication study. *International Journal of Eating Disorders, 36*, 1-11.

McVey, G., Gusella, J., Tweed, S., & Ferrari, M. (2009). A controlled evaluation of web-based training for teachers and public health practitioners on the prevention of eating disorders. *Eating Disorders: Journal of Treatment and Prevention, 17*, 1-26.

McVey, G. L., Kirsh, G., Maker, D., Walker, K., Mullane, J., Laliberte, M., Ellis-Claypool, J., Vorderbrugge, J., Burnett, A., Cheung, L., Banks, L. (2010). Promoting positive body image among university students: A collaborative pilot study. *Body Image, 7*, 200-204.

McVey, G. L., Lieberman, M., Voorberg, N., Wardrope, D., & Blackmore, E. (2003a). School-based peer support groups: A new approach to the prevention of eating disorders. *Eating Disorders: Journal of Treatment and Prevention, 11*, 169-185.

McVey, G. L., Lieberman, M., Voorberg, N., Wardrope, D., Blackmore, E., & Tweed, S. (2003b). Replication of a peer support prevention program designed to reduce disordered eating: Is a life skills approach sufficient for all middle school students? *Eating Disorders: Journal of Treatment and Prevention, 11*, 187-195.

McVey, G. L., Tweed, S., & Blackmore, E. (2007). Healthy Schools-Healthy Kids: A controlled evaluation of a comprehensive universal eating disorder prevention program. *Body Image, 4*, 115-136.

McVey, G. L., Tweed, S., & Ferrari, M. (2005). *The role of teachers in the prevention of eating disorders: Findings from a school-based prevention program* (poster presented at the meeting of Eating Disorder Research Society Annual Meeting, Toronto, ON).

Menzel, J., & Levine, M. P. (2010). Competitive athletics as a context for embodying experiences and the promotion of positive body image. In R. Calogero, S. Tantleff-Dunn, & J. K. Thompson (Eds.), *Self-objectification in women: Causes, consequences, and counteractions* (pp. 163-186). Washington, DC: American Psychological Association.

Neumark-Sztainer, D., Levine, M. P., Paxton, S. J., Smolak, L., Piran, N., & Wertheim, E. H. (2006). Prevention of body dissatisfaction and disordered eating: What next? *Eating Disorders: Journal of Treatment and Prevention, 14,* 265-285.

Neumark-Sztainer, D., Wall, M. M., Haines, J. I., Story, M. T., Sherwood, N. E., & van den Berg, P. A. (2007). Shared risk and protective factors for overweight and disordered eating in adolescents. *American Journal of Preventive Medicine, 33,* 359-369.

O'Dea, J. A. (2005). School-based health education strategies for the improvement of body image and prevention of eating problems: An overview of safe and effective interventions. *Health Education, 105,* 11-33.

O'Dea, J. A., & Abraham, S. (2000). Improving the body image, eating attitudes, and behaviors of young male and female adolescents: A new educational approach that focuses on self-esteem. *International Journal of Eating Disorders, 28,* 43-57.

O'Dea, J. A., & Maloney, D. (2000). Preventing eating and body image problems in children and adolescents using the health promoting schools framework. *Journal of School Health, 70,* 18-21.

Perez, M., Becker, C. B., & Ramirez, A. (2010). Transportability of an empirically supported dissonance-based prevention program for eating disorders. *Body Image, 7,* 179-186.

Perry, C. L. (1999). *Creating health behavior change: How to develop community-wide programs for youth.* Thousand Oaks, CA: Sage.

Piran, N. (1995). Prevention: Can early lessons lead to a delineation of an alternative model? A critical look at prevention with schoolchildren. *Eating Disorders: Journal of Treatment and Prevention, 3,* 28-36.

Piran, N. (1998). A participatory approach to the prevention of eating disorders in a school. In W. Vandereycken & G. Noordenbos (Eds.), *The prevention of eating disorders* (pp. 173-186). London: Athlone.

Piran, N. (1999a). Eating disorders: A trial of prevention in a high-risk school setting. *Journal of Primary Prevention, 20,* 75-90.

Piran, N. (1999b). On the move from tertiary to secondary and primary prevention: Working with an elite dance school. In N. Piran, M. P. Levine, & C. Steiner-Adair (Eds.), *Preventing eating disorders: A handbook of interventions and special challenges* (pp. 256-269). Philadelphia, PA: Brunner/Mazel.

Piran, N. (1999c). The reduction of preoccupation with body weight and shape in schools: A feminist approach. In N. Piran, M. P. Levine, & C. Steiner-Adair

(Eds.), *Preventing eating disorders: A handbook of interventions and special challenges* (pp. 148-159). Philadelphia, PA: Brunner/Mazel.

Piran, N. (2001). Re-inhabiting the body from the inside out: Girls transform their school environment. In D. L. Tolman & M. Brydon-Miller (Eds.), *From subjects to Subjectivities: A handbook of interpretative and participatory methods* (pp. 218-238). New York: New York University Press.

Piran, N. (2004). Teachers: On "being" (rather than "doing") prevention. *Eating Disorders: Journal of Treatment and Prevention, 12,* 1-9.

Piran, N. (2005). Prevention of eating disorders: A review of outcome evaluation research. *Israel Journal of Psychiatry and Related Sciences, 42,* 172-177.

Piran, N. (2010). A feminist perspective on risk factor research and on the prevention of eating disorders. *Eating Disorders: Journal of Treatment and Prevention, 18,* 183-198.

Ranby, K. W., Aiken, L. S., MacKinnon, D. P., Elliot, D. L., Moe, E. L., McGinnis, W., & Goldberg, L. (2009). A mediation analysis of the ATHENA Intervention for female athletes: Prevention of athletic-enhancing substance use and unhealthy weight loss behaviors. *Journal of Pediatric Psychology, 34,* 1069-1083.

Reese, L. E., Wingfield, J. H., & Blumenthal, D. (2009). Advancing prevention, health promotion, and social justice through practical integration of preventive science and practice. In M. E. Kenny, A. M. Horne, P. Orpinas, & L. E. Reese (Eds.), *Realizing social justice: The challenge of preventive interventions* (pp. 37-55). Washington, DC: American Psychological Association.

Rose, G. (2001). Sick individuals and sick populations. *International Journal of Epidemiology, 30,* 427-432.

Rosskam, E. (2009). Using participatory action research methodology to improve worker health. In P. L. Schnall, M. Dobson, & E. Rosskam (Eds.), *Unhealthy work: Causes, consequences, cures* (pp. 211-228). Amityville, NY: Baywood.

Russell-Mayhew, S., Arthur, N., & Ewashen, C. (2007). Targeting students, teachers and parents in a wellness-based prevention program in schools. *Eating Disorders: Journal of Treatment and Prevention, 15,* 159-181.

Shepard, J., & Carlson, J. S. (2003). An empirical evaluation of school-based prevention programs that involve parents. *Psychology in the Schools, 40,* 641-656.

Sinton, M. M., & Taylor, C. B. (2010). Prevention: Current status and underlying theory. In W. S. Agras (Ed.), *Oxford handbook of eating disorders* (pp. 307-330). New York: Oxford University Press.

Smolak, L., & Levine, M. P. (1996). Developmental transitions at middle school and college. In L. Smolak, M. P. Levine, & R. H. Striegel-Moore (Eds.), *The developmental psychopathology of eating disorders: Implications for research, prevention, and treatment* (pp. 207-233). Hillsdale, NJ: Lawrence Erlbaum Associates.

Smolak, L., & Murnen, S.K. (2007). Feminism and body image. In V. Swami & A. Furnham (Eds.), *The body beautiful: Evolutionary and socio-cultural perspectives* (pp. 236-258). London: Palgrave Macmillan.

Smolak, L., Murnen, S. K., & Ruble, A. E. (2000). Female athletes and eating disorders: A meta-analysis. *International Journal of Eating Disorders, 27,* 371-381.

Society for Prevention Research. (2004). *Standards of evidence: Criteria for efficacy, effectiveness and dissemination.* Retrieved from http://www.prevention research.org/StandardsofEvidencebook.pdf

Steiner-Adair, C. (1994). The politics of prevention. In P. Fallon, M. A. Katzman, & S. C. Wooley (Eds.), *Feminist perspectives on eating disorders* (pp. 381-394). New York: Guilford Press.

Steiner-Adair, C., Sjostrom, L., Franko, D. L., Pai, S., Tucker, R., Becker, A. E., & Herzog, D. B. (2002). Primary prevention of eating disorders in adolescent girls: Learning from practice. *International Journal of Eating Disorders, 32,* 401-411.

Stice, E., Shaw, H., & Marti, C. N. (2007). A meta-analytic review of eating disorder prevention programs: Encouraging findings. *Annual Review of Clinical Psychology, 3,* 207-231.

Thompson, R. A., & Sherman, R. T. (2010). *Eating disorders in sport.* New York: Routledge.

Tobler, N. S., Roona, M. R., Ochshorn, P., Marshall, D. G., Streke, A. V., & Stackpole, K. M. (2000). School-based adolescent prevention programs: 1998 meta-analysis. *Journal of Primary Prevention, 20,* 275-336.

Trost, A. S. (2007). The Healthy Image Partnership (HIP) parents program: The role of parental involvement in eating disorder prevention. *Dissertation Abstracts International, 61*(12), 2327.

Weissberg, R. P., Kumpfer, K. L., & Seligman, M. E. P. (Eds.). (2003). Prevention that works for children and youth. [Special issue]. *American Psychologist, 58*(6-7).

Wilksch, S. M., & Wade, T. D. (2009). School-based eating disorder prevention. In S. Paxton & P. Hay (Eds.), *Interventions for body dissatisfaction and eating disorders: Evidence and practice. Melbourne* (pp. 7-22). Australia: IP Communications.

Yager, Z., & O'Dea, J. A. (2008). Prevention programs for body image and eating disorders on university campuses: A review of large, controlled interventions. *Health Promotion International, 23,* 173-189.

CHAPTER TWO

Prevention of Disordered Eating through Structural Change: The Population Health Framework and Lessons from Case Studies in Intensive Community-Based Intervention

Lindsay McLaren, *University of Calgary*
Niva Piran, *Ontario Institute for Studies in Education, University of Toronto*

Body dissatisfaction, disordered eating behaviour, and eating disorders have been linked with numerous correlates or risk factors operating at various levels, including the individual level (e.g., the internalization of thinness, body dissatisfaction, perfectionism; see Stice, 2001); the level of one's family or peer group (e.g., critical comments about body weight/shape from parents or peers, see McLaren, Kuh, Hardy, & Gauvin, 2004; Wertheim, Paxton, & Blaney, 2004); and the broader socio-cultural environment (e.g., gender inequity, see Piran, 2001a; Piran, 2001b; Piran & Thompson, 2008; and weight prejudice and its intersection with classism or ethno-cultural bias, see Anderson-Fye & Becker, 2004; Bowen, Tomoyasu, & Cauce, 1999; Piran, 2001b).

One might expect this breadth of influences to translate into a similar breadth of targets for prevention strategies. In general, this is not the case. Although there is increasing recognition of the need for an ecological approach to preventing eating disorders (McVey, Tweed, Blackmore, 2007; Neumark-Sztainer, Sherwood, Coller, & Hannan, 2000; Neumark-Sztainer et al., 2006; Piran, 1995), whereby individual and contextual systems and their interaction are emphasized (Bronfenbrenner, 1979; McLaren & Hawe, 2005), the focus of most existing prevention efforts has ultimately been the individual, and it has typically entailed some variant of provision of information. To illustrate, Pratt and Woolfenden (2009) conducted a Cochrane systematic review of interventions (all evaluated using a randomized controlled design) to prevent eating disorders in the general population or in high-risk samples. Although socio-cultural factors (e.g., social pressures to be thin) were acknowledged by the study's authors, the intervention target in all twelve studies was the individual, who was the recipient—via didactic or interactive means—of health promotion messages around healthy eating, coping skills, and media literacy. In other words, the implicit or explicit approach was to build individuals' resistance to broader socio-cultural influences rather than to tackle these broader influences themselves—either directly or indirectly by articulating a process through which individual knowledge/skills may translate into broader socio-cultural change.

Pratt and Woolfenden (2009, p. 16) concluded their review by stating that "there is insufficient support for the effectiveness of any specific type of eating disorder prevention program for children and adolescents." By way of explanation, the authors commented that "the impact of the media and the peer group on a developing adolescent's belief systems are very strong and appear quite resistant to short-term individual or small group therapeutic intervention," a sentiment that has been echoed elsewhere (Neumark-Sztainer et al., 2006). A tendency to revert to the individual level as the target for prevention strategies is not unique to the eating disorders field and, in fact, is apparent in many areas of health, where intervention effectiveness is similarly low, such as obesity prevention (for example, Summerbell et al., 2006). In their important article entitled "Prevention of body dissatisfaction and disordered eating: What next?" Neumark-Sztainer and colleagues (2006, p. 267) comment that, given the important contribution of cultural factors to the development of body dissatisfaction and disordered eating, "efforts to change the environment are likely to be critical." The question is: how do we accomplish this? Some guidance is needed.

The population health framework can provide this guidance, and the objective of the present chapter is to convey the framework's implications for the prevention of eating disorders and related outcomes (e.g., disordered eating). The chapter is divided into two major sections. In the first section, we introduce the population health framework and identify how it could apply to disordered eating prevention. In the second section, which looks towards bridging the population health framework with the existing research literature on disordered eating prevention, we consider an initiative that has elements of a population health approach and that has produced notable and sustained preventive effects in a school setting. We conclude by offering several suggestions for achieving such a pronounced and longer-term impact from disordered eating prevention efforts.

Population Health Framework

Perhaps the best way to introduce the population health framework is to provide a vignette contained in the 1999 report of Canada's Federal-Provincial-Territorial Committee on Population Health (Public Health Canada, 1999):

> *Why is Jason in the hospital?*
> Because he has a bad infection in his leg.
> *But why does he have an infection?*
> Because he has a cut on his leg and it got infected.
> *But why does he have a cut on his leg?*
> Because he was playing in the junkyard next to his apartment building and there was some sharp, jagged steel there that he fell on.
> *But why was he playing in a junkyard?*
> Because his neighbourhood is kind of run down. A lot of kids play there and there is no one to supervise them.
> *But why does he live in that neighbourhood?*
> Because his parents can't afford a nicer place to live.
> *But why can't his parents afford a nicer place to live?*
> Because his Dad is unemployed and his Mom is sick.
> *But why is his Dad unemployed?*
> Because he doesn't have much education and he can't find a job.
> *But why...*

As illustrated in the vignette, the determinants of health are complex and interrelated. One could continue to ask "but why..." when unravelling the multiple layers of influence on Jason's health. The infection in his leg is only one part of the story, and there are several points at which one could intervene: antibiotics for the infection; municipal, private sector, or grassroots efforts to clean up the junk yard; and provincial and/or federal social policy to support families. In the following example, we offer an adaptation of the vignette suitable to the chapter at hand:

> *Why is Julie in the hospital?*
> Because she has anorexia nervosa that has become life threatening.
> *But why has her illness become life threatening?*
> Because prolonged starvation has caused her body systems to begin to shut down.
> *But why has Julie engaged in prolonged starvation?*
> Because she wanted very much to be thin.
> *But why did she want to be thin?*

In part, because of comments about her weight made by members of her
family and peer group.

But why did her family and friends make these comments?

Such comments often reflect the enormous value placed on thinness in
the society in which Julie lives and equating thinness with moral
virtue, particularly in women.

But why is this the case and why is it unique to women?

Because of broader issues that our society grapples with, such as gender
inequity, weight prejudice, and their intersection with classism and
ethno-cultural biases.

But why...

Clearly, a biomedical model of health, whereby health is equated with the
absence of disease, is insufficient to embrace these myriad determinants.
A broader definition of health is required, which embraces mental and
social as well as physical dimensions of health and which views health
as a resource for living rather than as a static end state (Health and Welfare Canada, 1986; World Health Organization, 1948). Life-threatening
anorexia nervosa clearly necessitates urgent medical intervention; however,
if the goal is to avoid future cases such as Julie's, one must look beyond the
medical setting. As with Jason's story, intervention in Julie's vignette could
conceivably occur at several levels: the family, the school or work environment, the community, and — crucially — broader societal processes and
institutions that profit from the commodification of women's bodies.

As a more formal definition, the Public Health Agency of Canada (2004,
para. 1) defines population health as an approach to health that aims to
"improve the health of the entire population [and to] reduce health inequities among population groups." To achieve these objectives, the population
health approach necessitates looking at and acting on the broad range of
factors and conditions that have a strong influence on our health (ibid.).
Health inequities refer to variation in health outcomes that occurs within
and between countries, which reflect variations in economic and social circumstances that are unjust or avoidable (Commission on the Social Determinants of Health, 2008; Whitehead, 1992). The topic of socio-economic
inequalities in weight-related health issues is addressed in Chapter 10 of
this volume. In this chapter, we focus on other aspects of a population
health approach.

A focus on populations means that we are not focusing just on those who
are sick or who are at risk of becoming sick. In this way, population health
embraces prevention, including not only primary prevention (prevention of
ill health in those who are currently healthy or at least asymptomatic) but

also primordial prevention, which is about preventing risk factors, reducing the risk of risk, and acting on the causes of causes (Kaplan & Lynch, 1999; Last, 2001; Marmot, 2007). A useful concept in this case is upstream:

> There is an old story about a man who sees someone drowning in a river and jumps in to save him. As soon as he does this, he notices even more people in the river in danger of drowning. He dives in again and again to help. He quickly becomes exhausted from rescuing everyone and he begins to wonder what is happening upstream to get people into difficulties in the river in the first place, and what can be done to keep them out of it.
>
> It turns out that further upstream there are two communities, one on each side of the river. To get from one community to another, people have to wade across the river because there is no bridge. But the water is fast flowing and quite deep, not everyone can swim, and only a few people can afford boats.
>
> In population health, the idea is that the further "upstream" an action is directed, the greater the potential for improving population health. In the case of the people in the river, for example, the population health approach would be to build a bridge between the two communities and also to make sure that as many people as possible learned to swim. (Canadian Population Health Initiative, 2007)

Returning to the earlier story of Julie, inserting a feeding tube to enable caloric intake or a mechanical device to keep her heart beating would be a downstream approach, analogous to pulling drowning people out of the river. Intervening in an upstream manner would involve efforts to achieve a socio-cultural environment that facilitates—rather than detracts from—desired outcomes such as body acceptance and gender equity. Such efforts, discussed in further detail later in this chapter, could help to prevent Julie—and others like her—from entering the hospital in the first place.

The Causes of Cases and the Causes of Incidence: Introducing Rose

When thinking about populations, it is necessary to have an understanding of cause that applies to whole populations as a unit of analysis. For this, we draw on the work of British epidemiologist Geoffrey Rose (1985, 1992), who made the simple but important distinction between the *causes of cases* (that is, reasons why one individual gets sick while another remains healthy) and the *causes of incidence* (i.e., reasons why the prevalence of some illness differs between two populations or changes across a population over time). The reason this distinction is important is because causes at the two levels may be different. For example, certain personality traits (e.g., neuroticism) or psychological attributes (e.g., self-esteem) may cause (or constitute risk factors for) body dissatisfaction at the individual level; while the "causes" of a higher prevalence of body dissatisfaction in one population (e.g., a country, a city, a community, or a school) than in another may include social norms and expectations around the status of women and body shape and size that are unique to that population.

Understanding both types of causes is important, and exclusive focus on one or the other can lead to an incomplete understanding of a phenomenon. For example, a particular personality trait may emerge as an important risk factor for body dissatisfaction within a population and provide important clues about vulnerability within that population, but it may not register as a risk factor when comparing one country to another. Likewise, differential impact of the media may be difficult to detect within a media-saturated society, but it may emerge quite prominently when comparing two populations or one population at two points in time.[1] An example of the latter scenario is Becker's (2004; see also Becker, Burwell, Gilman, Herzog, & Hamburg, 2002) investigation of eating attitudes and behaviours in ethnic Fijian schoolgirls prior to, and three years following, the introduction of Western television. Within this context of rapid social change from a media-naive culture that did not traditionally value thinness, marked increases in disordered eating attitudes and behaviours were observed. For example, the percentage of girls with eating attitude-related questionnaire scores (EAT-26) beyond the recommended cutoff was 12.7% in 1995 versus 29.2% in 1998. Reported vomiting to control weight was non-existent in 1995 and 11.3% in 1998. Girls' narratives revealed an interest in weight loss that reflected a desire to emulate television characters.

High-Risk and Population Approaches to Prevention

Rose (1985, 1992) outlined two prevention strategies corresponding to the two aforementioned levels of cause.[2] The high-risk strategy, analogous to a selected approach, involves identifying individuals who are at risk of developing a health problem and targeting them in a specific way (e.g., Stice, Shaw, & Marti, 2007). In the population strategy, analogous to a universal approach, individuals are not singled out based on risk status; rather, a population as a whole is targeted (e.g., Stice et al., 2007). Taking body dissatisfaction as a proximal risk factor for disordered eating (Stice et al., 2007; Striegel-Moore & Bulik, 2007), an example of a high-risk approach would be identifying individuals with elevated body dissatisfaction and providing education and support to help them accept their bodies and become critical consumers of unrealistic images presented in visual mass media. An example of a population-level approach would be to target the harmful messages themselves (i.e., messages that convey "Western" culture's unrealistically thin female beauty ideal and the objectification of the female body, which, in turn, influence or constitute a risk factor for body dissatisfaction and disordered eating; Levine & Murnen, 2009; Striegel-Moore & Bulik, 2007), through efforts by industry and/or government to downplay an emphasis on physical appearance or to present a diversity of body sizes among fashion models and other beauty icons.

The high-risk strategy is the conventional approach in the medical profession and is intuitively appealing in that the intervention is delivered to those who need it most or who would be expected to benefit most (Rose, 1992). Correspondingly, high-risk interventions can also be effective in a limited sense. For example, in a meta-analysis of eating disorder prevention programs evaluated using a controlled design, Stice, Shaw, and Marti (2007) observed that the risk status of participants was an important moderator of program effectiveness, such that selected programs (targeting high-risk participants) were more effective than universal programs.

However, there are significant limitations associated with the high-risk strategy (Rose, 1985, 1992). Most prominently, the approach is by nature temporary and palliative. According to Rose (1992, p. 47), the high-risk approach "does not seek to alter the situations which determine exposure, nor to attack the underlying reasons why the particular health problem exists." Encouraging young women to become critical consumers of harmful messages conveyed through fashion media does nothing (in and of itself) to change or reduce the harmful messages themselves, and, thus, prevention efforts for these high-risk individuals would have to continue indefinitely (that is, a one-time approach is inherently insufficient). Further, because the root causes of the problem (that is, our society's unrealistically thin female beauty ideal and objectification of the female body, generally speaking) have not been addressed, new "high-risk" individuals (for example, individuals with elevated body dissatisfaction) will continue to emerge, and they too will require ongoing prevention. In short, the high-risk approach works against the grain, which leads to the observation made by Stice and his colleagues (2007, p. 222), among others, that "prevention effects tend to fade over time, which may be unavoidable given the ubiquitous pressures for thinness in our culture."

Another potential drawback of the high-risk approach has to do with the feasibility of identifying those at risk (Rose, 1992). Such efforts (e.g., screening) can be time intensive and resource intensive, and the results are not always clear. Risk is often appropriately characterized as existing on a continuum, as opposed to clear categories of presence versus absence (Rose, 1992). In such a situation, a designated clinical cutoff may be somewhat arbitrary, and the question arises of what to do with those at a borderline level of risk. However, even if we were capable of perfectly accurate identification

TABLE 1: INCIDENCE OF DOWN'S SYNDROME ACCORDING TO MATERNAL AGE

Maternal age (years)	Risk of Down's syndrome per 1,000 births	Total births in age group (as percentage of all ages)	Percentage of total Down's syndrome age occurring in age group
<30	0.7	78	51
30-34	1.3	16	20
35-39	3.7	5	16
40-44	13.1	0.95	11
≥45	34.6	0.05	2
All ages	1.5	100	100

Source: Reproduced from Rose (2001). Used with the permission of Oxford University Press.

of high-risk individuals, and even if a high-risk prevention strategy existed that was 100% effective, an important limitation remains: the difficulty of achieving a population-level impact. A reason for this difficulty was articulated by Rose (1992, p. 24) in his assertion that "a large number of people exposed to a small risk may generate many more cases than a small number exposed to a high risk," and this theory is illustrated in Table 1, which relates the occurrence of Down's syndrome births to maternal age. Although older mothers have a higher risk of this outcome than younger mothers, the number of older mothers is far exceeded by the number of younger mothers and, thus, a large proportion (in this case, approximately half) of Down's syndrome births occur in younger mothers, simply because there are so many of them. Earlier, we commented on the effectiveness "in a limited sense" of high-risk approaches. The limited view of effectiveness is herein illustrated—an effective high-risk approach may not register as change when population level indicators (e.g., prevalence) are considered to be the barometer of impact.

This phenomenon (a large number of people at small risk may give rise to more cases of disease than the small number at high risk) has been observed for a wide range of risk factors that are continuous in nature (i.e., for which a range of risk is possible) and that show a population frequency distribution that is unimodal and/or normal—examples include blood cholesterol and blood pressure (risk for cardiovascular disease),[3] intraocular pressure (risk for glaucoma), and bone health (risk for fractures) (Khaw & Marmot, 2008; Rose, 1992). As an extension of this work, Austin (2001) examined dieting frequency as a risk factor for disordered eating (specifically purging behaviour), using population-based data from US adolescents. After confirming that dieting frequency constituted a risk

FIGURE 1: PERCENTAGE OF PURGING CASELOAD OCCURRING IN EACH DIETING FREQUENCY CATEGORY, BASED ON DATA FROM FRENCH ET AL. (1995) PUBLISHED BY AUSTIN (2001)

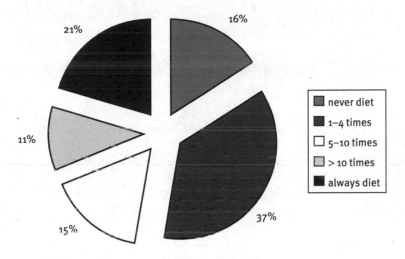

Source: Reprinted from Austin (2001). Used with permission from Elsevier.

factor for purging at the individual level (i.e., those who reported frequent dieting were more likely to purge than those who dieted less frequently), Austin demonstrated that while 21% of "cases" (those who purge) were in the highest dieting frequency group (the high risk group), a much greater proportion (63%) of purgers were found among girls who dieted less frequently (the lower risk group), as illustrated in Figure 1.

The implication is that, in order to have an impact on population-level indicators such as prevalence, it is insufficient to only target those at elevated risk. Rose's population strategy aims to shift a population's frequency distribution of risk, in the direction of lower risk (see Figure 2). As illustrated in Figure 2, this approach can theoretically have a major impact on the proportion in the high-risk range. The potentially large impact of the population strategy has to do with the features of a normal distribution: the mean (average) of the distribution is closely related to the proportion of deviance (e.g., the proportion of young women with "clinical" levels of body dissatisfaction is associated with [determined by] the mean level of body dissatisfaction in that population). If the distribution as a whole shifts to the left, the proportion falling beyond the clinical cutoff (beneath the curve, to the right of the dotted line) is, by definition, reduced, potentially by a remarkable magnitude.

**FIGURE 2: DEPICTION OF THE HYPOTHETICAL IMPACT OF A POPULATION-LEVEL
INTERVENTION, ACHIEVED BY SHIFTING THE FREQUENCY DISTRIBUTION IN A
DIRECTION OF LOWER RISK**

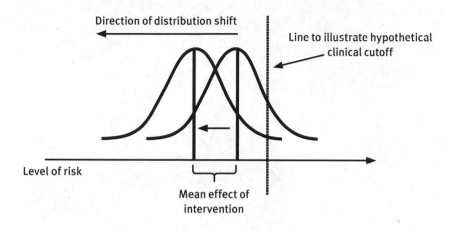

Population-Level Prevention of Disordered Eating

Shifting the population distribution of dieting or other risk factors such as
body dissatisfaction could be a powerful way to reduce the prevalence of
disordered eating (Austin, 2001). How would we actually go about doing
this? According to Rose (1985, 1992), and subsequently built on by others (McLaren et al., 2010), a population-level approach can take varying
forms: some are superficial/agentic in nature, while others are more radi-
cal/structural. Although in both cases the target is a population (which
may be interpreted variably as a geographic area, a group, a jurisdiction,
an institution, and so on) without regard to variation in risk status within,
the approaches differ from one another in an important regard. Interventions of a superficial or agentic nature aim to change individuals' attitudes
or behaviours through encouragement or persuasion (Rose, 1992) — for
example, a health information campaign or classroom curriculum. This
approach, though population-wide, would not be expected to have a major
impact on prevalence because it is (typically) blind to structural (e.g.,
social, cultural, and economic) barriers to change (McLaren et al., 2010;
Rose, 1992). For example, encouraging young women to accept their bodies, by increasing their awareness of the unrealistic depiction of women
in fashion media, is insufficient on its own to achieve large-scale change
in attitudes or behaviours in a context where opposing messages domi-
nate. Drawing from the diffusion of innovations theory, such an approach
may work for some (i.e., the innovators and early adopters, who may also

embody attributes that are protective against disordered eating such as self-esteem and internal locus of control), but it is unlikely to yield population-level impact. The theory predicts that variation in uptake is to be expected such that later adopters (those for whom intervention impact is delayed or not forthcoming, perhaps because they are more vulnerable to the harmful messages) "may require special efforts to overcome barriers" (Oldenburg & Parcel, 2002, p. 317).

Another type of population approach, which can offset some of the limitations of a superficial approach, is radical (Rose, 1992) or structural (McLaren et al., 2010) in nature. It aims to "remove the underlying impediments to healthier behaviour, or to control adverse pressures" (Rose, 1992, p. 134). In other words, the target of change is the conditions in which behaviours occur rather than the behaviours themselves (McLaren et al., 2010). Well-known examples of radical/structural population strategies of prevention exist outside of the eating disorders realm, such as the fluoridation of drinking water and mandatory seatbelt laws. These interventions are structural in that they contribute to creating a context in which the desired outcome (oral fluoride exposure, seatbelt use) is facilitated, such that an individual does not have to "go against the grain" to benefit from the intervention. Through a radical/structural approach, the issue of differential uptake (a built-in limitation of the superficial/agentic approach) is largely obviated because the desired behaviour or outcome has become the easy, or the default, choice. The two interventions mentioned (drinking water fluoridation and mandatory seatbelt laws) have contributed to important population-level improvements in the desired outcomes: a reduction in dental caries (McDonagh et al., 2000) and a reduction in traffic fatalities and crash-related serious injuries (Carpenter & Stehr, 2008), respectively. An added benefit of these radical/structural population strategies is that the impact can be ongoing. Once these interventions have been implemented, subsequent implementation costs (economic and social) may be few. For example, once the infrastructure for municipal water fluoridation has been built, the subsequent costs become minimal, and mandatory seatbelt laws with enforcement may contribute to seatbelt use becoming a social norm, such that non-use becomes the (potentially stigmatized) exception.

Importantly, although the intervention "types" described earlier convey a dichotomy, it is more appropriate to view superficial/agentic and radical/structural as falling along a continuum (McLaren et al., 2010). The intervention ladder shown in Figure 3 outlines a range of public health intervention approaches that vary in terms of their level of intrusiveness on individuals' lives. Generally speaking, superficial/agentic interventions

FIGURE 3: PUBLIC HEALTH INTERVENTION LADDER

Eliminate Choice. Regulate in such a way as to entirely eliminate choice, for example through compulsory isolation of patients with infectious diseases.
Restrict Choice. Regulate in such a way as to restrict the options available to people with the aim of protecting them, for example removing unhealthy ingredients from foods, or unhealthy foods from shops or restaurants.
Guide choice through disincentives. Fiscal and other disincentives can be put in place to influence people not to pursue certain activities, for example through taxes on cigarettes, or by discouraging the use of cars in inner cities through charging schemes or limitations on parking spaces.
Guide choices through incentives. Regulations can be offered that guide choices by fiscal and other incentives; for example, offering tax breaks for the purchase of bicycles that are used as a means of travelling to work.
Guide choices through changing the default policy. For example, in a restaurant, instead of providing chips as a standard side dish (with healthier options available), menus could be changed to provide a more healthy option as a standard (with chips as an option available).
Enable choice. Enable individuals to change their behaviours, for example by offering participation in an NHS "stop smoking" program, building cycle lanes, or providing free free fruit in schools.
Provide information. Inform and educate the public, for example as part of campaigns to encourage people to walk more or eat five portions of fruit and vegtables per day.
Do nothing or simply monitor the current situation.

Source: Nuffield Council on Bioethics (2007).

(e.g., the provision of information) are located towards the bottom of the ladder, while radical/structural strategies appear as one moves up the ladder, which place increasing emphasis on creating conditions that guide, facilitate, or mandate the desired outcome. We have previously argued in this chapter that many existing eating disorder prevention programs emphasize the provision of information targeted at individuals, thus falling towards the bottom of the intervention ladder. However, examples of approaches falling higher on the ladder exist. For example, in 1999, the Spanish federal government proposed legislation requiring that fashion models not be too thin (Bosch, 1999, 2000). In response to an estimated 15 percent increase in the incidence of anorexia nervosa per year, the opposition government initiated dialogue with advertisers and marketing companies persuading them to use models who are not unrealistically thin. More recently, these sentiments were echoed by the Madrid regional government, which, prompted by catwalk models during Spanish Fashion Week 2006, demanded that models have a body mass index of at least 18 kilograms per square metre (the body mass index range considered to be "normal" is 18.5-24.9 kilograms per square metre).

Assuming that the aim of these Spanish initiatives was to reduce the visibility of (and hence exposure to) visual images that convey harmful messages, these examples might be characterized as "restrict choice" on the intervention ladder, in that the visual images are "regulate(d) in such a way as to restrict the options available to people [i.e., reduce or eliminate options that are unrealistically thin] with the aim of protecting them [from the effects of such exposure]" (Nuffield Council on Bioethics, 2007, p. 42). Notwithstanding ethical and ideological resistance to "intrusive" health interventions, we assert the following: to the extent that the size of fashion models taps into broader social influences on (causes of) disordered eating, such intervention approaches could plausibly contribute to population-wide and sustained impacts on disordered eating prevalence and/or incidence. Unfortunately, the details pertaining to the implementation of these initiatives do not appear to be available, nor is there any information about their impact, if any.

The intervention ladder provides other suggestions that could be incorporated into disordered eating prevention efforts, towards the achievement of a sustained population-level impact. To begin to integrate these ideas, however, we must first embrace the fact that the unrealistic aspect of the idealized thin female physique is what makes it desirable and thus profitable in our capitalist economy, which, in turn, makes it ubiquitous (e.g., Campos, 2005; Shilling, 2005). Thus, intervention efforts would need to break the link so that it is no longer profitable for companies, institutions, and individuals to promote (and thereby benefit from the promotion of) the unrealistically thin ideal and the objectification of women. One approach could be pricing (dis)incentives to guide consumer behaviour. For example, if magazines that promoted an unrealistically thin ideal/ objectification of women were more expensive to purchase than others, their profitability would decline and they may ultimately disappear (notwithstanding the complexities associated with free publications on the Internet). Another approach could involve incentives (e.g., tax breaks and merit awards) for companies, institutions, and others to promote a healthier, more equitable ideal. Such efforts have been undertaken voluntarily (e.g., the Dove campaign for real beauty).[4] Interventions such as these are large scale, complex, and likely to carry unanticipated or unintended consequences. Thus, to accompany incentive-based interventions, it would be essential to support efforts to rigorously evaluate their implementation and impact, such as devoted research grant opportunities. Such opportunities would need to embrace the methods (e.g., a natural [quasi-] experimental case study) and partnerships (e.g., academic-private sector or academic-government [municipal/provincial/federal] sector) that are unique to these types of research questions (for an example of this type of funding opportunity, see the Institute of Population and Public Health within the Canadian Institutes of Health Research).[5]

In the previous paragraphs, we introduced a population health framework and asserted its potential utility for achieving sustained, population-level prevention of disordered eating. In a number of ways, this approach departs from current eating disorder prevention initiatives. Specifically, the population health approach emphasizes environmental change through action on underlying causes and its population-level impact. In contrast, many existing eating disorder prevention programs emphasize individual change and impact within the group being studied (e.g., Pratt & Woolfenden, 2009). Further, much eating disorder prevention takes place among youth within school settings, while the population health approach is potentially much broader in scope. We thus need to find a way to bridge the two arenas. By way of offering such a bridge, we now turn to existing work in eating disorder prevention that accommodates features of a population health approach (i.e., environmental change, action on the underlying causes, and an evaluation of population-level impact) but that retains practices widely accepted in the eating disorder prevention literature (i.e., a focus on youth in school settings and curriculum change). Importantly, the work we discuss in the following section shows evidence of a significant, sustained population-level impact and, as such, attests to the potential utility of the population health approach as applied to eating disorder prevention.

Intervening at the Community Level: A Possible Bridge between the Radical/Structural and the Individual-Level Approaches

We would like to propose that community-based interventions with certain attributes may provide a possible path to sustained, population-level prevention of eating disorders in youth. In this way, school communities or sororities, for example, can become the target of intervention that aims at changing adverse structural factors in these communities such as weight prejudice (as it often intersects with social class prejudice), gender, or other forms of inequity. In these community-based approaches, individual members work constructively to transform their community, informed by their ecological understanding of body weight and shape preoccupation and disordered eating patterns.

One model for such interventions in schools is the Health-Promoting School Model of the European Network of Health-Promoting Schools (Burgher, Rasmussen, & Rivett, 1999). In this model, the school community becomes a target of intervention aimed at enhancing the physical, social, psychological, and intellectual health of students. In response to a health challenge, the school system initiates a comprehensive approach to health enhancement that addresses three main elements: the school environment, the community, and the classroom curriculum. Student empowerment and the active engagement of all stakeholders of the school community (administrators, teachers, parents, and students) are pivotal elements of the program. Addressing issues of diversity and equity are also key elements of this approach to health. A health initiative in a health-promoting school typically involves the implementation of relevant policies and procedures, physical and organizational changes in the school environment, staff training, and curriculum changes. Professionals working in the field of eating disorder prevention have called for adopting this model in efforts to prevent eating disorders among school children (O'Dea & Maloney, 2000; Piran, 1999a). O'Dea and Maloney (2000), for instance, give an example of a high school in Australia in which a problem of laxative abuse was found among a sizable minority of students. With input from all of the stakeholders of the school community, the relevant curriculum was changed from including a unit on symptoms of eating disorders to a focus on social expectations of women, the media, and coping strategies. Similarly, teachers scrutinized their attitude towards diverse body shapes, thereby contributing to a school ethos that was more favourable to the development of healthy attitudes around weight and food (see also Piran, 2004, for a discussion of the role of teachers in changing the school environment). Changes to the selection of foods available in the school cafeteria represented a change in the physical environment of the school. The collaboration among different stakeholders in the school community around the issue of laxative consumption and the enhanced links with community-based health resources represented structural changes to the school mode of operation. While no data were provided regarding changes in the prevalence of laxatives among students, it is important to emphasize that ecological approaches to change highlight different levels of outcome, from more immediate outcomes (system change such as establishing a relevant committee or shifting the allocation of resources), to intermediate outcomes (such as changes to policies, norms, and the school environment), to an ultimate outcome (such as changes in individuals' behaviours) (e.g., Green & Kreuter, 1991). In their article, O'Dea and Maloney (2000) delineate immediate and intermediate changes, without reporting on students' behaviours.

The emphasis on school culture, on issues of gender equity, and on weight prejudice has been highlighted by Piran in her prevention work in schools (e.g., Piran, 2001b, 2004). Piran (2001b) has applied a participatory-action approach to the prevention of eating disorders in a competitive residential dance school. This program followed the Health-Promoting School Model in its emphasis on implementing changes in all aspects of the school environment, empowering students, examining issues of equity, and intervening with all of the stakeholders in the school community, with a particular emphasis on staff education and teacher training. However, the prevention program was also informed by the theory of the participatory action paradigm described in detail in the intensive case study analysis of the dance school intervention (Piran, 2001b). In the dance school program, students were continually invited to examine in focus groups the factors that made them want to alter their body weight and shape, the changes they wanted to see in their school environment, and the tasks they wanted to take on in changing their school environment. The participatory action prevention project was found to be associated with significant and sustained population-level changes in students' body esteem and eating patterns (Piran, 1999a). Specifically, over a 10-year period, during which three different cohorts of same-aged girls were studied, remarkable declines in the prevalence of disordered eating and body dissatisfaction were documented (Piran, 1999a). For example, among students in grades 10-12, the prevalence of disordered eating (based on the EAT-26 scale) declined from approximately 48% in 1987 to approximately 16% in 1996. Although there was no control group, there was certainly no evidence of such a reduction in disordered eating across the general population during the same time period or in the changed standards of thinness in the ballet world, suggesting that the effects reflect circumstances within the school to at least some extent. Beyond the association of the program with significant and sustainable reductions in disordered eating patterns, the program has shed new light on the understanding of eating disorders as well as on the processes of change involved in the prevention of eating disorders in schools.

In the domain of theory construction, an analysis of the students' group discussions revealed that students' critical reflections about the social forces that adversely affected their body experiences at the school related to social power, equity, and worth (Piran, 2001b). These experiences were shaped by the "macro," population-wide, social factors of gender, ethno-cultural, or socio-economic group membership. In terms of gender, for example, being a girl at the school made it more likely that a student would be exposed to experiences that compromised her sense of ownership over her physical body, that she would be subjected to (often bodily) demeaning prejudices (such as being teased about being a "fat cow"), and that she would be expected to fit "feminine" moulds of being "good" or "demure." All of these experiences adversely affected the girls' embodied experiences. The innovative understanding derived in the participatory action project of the multiple ways in which gender shapes experiences that may contribute to the development of eating disorders was later confirmed using quantitative studies. Specifically, structural equation modelling with two different large samples of young women—a university sample and a community sample—confirmed a model that proposed that violations of body ownership, as well as experiences of exposure to prejudicial treatment, exerted a direct influence on the development of disordered eating patterns (Piran & Thompson, 2008). Similarly, internalized social constructions of "femininity" were found to be associated with disordered eating patterns (Piran & Cormier, 2005). Indeed, in line with Kraemer, Tebes, Kaufman, and Connell's (2003) suggestions, in addition to Fishman's (1999) ideas, the intensive case study analysis of the community-based, participatory prevention program has led to advances in theory construction of body weight and shape preoccupation and disordered eating patterns.

Also relevant to the theoretical understanding of disordered eating patterns is a discussion of the relationship between population-based "macro"-level and individual-level risk factors. Students' narratives in the participatory action prevention project suggest a connection between "macro"-level social factors and individual-level factors. This scenario is reflected, for example, in a quotation from a girl group's discussion of their own teasing behaviour, which precipitated a rapid weight loss in their peer: "We call her 'butch' because she has such strong muscles, she can lift a guy...A girl is not supposed to be stronger than guys, she is supposed to be smaller...Guys don't like it when you are too strong, like too opinionated or something...Girls can't have too much power" (Piran, 2001b, p. 226). This quotation is one of many in the study that demonstrates the inherent connection between "macro" social factors, such as gender, and individual-level experiences in students' narratives. Similarly, an African-Canadian student in the dance school shared the important advice she received at home, grounded in her family members' experiences of pervasive exposure to heritage-based prejudicial treatment: "You have to stay really skinny; it's your only chance to make it" (see Nichter, Vuckovic, & Parker, 1999, for a discussion of body image dissatisfaction among African-American women who internalize white women's ideals of beauty). A large-scale prospective qualitative study of girls and a life history study of young women have similarly confirmed girls' critical understanding of the connection between social privilege and daily body-anchored experiences (e.g., Piran, Carter, Thompson, & Pajouhandeh, 2002; Piran et al., 2006). Piran (2010) has suggested that individual-level risk factors such as the internalization of thinness and social comparisons be seen as epiphenomena of higher-level risk factors, such as gender. In this context, it is important to point out that, coming full circle from our introduction, almost all prevention programs to date have not included a discussion of the social issues related to gender, ethno-cultural heritage, or socio-economic factors in relation to body image and disordered eating patterns (Piran, 2001a, 2001b). Clearly, the observation that girls' own reflections about their body-anchored experiences include direct references to these macro-level factors begs the question of whether prevention programs often silence the critical understanding of students (Piran, 1995, 2001b).

The intensive case study analysis of the dance school participatory action prevention project was also informative in understanding processes of change contributory to sustained changes in students' well-being (Piran, 2001b). This was the first prevention program for eating disorders that focused on systemic changes in line with the health-promoting school and participatory action approaches. A central component of the participatory action approach in the school was that actions aimed at changing the school environment were reflected upon, initiated, and guided by the students. It is therefore instructive to examine the facets of the school environment that were changed following the implementation of the program and their sequencing. The centrality of peer experience for the students was reflected by their choice of peer group norms as the first domain of change. In the process of creating a safety base for school-wide changes, students worked first to establish peer norms that were constructive to their self and body experiences, such as agreeing among themselves to generate no evaluative comments on each other's body shape or characteristics and to avoid peer teasing (related to weight, gender, ethno-cultural group membership, or other factors) (Piran, 1999b, 2001b). Indeed, professionals working in the field of the prevention of eating disorders have noted the constructive potential of positive group norms (e.g., Paxton, 1999). Further, other prevention programs have also emphasized peer norms in prevention work. For example, in utilizing a participatory paradigm, Haines, Neumark-Sztainer, Perry, Hannan, & Levine (2006) followed students' guidance in focusing on peer weight and appearance teasing in their aim to prevent eating disorders. McVey, Lieberman, Voorberg, Wardrope, and Blackmore (2003) conducted self-selected peer groups in a prevention program for eating disorders. Becker, Ciao, and Smith (2008) similarly used peer facilitators in sororities to establish constructive peer norms in these settings, using a collaborative approach. In the dance school program, the creation of greater safety within peer groups allowed the students to pursue, usually in groups, discussions with other stakeholders in the school community about needed changes in the larger school environment.

Following the establishment of more constructive peer norms, students, with the support of school personnel and the group's facilitator, pursued changes in the dance school environment (Piran, 2001b). The domains of the school that were addressed included the school training curriculum, staff training, hiring, and replacement, new school policies (such as anti harassment policy), norms, procedure, staff-student committees, and the physical setting. Clearly, establishing a school environment that is more constructive to body and self experiences requires multiple changes in the school community. Indeed, other school-wide initiatives to change the school environment conducted thus far in eating disorder prevention have similarly included staff training and parent education (McVey et al., 2007), changes to the physical environment such as new posters in the school corridors (McVey et al., 2007), or curriculum changes (O'Dea & Maloney, 2000). The combined impact of changing multiple components of the school environment should be emphasized: curricular changes, special group meetings, school plays, teacher and parent training, poster campaigns, and other avenues of influence (McVey et al., 2007). It is important to note that preventive gains in a program that utilizes environmental change are more likely to be sustained (Piran, 1999a, 2001b, 2010). To date, even prevention programs that have shown a strong short-term change have tended to "fade" over time (Becker, Bull, Schaumberg, Cauble, & Franco, 2008). It is still uncommon for prevention programs to utilize a community-based systemic approach to prevention. Initial results, however, support the power of systemic changes in leading to sustained preventative gains.

Conclusions

Experts in the field of disordered eating prevention have acknowledged that, to achieve important and sustained preventive impact, efforts to change the environment are needed (Neumark-Sztainer et al., 2006). The population health framework can provide guidance in this regard, and the demonstrated impact of existing initiatives that embrace aspects of the population health framework attest to the utility of this framework for the prevention of disordered eating. We conclude by articulating the following key points, suggestions, and recommendations stemming from this chapter's content.

- When developing prevention initiatives, the population health framework emphasizes the need to take action on underlying causes towards the creation of circumstances that facilitate—rather than detract from—the desired outcome.
- To take action on underlying causes, we need continued, high-quality research on the underlying causes: what they are, how they work, and—considering that these are likely to be complex and deeply rooted social phenomena—what are the optimal proxy or indicator variables that allow us to monitor them over time at a population level.
- To identify intervention strategies that move beyond individuals as targets and that aim to create circumstances that facilitate desired outcomes, experts working in disordered eating prevention might consider using the public health intervention ladder as a guide (see Figure 3).
- Notwithstanding ethical and ideological opposition to strategies located towards the top of the intervention ladder, it is worthwhile to consider a role for these more intrusive interventions in comprehensive disordered eating prevention, based on their pronounced positive impact in other areas of public health (e.g., drinking water fluoridation and mandatory seatbelt laws).
- To complement the "top-down" approach conveyed by the intervention ladder, change to the social and physical environment can also ensue from a "bottom-up" approach that emphasizes local priorities and empowerment. As illustrated in Piran's ballet school research, this approach can also yield pronounced impact within particular settings.
- To achieve sustained preventive impact in the general population, a combination of top-down and bottom-up approaches will likely be required. While significant and sustained impact within a particular setting (for example, a school) is highly desirable, it is important to keep the broader context in mind. The impact of even the most highly effective school intervention will be diluted or offset if the out-of-school environment remains toxic.
- To facilitate the basic intervention research implied in these recommendations, including possible unintended consequences of population-level interventions, dedicated funding opportunities are needed.

Notes

1 Notwithstanding the numerous within-population studies that have demonstrated, using experimental design, a negative impact of mass media images on body image in girls and young women (see the meta-analyses by Groesz, Levine, and Murnen, 2002; Grabe, Ward, and Hyde, 2008).
2 Please note that Rose's work did not focus on eating disorders; thus our examples represent an extrapolation of his ideas.
3 More recently, this assertion has been questioned by authors in the field of cardiovascular medicine, in light of notable improvements in risk identification for those at risk of cardiovascular events (Manuel et al., 2006; Zulman, Vijan, Omenn, and Hayward, 2008). Nonetheless, the argument that high-risk approaches are temporary and palliative remains valid (McLaren, McIntyre, and Kirkpatrick, 2010).
4 Dove campaign for real beauty. Retrieved from http://www.campaignforreal beauty.com.
5 Institute of Population and Public Health within the Canadian Institutes of Health Research. Retrieved from http://www.cihr-irsc.gc.ca/e/13777.html.

References

Anderson-Fye, E. P., & Becker, A. E. (2004). Sociocultural aspects of eating disorders. In J.K. Thompson (Ed.), *Handbook of eating disorders and obesity* (pp. 565-589). Hoboken, NJ: John Wiley and Sons.

Austin, S. B. (2001). Population-based prevention of eating disorders: An application of the Rose prevention model. *Preventive Medicine, 32*, 268-283.

Becker, A. (2004). Television, disordered eating, and young women in Fiji: negotiating body image and identity during rapid social change. *Culture Medicine and Psychiatry, 28*, 533-559.

Becker, C. B., Bull, S., Schaumberg, K., Cauble, A., & Franco, A. (2008). Effectiveness of peer-led eating disorders prevention: A replication trial. *Journal of Consulting and Clinical Psychology, 76*, 347-354.

Becker, A., Burwell, R. A., Gilman, S. E., Herzog, D. G., & Hamburg, P. (2002). Eating behaviours and attitudes following prolonged exposure to television among ethnic Fijian adolescent girls. *British Journal of Psychiatry, 180*, 509-514.

Becker, C. B., Ciao, A. C., & Smith, L. M. (2008). Moving from efficacy to effectiveness in eating disorder prevention: The Sorority Body Image Program. *Cognitive and Behavioural Practice, 15*, 18-27.

Bosch, X. (1999). Spain tackles eating disorders. *British Medical Journal, 318*, 960.

Bosch, X. (2000). Please don't pass the paella: eating disorders upset Spain. *Journal of the American Medical Association, 283*, 1405-1410.

Bowen, D. J., Tomoyasu, N., & Cauce, A. M. (1999) The triple threat: A discussion of gender, class, and race differences in weight. In L. A. Peplau, S. C. DeBro, R. C. Veniegas, & P. L. Taylor (Eds.), *Gender, culture, and ethnicity* (pp. 291-306). Mountain View, CA: Mayfield.

Bronfenbrenner, U. (1979). *The ecology of human development: Experiments by nature and design.* Cambridge, MA: Harvard University Press.

Burgher, M. S., Rasmussen, V. B., & Rivett, D. (1999). *The European network of health promoting schools.* Retrieved from European Network of Health Promoting Schools, http://www.schoolsforhealth.eu/upload/TheENHPStheallianceof educationandhealth.pdf

Canadian Population Health Initiative. (2007). *An introduction to population health* (E-Learning Course). Online: http://www.cihi.ca

Campos, P. (2005). *The diet myth* [previously published as *The obesity myth*]. New York: Gotham Books.

Carpenter, C. S., & Stehr, M. (2008). The effects of mandatory seatbelt laws on seatbelt use, motor vehicle fatalities, and crash-related injuries among youths. *Journal of Health Economics, 27,* 642-662.

Commission on the Social Determinants of Health. (CSDH). (2008). *Closing the gap in a generation: Health equity through action on the social determinants of health* (Report of the CSDH). Geneva: World Health Organization.

Fishman, D. B. (1999). *The case for pragmatic psychology.* New York: New York University Press.

Grabe, S., Ward, L. M., & Hyde, J. S. (2008). The role of the media in body image concerns among women: A meta-analysis of experimental and correlational studies. *Psychological Bulletin, 134,* 460-476.

Green, L. W., & Kreuter, M. W. (1991). *Health promotion planning: An educational and environmental approach* (2nd edition). Mountain View, CA: Mayfield Publishing.

Groesz, L. M., Levine, M. P., & Murnen, S. K. (2002). The effect of experimental presentation of thin media images on body satisfaction: A meta-analytic review. *International Journal of Eating Disorders, 31,* 1-16.

Haines, J., Neumark-Sztainer, D., Perry, C. L., Hannan, P. J., & Levine, M. P. (2006). V.I.K. (Very Important Kids): A school-based program designed to reduce teasing and unhealthy weight-control behaviours. *Health Education Research, 21,* 884-895.

Health and Welfare Canada. (1986). *Ottawa Charter for Health Promotion.* Retrieved from http://www.who.int/hpr/NPH/docs/ottawa_charter_hp.pdf

Kaplan, G. A., & Lynch, J. W. (1999). Socioeconomic considerations in the primordial prevention of cardiovascular disease. *Preventive Medicine, 29,* S30-S35.

Khaw, K. T., & Marmot, M. (2008). Commentary. In G. Rose (Ed.), *Rose's strategy of preventive medicine* (pp. 1-31). Oxford: Oxford University Press.

Kraemer Tebes, J., Kaufman, J. S., & Connell, C. M. (2003). The evaluation of prevention and health promotion programs. In T. P. Gullotta & M. Bloom (Eds.), *Encyclopedia of Primary Prevention and Health Promotion* (pp. 42-61). New York: Kluwer Academic/Plenum Publishers.

Last, J. M. (Ed). (2001). *A dictionary of epidemiology* (4th edition). Oxford: Oxford University Press.

Levine, M. P., & Murnen, S. K. (2009). "Everybody knows that mass media are / are not [pick one] a cause of eating disorders": A critical review of evidence for a causal link between media, negative body image, and disordered eating in females. *Journal of Social and Clinical Psychology, 28,* 9-42.

Manuel, D. G., Lim, J., Tanuseputro, P., Anderson, G. M., Alter, D. A., Laupacis, A., & Mustard, C. A. (2006). Revisiting Rose: Strategies for reducing coronary heart disease. *British Medical Journal, 332,* 659-662.

Marmot, M. (2007). Achieving health equity: From root causes to fair outcomes. *Lancet, 370,* 1153-1163.

McDonagh, M. S., Whiting, P. F., Wilson, P. M., Sutton, A. J., Chestnutt, I., Cooper, J., Misso, K., Bradley, M., Treasure, E., & Kleijnen, J. (2000). Systematic review of water fluoridation. *British Medical Journal, 321,* 855-859.

McLaren, L., & Hawe, P. (2005). Ecological perspectives in health research. *Journal of Epidemiology and Community Health, 59,* 6-14.

McLaren, L., Kuh, D., Hardy, R., & Gauvin, L. (2004). Positive and negative body-related comments and their relationship with body dissatisfaction in middle-aged women. *Psychology and Health, 19,* 261-272.

McLaren, L., McIntyre, L., & Kirkpatrick, S. (2010). Rose's population strategy of prevention need not increase social inequalities in health. *International Journal of Epidemiology, 39,* 372-377.

McVey, G. L., Lieberman, M., Voorberg, N., Wardrope, D., & Blackmore, E. (2003). School-based peer support groups: A new approach to the prevention of disordered eating. *Eating Disorders, 11,* 169-186.

McVey, G., Tweed, S., & Blackmore, E. (2007). Healthy schools-healthy kids: A controlled evaluation of a comprehensive universal eating disorder prevention program. *Body Image, 4,* 115-136.

Neumark-Sztainer, D., Levine, M. P., Paxton, S. J., Smolak, L., Piran, N., & Wertheim, E. H. (2006). Prevention of body dissatisfaction and disordered eating: What next? *Eating Disorders, 14,* 265-285.

Neumark-Sztainer, D., Sherwood, N. E., Coller, T., & Hannan, P. J. (2000). Primary prevention of disordered eating among preadolescent girls: Feasibility and short-term effect of a community-based intervention. *Journal of the American Dietetic Association, 100,* 1466-1478.

Nichter, M., Vukovic, N., & Parker, S. (1999). The Looking Good, Feeling Good Program: A multi-ethnic intervention for healthy body image, nutrition, and physical activity. In N. Piran, M. Levine, and C. Steiner-Adair (Eds.), *Preventing eating disorders: A handbook of interventions and special challenges* (pp. 175–93). Philadelphia, PA: Brunner/Mazel.

Nuffield Council on Bioethics. (2007). *Public health: ethical issues.* London: Nuffield Council on Bioethics. Retrieved from http://www.nuffieldbioethics .org/publichealth.

O'Dea, J., & Maloney, D. (2000). Preventing eating and body image problems in children and adolescents using the Health Promoting Schools Framework. *Journal of School Health, 70,* 18-21.

Oldenburg, B., & Parcel, G. S. (2002). Diffusion of innovations. In K. Glanz, B. K. Rimer, & F. M. Lewis (Eds.), *Health Behavior and Health Education:*

Theory, Research, and Practice (3rd edition; pp. 312-334). San Francisco, CA: Jossey-Bass.

Paxton, S. J. (1999). Peer relations, body image, and disordered eating in adolescent girls: Implications for prevention. In N. Piran, M. P. Levine, & C. Steiner-Adair (Eds.). *Preventing eating disorders: A handbook of interventions and special challenges* (pp. 134-147). Philadelphia, PA: Brunner/Mazel (Taylor and Francis Group).

Piran, N. (1995). Prevention: Can early lessons lead to a delineation of an alternative model? A critical look at prevention with schoolchildren. *Eating Disorders, 3,* 28-36.

Piran, N. (1999a). Eating disorders: A trial of prevention in a high risk school setting. *Journal of Primary Prevention, 20*(1), 75-90.

Piran, N. (1999b). The reduction of preoccupation with body weight and shape in schools: A feminist approach. In N. Piran, M. P. Levine, & C. Steiner-Adair (Eds.), *Preventing eating disorders: A handbook of interventions and special challenges* (pp. 148-150). Philadelphia, PA: Brunner/Mazel (Taylor and Francis Group).

Piran, N. (2001a). A gendered perspective on eating disorders and disordered eating. In J. Worell (Ed.), *Encyclopedia of gender* (pp. 369-378). San Diego, CA: Academic Press.

Piran, N. (2001b). Re-inhabiting the body from the inside out: Girls transform their school environment. In D. L. Tolman & M. Brydon-Miller (Eds.), *From subjects to subjectivities: A handbook of interpretive and participatory methods* (pp. 218-238). New York: New York University Press.

Piran, N. (2004). Teachers: On "being" prevention. *Eating Disorders, 12,* 1-9.

Piran, N. (2010). A feminist perspective on risk factor research and on the prevention of eating disorders. *Eating Disorders: Journal of Treatment and Prevention, 18*(3), 183-198.

Piran, N., Antoniou, M., Legge, R., McCance, N., Mizevich, J., Peasley, E., & Ross, E. (2006). On girls' disembodiment: The complex tyranny of the "ideal girl." In D. L. Gustafson & L. Goodyear (Eds.), *Women, Health, and Education: CASWE Sixth Bi-Annual International Institute Proceedings* (pp. 224-229). St. John's, NL: Memorial University.

Piran, N., Carter, W., Thompson, S., & Pajouhandeh, P. (2002). Powerful girls: A contradiction in terms? Young women speak about the experience of growing up in a girl's body. In S. Abbey (Ed.), *Ways of knowing in and through the body: Diverse perspectives on embodiment* (pp. 206-210). Welland, ON: Soleil Publishing.

Piran, N., & Cormier, H. (2005). The social construction of women and disordered eating patterns. *Journal of the Counselling Psychologist, 52*(4), 549-558.

Piran, N., & Thompson, S. (2008). A study of the adverse social experiences model to the development of eating disorders. *International Journal of Health Promotion and Education, 46*(2), 65-71.

Pratt, B. M., & Woolfenden, S. R. (2009). Interventions for preventing eating disorders in children and adolescents. *Cochrane Database of Systematic Reviews* 2, Article no. CD002891, doi: 10.1002/14651858.CD002891

Public Health Agency of Canada. (1999). *Toward a healthy future: Second report on the health of Canadians.* Retrieved from http://www.phac-aspc.gc.ca/ph-sp/report-rapport/toward/pdf/toward_a_healthy_english.PDF

Public Health Agency of Canada. (2004). *What is the population health approach?* Retrieved from http://www.phac-aspc.gc.ca/ph-sp/approach-approche/index-eng.php

Rose, G. (1985). Sick individuals and sick populations. *International Journal of Epidemiology, 14,* 32-38.

Rose, G. (1992). *The strategy of preventive medicine.* Oxford: Oxford University Press.

Shilling, C. (2005). *The body and social theory* (2nd edition). London: Sage.

Stice, E. (2001). Risk factors for eating pathology: Recent advances and future directions. In R. H. Striegel-Moore & L. Smolak (Eds.), *Eating disorders: Innovative directions in research and practice* (pp. 51-73). Washington, DC: American Psychological Association.

Stice, F., Shaw, H., & Marti, C. N. (2007). A meta-analytic review of eating disorder prevention programs: Encouraging findings. *Annual Review of Clinical Psychology, 3,* 207-231.

Striegel-Moore, R. H., & Bulik, C. M. (2007). Risk factors for eating disorders. *American Psychologist, 62,* 181-198.

Summerbell, C. D., Waters, E., Edmunds, L. D., Kelly, S., Brown, T., & Campbell, K. J. (2006). Interventions for preventing obesity in children (Systematic Review). *Cochrane Database of Systematic Reviews,* 1, Article no. CD001872.

Wertheim, E. H., Paxton, S. J., & Blaney, S. (2004). Risk factors for the development of body image disturbances. In J. K. Thompson (Ed.), *Handbook of eating disorders and obesity* (pp. 463-494). Hoboken, NJ: John Wiley and Sons.

Whitehead, M. (1992). The concepts and principles of equity and health. *International Journal of Health Services, 22,* 429-445.

World Health Organization. (1948). *WHO definition of health.* Retrieved from http://www.who.int/about/definition/en/print.html

Zulman, D. M., Vijan, S., Omenn, G. S., & Hayward, R. A. (2008). The relative merits of population-based and targeted prevention strategies. *Millbank Quarterly, 86,* 557-580.

CHAPTER THREE

Public Health Interventions for Body Dissatisfaction and Eating Disorders: Learning from Victoria

Susan J. Paxton, *La Trobe University*

The need for the prevention of body image and eating disorders using a public health approach has been increasingly recognized as the extent of the burden of these disorders is better understood. If an effective population-based means of preventing body image and eating disorders could be identified and implemented, much pain and suffering would be alleviated. However, only in a few countries has the attention of public health policy-makers turned to this task. This chapter will first consider the history and rationale for public health approaches to prevention and then explore possible targets for public health intervention. The state of Victoria in Australia is one place in which serious attention has been given to public health initiatives to reduce body image and eating disorders, and approaches that have been explored in Victoria will next be described. The final section of this chapter explores future challenges for public health interventions in this field.

Public Health Approaches to Prevention

Public health is evolving, but at its core it emphasizes the health of populations rather than of individuals—that is, public health interventions endeavour to improve health through population-level interventions rather than through interventions targeting specific individuals at the highest risk of disease (Baum, 2008). In her exploration of the history of developments in public health, Baum (2008) proposes that the 1970s and 1980s saw a growth in the recognition of the role of lifestyle in influencing health and illness, with Canada being the first country to incorporate notions of a healthy lifestyle into its health policy (Lalonde, 1974). There followed campaigns that aimed to increase health-promoting behaviours such as increasing physical activity and quitting smoking. Baum (2008) proposes, however, that at the heart of many of these interventions was the assumption that individuals were responsible for making their own healthy lifestyle choices.

The 1986 *Ottawa Charter for Health Promotion* introduced the "new public health" orientation, marking a turning point in the focus of public health.[1] In this charter, factors outside individual control were viewed as playing critical roles in health. Factors noted as particularly influential were government policies such as those related to education, wealth distribution, and social environments. The charter recommended the creation of social, economic, and physical environments that would support health.

Thus, implementation of new public health policies clearly required government endorsement and active involvement. However, in Australia, as in other countries, practical government support for new public health philosophies has been inconsistent. In Australia, the Conservative national government under Prime Minister John Howard (1996-2007) promoted policies that supported individualism, personal responsibility, and private health care rather than community development based on new public health goals (Baum, 2008). In addition, as Baum (2008, p. 41) has noted, new public health goals are frequently contrary to those of business and require "an oppositional position in regard to the profit-making activity of many other sectors." Not surprisingly, governments across the Liberal-Conservative spectrum are frequently reluctant to take on such interests.

However, government involvement in public health interventions is highly desirable, as governments have at their disposal a number of tools to bring about changes that may promote healthy social and physical environments. Governments can, for example, legislate for change. Prominent examples of the effectiveness of this approach have been the legislation for the compulsory use of seatbelts in cars and helmets on bicycles and of smoking bans in public places. Taxation policies are another tool that may promote healthy behaviours, such as having no taxes on fresh foods but high taxes on tobacco (World Bank, 1999). Governments may also promulgate and monitor non-binding codes of conduct that outline responsible industry behaviour. Importantly, governments can provide public funds for the development, evaluation, refinement, and dissemination of health-promoting activities such as community-based and school-based prevention activities and for universal health promotion campaigns such as media and billboard advertising. Interventions of this kind may be designed and delivered by governments, government instrumentalities (e.g., public schools and community centres), or by private bodies that receive government funding for this purpose (e.g., private schools and church groups). Examples include advertising campaigns raising awareness of the dangers of binge drinking, gambling, and driving under the influence of alcohol or other drugs. Finally, governments may also provide co-ordination across government departments to try to ensure a consistency in messages across health campaigns.

Despite some opposing political and economic pressures, there have been some notable and successful public health interventions, especially at the state government level, which is the level of government largely responsible for the provision of health services in Australia. For example, in 1987 in the state of Victoria, the Victorian Health Promotion Foundation (VicHealth) was established. It was funded using tobacco tax revenues and had the goal of eliminating smoking throughout the population (initially 31.5% of people smoked, and now this figure is at 17%). The role of VicHealth has widened to include a range of public health interventions to address: the creation of a socially inclusive society, discrimination, physical inactivity, and overweight and obesity, among others (VicHealth, 2010). In the mental health area of depression, Beyondblue (2008), an independent project with both state and federal funding, was established in 2000 and has had considerable success in raising awareness about, and reducing stigmatization surrounding, depression.

It is against this background that the first tentative steps towards public health interventions for body image and eating disorders have taken place in Victoria. The first step in the development of a public health intervention is the identification of appropriate public health intervention targets, specifically the risk factors for body image and eating problems. These factors will be discussed in the next section.

Identifying Possible Public Health Intervention Targets

Body image and eating disorders may be viewed as lying on a continuum from healthy body image and eating behaviours, to moderate body dissatisfaction and disordered eating, to severe body dissatisfaction and eating disorders (Levine & Smolak, 2006). The task of public health interventions in this field is to prevent movement up this continuum. This task requires a firm understanding of the causal risk factors that contribute to the development of body image and eating disorders since the reduction of these risk factors might be anticipated to break the developmental sequence (Jacobi, Hayward, de Zwaan, Kraemer, & Agras, 2004). Furthermore, the task requires the identification of modifiable and influential risk factors that are open to public health intervention. In order to translate etiologic theory into community health interventions, it is essential to identify key leverage points or those points that are amenable to, and feasible for, public health intervention (Austin, 2001; Stokols, 1996). Although our knowledge of risk factors of this kind is by no means complete, we now have an extensive body of knowledge about risk factors for eating disorders on which to draw when considering targets for public health intervention (see Chapter 6 in this volume).

Dieting and the use of extreme weight loss behaviours are consistently observed to be prospective risk factors for the development of eating disorders (e.g., Austin, 2001; Neumark-Sztainer et al., 2006a). Notably, the use of extreme weight loss behaviours also predicts the development of overweight and obesity, which is another one of the Australian government's current concerns (e.g., Neumark-Sztainer et al., 2006a). Thus, a reduction of dieting in the community, especially the use of extreme weight loss behaviours frequently known as fad diets or crash diets, can be anticipated to reduce the incidence of eating disorders and therefore would be an appropriate target for public health intervention (Austin, 2001).

However, it is valuable to consider the causal risk factors for dieting. Body dissatisfaction is a consistently observed prospective risk factor for dieting and eating pathology (e.g., Neumark-Sztainer, Paxton, Hannan, Haines, & Story, 2006b; Stice, 2002). Taking a further step back in the causal chain, having a high internalization of the thin socio-cultural ideal (i.e., placing a high value on thinness) and a high tendency to compare one's body with others are predictors of the development of body dissatisfaction and are likely to be causal risk factors (e.g., Cafri, Yamamiya, Brannick, & Thompson, 2005; Durkin, Paxton, & Sorbello, 2007; Jones, 2004). These attitudes and behaviours may also be targets for public health intervention.

Finally, additional causal risk factors for body dissatisfaction, for which there is strong support, either directly connected or mediated by the internalization of the thin ideal or body comparison, include a high body mass index (BMI); perceived pressure to be thin from media, family, and friends; and low self-esteem, negative affect, and perfectionism (e.g., Cafri et al., 2005; Dohnt & Tiggemann, 2006; Field et al., 2004; Paxton, Eisenberg, & Neumark-Sztainer, 2006; Stice, 2002).

In Australia, of these risk factors for body image and eating disorders, pressure from media to be extremely thin and to conform to an unrealistic ideal has received the most attention as a target of public health interventions. External social pressures are potentially modifiable, although public health interventions have yet to address the pressures from family and friends. A high BMI has been the target of public health interventions in the context of obesity prevention. If addressed appropriately, this factor could have an impact on body dissatisfaction and eating disorders.

The Development of Public Health Interventions for Body Image and Eating Disorders in Victoria, Australia

Historical Background

Although numerous groups and individuals have previously recognized the need for public health prevention interventions, the first organization funded specifically to adopt a public health approach to improving body image and reducing the incidence of eating disorders in Victoria was Body Image and Health Incorporated (BIH). Funded by VicHealth from 1993 to 2001, BIH's mission was to work for social change so that people of all shapes and sizes could feel good about, and care for, their bodies and themselves (Body Image and Health, 2001). Its goal was to change the social environments that encouraged the endorsement of an unhealthy body ideal and weight loss practices, with a focus on the fashion industry and media.

Among other activities, BIH worked with media and fashion houses in Victoria to promote models with a wider range of body types as well as the creation and marketing of designer clothes in all sizes. BIH also introduced International No Diet Day to Australia and, through it, publicized the dangers of displaying extreme weight loss behaviours. It also worked with health educators and fitness centres to alert them to the promotion of unrealistically thin ideals and dangerous diets. BIH adopted an evidence-based approach to its activities and supported research through an annual conference. Working with the Victoria Department of Human Resources (2002), BIH produced *Shapes: Body Image Program Planning Guide*, a still widely used resource guide for school-based body dissatisfaction prevention interventions.

In 2002, the Victoria Centre of Excellence in Eating Disorders (VCEED) was established by the Victoria government. Initially, the VCEED's aim was to improve health care, prevention, early intervention, and treatment for people with eating disorders in Victoria, and it focused on providing education, training, and consultation. The VCEED (2004) produced a valuable manual for schools to guide them in the early detection of eating disorders. However, in general, it did not adopt a strong public health stance but, rather, provided resources for treatment. Recently, its role in supporting eating disorder treatment services has been enhanced, while its prevention role has been diminished. However, along with the Eating Disorders Foundation of Victoria (EDFV), a government-funded agency that provides support for sufferers of eating disorders and their family and friends, the

VCEED played an important role in raising the profile within the Victorian government of the needs of individuals with eating disorders.

Within an environment in which distress associated with body image and eating disorders has been recognized but in which support for a public health approach to tackle the problem has faded, the minister for employment and youth affairs in the Victorian state government took a bold stand. Having listened to youth in her electorate speaking about their problems associated with body image, she supported in 2003 the establishment of a parliamentary inquiry "into issues relating to body image among young people and associated effects on their health and wellbeing." Following widespread consultation, the Family and Community Development Committee (2005) issued their report. Two recommendations specifically addressed public health interventions for body image. It was recommended that "a code of conduct for the media industry be developed, recognizing the media's social responsibility to display images that are representative of the community" (p. x) and "that the Department of Education consider the development and promotion of programs that develop skills in media literacy" (p. xiii).

This inquiry provided impetus to reignite public health approaches to address areas that have been identified as risk factors for body image and eating disorders. The Victorian government has made some inroads into implementing both recommendations. In particular, they have funded a campaign entitled Fad Diets Won't Work; developed the Voluntary Media Code of Conduct on Body Image; initiated a teacher training program on body image and self-esteem entitled BodyThink; and started a body image community grant scheme.

Media Advertising
The first response to the parliamentary inquiry addressed the Fad Diets Won't Work campaign. This campaign was conducted within the context of a wider campaign, Go for Your Life, which was essentially a healthy eating and physical activity campaign that aims to combat obesity. Drawing on research (for example, Neumark-Sztainer, 2005) that shows that the use of extreme weight loss behaviours is a risk factor for body dissatisfaction and disordered eating as well as for overweight and obesity, this campaign endeavoured to educate the public about the negative impact of fad dieting, including physical and psychological problems and, in particular, weight gain. The campaign featured a series of advertisements in which a young woman is shown saying: "Fad dieting helped me go from a size 14 to a size 12, back to a size 16: Over the long term fad diets won't work" and

"Fad diets turned me into a new person—a much crankier one: Over the long term fad diets won't work." These advertisements appeared on billboards and public transport around Victoria in 2007 for approximately one month. Additional information about healthy weight management and body image problems was also provided on the Department of Human Services website.

This campaign was a universal public health intervention with adolescent girls and young women as the target audience. The goal of reducing unhealthy dieting as a prevention intervention for eating disorders appears to be an appropriate one (e.g., Stice, 2002). The messages were clear and most likely of interest to women. In addition, including this campaign as part of the Go for Your Life campaign was a practical way of obtaining funding by drawing on substantial financial support for an anti-obesity campaign. The major drawback of the campaign was that the public exposure was of such a short duration and its impact was not evaluated. The information remains on a government website, but it is unlikely that the public would access it from this source. Not only does this mean that the public does not benefit, but it is also a waste of the resources invested in the campaign.

A further innovative advertising campaign to prevent body image and eating disorders by challenging the internalization of media body ideals was conducted in 2009 (Victoria, Department of Planning and Community Development, 2009). This campaign was entitled Real Life Doesn't Need Retouching and depicted images of idealized media images of beauty, love, and friendship juxtaposed with images of real young people that displayed these characteristics. It concluded with the tag "Real life doesn't need retouching" and "Take a stand against digital manipulation." The advertisement was displayed on the social networking site MySpace for a month. Again, this advertisement was based on risk factor research and had a clear and compelling message. However, it was not widely displayed and was only presented for one month. Consequently, the reach was only very limited, and greater exposure will be required in the future in order for it to have a significant effect.

Voluntary Media Code of Conduct on Body Image

In 2007, the state government of Victoria established a committee comprising representatives from media and fashion groups, body image and eating disorder groups, and government representatives, charged with the task of developing a voluntary media code of conduct on body image issues. In 2008, the Voluntary Media Code of Conduct on Body Image was released. The code is:

Designed to encourage the fashion, media and advertising industries to place greater emphasis on diversity, positive body images and a focus on health rather than body shape. In doing so, the Code aims to decrease young people's vulnerability to feelings of low self-esteem, disordered eating and negative body image associated with exposure to idealised, unrealistic images in the media and advertising. (Office of Youth, 2008a)

The code has four recommendations for the media:

- *Altered and enhanced images:* The use of unachievable and unrealistic digitally-manipulated images of people in the media is discouraged. If such alteration has occurred, digitally altered images should be disclosed and accompanied by a tag stating that "this image has been digitally altered" to help young people make a balanced appraisal.
- *Diversity in shapes:* Consideration should be given to the inclusion of a variety of body shapes in order to provide a fair representation in both editorial and advertising images.
- *Fair placement:* Consideration should be given to the editorial context in which diet, exercise, or cosmetic surgery advertising is placed.
- *Modelling health:* Glamorization of severely underweight models or celebrities is potentially dangerous. Effort should be made to depict people of healthy weight and size.

A number of influential media organizations have signed up to support the code, which has provided a focus for a range of events highlighting to the public the problems associated with digitally manipulated images in the media (see Chapter 4 in this volume). As a result, some fashion houses are using models of more diverse shapes, and magazines have occasionally labelled digitally enhanced images. However, the code does not appear to have had a major impact on the nature of the images of females or males presented in the media. Since it is voluntary, there is no obligation to sign up to the code, and it may be that, although some organizations are generally supportive of the code, they are reluctant to sign support in case this may be used against them at some point. Despite the shortcomings of a voluntary code, this document continues to serve an important role in raising awareness.

This innovative code has also served to prompt action at other government levels. Of particular interest, the national government has now recognized the negative impact of poor body image. It established a National Advisory Group on Body Image, which has made recommendations for a nationwide voluntary media code of conduct. This code is similar, but it would have a greater emphasis on the presentation of positive body image messages in the media (National Advisory Group on Body Image, 2009). The advisory group has also recommended other ways to engage in a positive way with industry such as giving awards for achievements in promoting positive body image, and it is important that additional strategies are identified.

School-Based Prevention Interventions

A further public health intervention strategy is the widespread dissemination of school-based prevention intervention programs. The Victoria government, along with philanthropic organizations, has provided funding for the training of teachers across Victoria in the delivery of the body image and self-esteem program BodyThink (Dove, 2006). BodyThink is a workshop program that is designed for a flexible delivery, but it is most appropriately delivered in about four classroom sessions. It is appropriate for co-educational middle- and high-school settings. By the end of 2008, the Butterfly Foundation (the national advocacy group for eating disorders) had provided training in the delivery of the program to over 900 professionals, and it is estimated that over 40,000 young people had participated in the program (Richardson, Paxton, & Thomson, 2009). A short-term follow up evaluation of BodyThink found that, in girls, media literacy and internalization of the thin ideal were improved and, in boys, media literacy and body satisfaction were improved (Richardson et al., 2009).

In addition to the widespread dissemination of a school-based prevention intervention, it is essential to identify the most effective prevention interventions and, to this end, government-funded research would be extremely valuable. It is notable that research does suggest that other short-term interventions may have a greater impact than BodyThink (e.g., Richardson & Paxton, 2010; Wilksch & Wade, 2009). It is also essential that funding support for such programs is continuous and reliable. Further, there is research support for whole-school approaches that not only reach students but also reach teachers and parents (e.g., McVey, Tweed & Blackmore, 2007; National Advisory Group on Body Image, 2009) (see Chapters 1 & 2 in this volume). It is very encouraging that in 2010 the Victoria government is exploring the integration of evidence-based prevention interventions in high-school curricula and environments as this is likely to be a powerful public health intervention approach.

Body Image Community Grant Scheme

The final public health initiative of the Victoria government has been the provision of $5,000 grants to 50 community organizations each year from 2007 to 2010. The purpose of these grants is to deliver projects that are aimed to "increase awareness of healthy weight and positive body image, and to enable practical support for young people to gain better understanding of positive body image messages" (Office for Youth, 2008b, pp. 1-2). The projects were very diverse and included group projects with the titles "e+body image" (an examination of body image in the context of the Internet), "Deconstructing Dolly" (a media literacy program for girls), and "Plastic Dream" (an animated story depicting body image issues for teenage boys). Although no formal evaluation was conducted, informal evaluation suggested that participants found the involvement to be very valuable. There was high demand for the grants, illustrating community need for initiatives in this area. Although it is likely that the participants gained from these projects, from a public health perspective, they reached a very small proportion of the population.

Conclusion

It is very encouraging that some governments have recognized the importance of public health interventions for body image and eating disorders. In Victoria, the importance of tackling the prevention of mental illness generally and of eating disorders in particular have been clearly articulated in forward-planning documents (Victoria, Department of Human Services, 2008). However, despite the impressive progress in Victoria and in many parts of Canada (see Chapters 1 & 2 in this volume), there is nowhere in the world where it could be said that there has been adequate public health intervention in this area. Thus, the first challenge is to increase recognition by governments of the need and benefits of public health action. In addition, it is insufficient for governments to "recognize" body image and eating disorders as significant problems warranting public health interventions. Governments must also see this issue as a high-priority need. This is the greater challenge. There is very high competition for the public health dollar and many other vocal and worthy interest groups.

Even within our own field, it is difficult to maintain a funding focus on public health intervention when treatment facilities are also so frequently under-resourced. Carers of patients with eating disorders are usually and understandably desperate to obtain appropriate treatment, and it is hard to argue for prevention interventions when the very immediate needs of patients and families are not being adequately met. Nonetheless, it is hoped that prevention interventions will ultimately reduce the need for treatment.

One area of public health intervention with which eating disorder prevention is particularly competing is obesity prevention. There is little doubt that an increase in the prevalence of obesity will bring about increased health challenges and that it is appropriate to support interventions that result in healthier eating and physical activity levels (Neumark-Sztainer, 2005). The difficulty with our field is that obesity prevention is typically seen as being contrary to body image and eating disorder prevention. As demonstrated earlier (Fad Diets Won't Work), this is not necessarily the case. However, many public health interventions for obesity do encourage extreme weight control behaviours that are likely to place individuals at a higher risk of both obesity and eating disorders. It is essential that we achieve greater co-operation across public health interventions that encourage healthy eating and body image to ensure that public health messages are consistent with eating disorder and anti-obesity goals (Neumark-Sztainer, 2009). In addition, for pragmatic reasons, co-operation is highly desirable to capitalize on the higher levels of funding in the obesity prevention area.

Although one-off public health initiatives may have some immediate impact, there is always going to be the need for ongoing funding and evolving program development. One campaign will never be sufficient, and, indeed, it may be a waste of public money if it is not followed up. In addition, in light of the inevitable limitations in funding, it is important that the public health interventions that are funded are those that maximize reach across the community. However, it is also essential to fund interventions that work. Further research is needed to identify the most effective public health interventions. Currently, governments are guided somewhat by the face value, including the political value, of an intervention rather than by research. Governments need to be encouraged to fund body image and eating disorder public health research and to evaluate carefully initiatives that are being adopted.

A further challenge facing public health interventions for body image and eating disorders is to ensure interventions are appropriately evaluated. It is essential that we identify effective interventions to provide further support for their more widespread dissemination. As well as the use of evaluation techniques matched to the particular public health intervention, such efforts will require substantial funding, which has not yet been forthcoming.

Finally, interventions that assist in preventing body image and eating disorders will generate commercial tensions. In particular, fearing a loss of interest in their "image" and their products, parts of the media and fashion industries are reluctant to make changes that will reduce the glamorization of extremely thin models. In addition, much of the advertising of unhealthy weight loss products is conducted by companies keen to sell their products. Public criticism of, and limitations on, these activities are not likely to be met favourably. Interests of this kind, including mass media, will need to be engaged in a very positive way to bring about change.

Although there are many challenges ahead for public health interventions to reduce body image and eating disorders, it is important to recognize that positive steps have been taken (see Chapters 1 & 2 in this volume). Awareness of the serious nature of eating disorders has increased in many governments, and there is a growing willingness to act and, indeed, a number of interventions that have been implemented. Professionals and researchers in the body image field need to continue to be vocal and active in advocating for public health action and to assist in the development of the evidence base for effective interventions.

Note

1 *Ottawa Charter for Health Promotion*, 21 November 1986, World Health Organization, Doc. WHO/HPR/HEP/95.1.

References

Austin, S. B. (2001). Population-based prevention of eating disorders: An application of the Rose Prevention Model. *Preventive Medicine, 32*, 268-283.

Baum, F. (2008). *The New Public Health* (3rd edition). Melbourne: Oxford University Press.

Beyondblue (2008). Retrieved from http://www.beyondblue.org.au/index.aspx?

Body Image and Health, Incorporated (2001). *Final Report to VicHealth* (Unpublished report) [on file with the author].

Cafri, G., Yamamiya, Y., Brannick, M., & Thompson, J. K. (2005). The influence of sociocultural factors on body image: A meta-analysis. *Clinical Psychology: Science and Practice, 12*, 421-433.

Dohnt, H., & Tiggemann, M. (2006). The contribution of peer and media influences to the development of body satisfaction and self-esteem in young children: A prospective study. *Developmental Psychology, 42*, 929-936.

Dove Self-Esteem Fund. (2006). *Body think: Building body confidence.* Melbourne, Australia: Unilever and Butterfly Foundation.

Durkin, S. J., Paxton, S. J. & Sorbello, M. (2007). An integrative model of the impact of exposure to idealized female images on adolescent girls' body satisfaction. *Journal of Applied Social Psychology, 37*, 1092-1117.

Family and Community Development Committee. (2005). *Inquiry into issues relating to the development of body image among young people and associated effects on their health and wellbeing.* Melbourne, Australia: State of Victoria.

Field, A. E., Camargo, C. A., Taylor, B., Berkey, C. S., Roberts, S. B., & Colditz, G. A. (2001). Peer, parent, and media influences on the development of weight concerns and frequent dieting among preadolescent and adolescent girls and boys. *Pediatrics, 107*, 54-60.

Jacobi, C., Hayward, C., de Zwaan, M., Kraemer, H. C., & Agras, W. S. (2004). Coming to terms with risk factors for eating disorders: Application of risk terminology and suggestions for a general taxonomy. *Psychological Bulletin, 130*, 19-65.

Jones, D. C. (2004). Body image among adolescent girls and boys: A longitudinal study. *Developmental Psychology, 40*, 823-835.

Lalonde, M. (1974). *A new perspective on the health of Canadians*. Ottawa: Ministry of National Health and Welfare.

Levine, M. P., & Smolak, L. (2006). *The prevention of eating problems and eating disorders: Theory, research and practice*. Mahwah, NJ: Lawrence Erlbaum.

McVey, G. L., Tweed, S., & Blackmore, E. (2007). Healthy schools—healthy kids: A controlled evaluation of a comprehensive eating disorder prevention program. *Body Image, 4*, 115-136.

National Advisory Group on Body Image. (2009). *A proposed national strategy on body image*. Canberra, Australia: Commonwealth of Australia. Retrieved from http://www.youth.gov.au/bodyImage/Documents/Proposed-National -Strategy-on-Body-Image.pdf

Neumark-Sztainer, D. (2005). Can we simultaneously work toward the prevention of obesity and eating disorders in children and adolescents? *International Journal of Eating Disorders, 38*, 220-227.

Neumark-Sztainer, D. (2009). Preventing obesity and eating disorders in adolescent girls: What can health care providers do? *Journal of Adolescent Health, 44*, 206-213.

Neumark-Sztainer, D., Levine, M., Paxton, S., Smolak, L., Piran, N., & Wertheim, E. (2006a). Prevention of body dissatisfaction and disordered eating: What next? *Eating Disorder: Journal of Treatment and Prevention, 14*, 265 285.

Neumark-Sztainer, D., Paxton, S. J., Hannan, P. J., Haines, J., & Story, M (2006b). Does body satisfaction matter? Five year longitudinal associations between body satisfaction and health behaviors in adolescent females and males. *Journal of Adolescent Health, 39*, 244-251.

Neumark-Sztainer, D., Wall, M., Guo, J., Story, M., Haines, J., Eisenberg, M. (2006). Obesity, disordered eating and eating disorders, in a longitudinal study of adolescents: How do dieters fare five years later? *Journal of American Dietetic Association, 106*, 559-568.

Office for Youth, Department of Planning and Community Development, Victorian State Government (2008a). *Voluntary media code of conduct*. Retrieved from http://www.youthcentral.vic.gov.au/News+%26+Features/ Body+Image/Media+Code+of+Conduct

Paxton, S. J., Eisenberg, M. E., & Neumark-Sztainer, D. (2006). Prospective predictors of body dissatisfaction in adolescent girls and boys: A five-year longitudinal study. *Developmental Psychology. 42*, 888-99.

Richardson, S. M., & Paxton, S. J. (2010). An evaluation of a body image intervention based on risk factors for body dissatisfaction: A controlled study with adolescent girls. *International Journal of Eating Disorders, 43*(2), 112-122.

Richardson, S. M., Paxton, S. J., & Thomson, J. S. (2009). Is *BodyThink* an efficacious body image and self-esteem program? A controlled evaluation with adolescents. *Body Image, 6*, 75-82.

Stice, E. (2002). Risk and maintenance factors for eating pathology: A meta-analytic review. *Psychological Bulletin, 128*, 825-848.

Stokols, D. (1996). Translating social ecological theory into guidelines for community health promotion. *American Journal of Health Promotions, 10,* 282-298.

VicHealth. (2010). Home page. Retrieved from http://www.vichealth.vic.gov.au/

Victoria, Department of Human Services. (2002). *Shapes: Body image program planning guide.* Retrieved from http://www.health.vic.gov.au/ healthpromotion/ quality/body_image.htm

Victoria, Department of Planning and Community Development. (2009). *Real life doesn't need retouching.* Retrieved from http://www.dpcd.vic.gov.au/

Victoria Centre of Excellence in Eating Disorder and Eating Disorders. (2004). *An eating disorders resource for schools: A manual to promote early intervention and prevention of eating disorders in schools.* Melbourne, Australia: Victoria Centre of Excellence in Eating Disorder and Eating Disorders.

Wilksch, S. M., & Wade, T. D. (2009). Reduction of shape and weight concern in young adolescents: A thirty-month controlled evaluation media literacy program. *Journal of American Academy of Child and Adolescent Psychiatry, 48,* 652-661.

World Bank. (1999). *Curbing the epidemic: Governments and the economics of tobacco control.* Retrieved from http://www1.worldbank.org/tobacco/

Mass Media 1: A Primer on Media Literacy's Role in the Prevention of Negative Body Image and Disordered Eating

Michael P. Levine, *Kenyon College*
Joe Kelly, *The Emily Program*

A great deal of research-based evidence supports the proposition that mass media and other socio-cultural factors play a causal role in creating and reinforcing the mediating factors that directly increase the probability of a spectrum of negative body image, disordered eating, and unhealthy methods of managing weight and shape (Grabe, Ward, & Hyde, 2008; Levine & Harrison, 2009; Levine & Murnen, 2009; Thompson, Heinberg, Altabe, & Tantleff-Dunn, 1999; see also Chapter 6 in this volume). Against this background, it is no surprise to see the development of prevention programs for eating disorders that focus on media literacy. Most assume that, since media messages can exert negative influences on individuals, people will be "inoculated" against, and thus protected from, these adverse messages if they learn about the media technologies and strategies used to create the messages. While this seems like a straightforward and logical assumption, it is frequently mistaken.

As with many other responses to the complex problem of eating disorders, what appears to be a simple and logical solution turns out to entail multiple challenges. After addressing some important definitional issues, the present chapter summarizes what is known about how media literacy can be effective in preventing or reducing body image and eating disorder problems. Then, in light of the challenges of responding to rapid technological advances, the chapter examines prevention efforts that go beyond media awareness and analysis. Based on this discussion, the chapter will suggest that the most effective prevention programs combine the skills of media "deconstruction" with other more complex strategies, known as the "five Cs of prevention." Finally, the chapter explores the dilemmas of living in an age dominated by media and marketing and discusses the remaining significant gaps in the evidence of prevention efficacy.

Media Literacy: Definition and Current Challenges

Media as Language

Mass media "generate messages designed for a very large, very heterogeneous, and essentially anonymous audience" (Levine & Smolak, 1996, pp. 236-237). These messages, including the basic practice of seeking out, "turning on," and spending time with a specific medium such as the Internet or television, serve many purposes. For creators and transmitters of mass media, the most important purpose is to deliver unfathomably large groups of potential consumers to paying advertisers. For consumers of mass media, the most important purposes are entertainment, education, socialization, identity development, politics, and the opportunity to be exposed to advertisers (Arnett, 1995; Comstock & Scharrer, 2007).

When analyzing mass media such as television, magazines, and cinema, it is helpful to think of each medium as a language analogous to English, French, or Chinese. Different media have their own vocabulary and grammar, although some media may have similar elements, in the same way that French and English have some similarities in sentence structure. Elements of other media are markedly different from one another. This analogy is especially important for adults trying to grasp the impact of today's prominent media—particularly the influential and quickly evolving "new" media such as Facebook, Twitter, tumblr, and YouTube. The accelerating development of increasingly sophisticated media poses ongoing challenges to effective media literacy training. A static media literacy program will never be able to keep up with these developments. Some studies now suggest that media literacy educators need to train children to create their own media using the relevant "language" (Marsh, 2006; Rentala & Korhonen, 2008; Van Bauwel, 2008). This is further evidence that analyzing media as language is a useful construct regardless of the particular medium.

To demonstrate the concept of media as language, consider a front cover of the mainstream magazine *Cosmopolitan*. A cover's success in using media "language" is critically important for ensuring off-the-newsstand sales. The cover's vocabulary (one aspect of a language's "semantics") consists of images, text, font, colours, and even the properties of the paper on which they are arrayed. The grammar (or "syntax") consists of how these "vocabulary" elements are arranged, altered, not altered, and/or manipulated (e.g., Photoshopping the model, placing the photo "over" part of the magazine's title, the variety of font style and size, the arrangement of words, the seductive expression on the model's face, and so on).

This combination of "vocabulary" and "grammar" is carefully, indeed painstakingly, designed to have particular effects on the audience of potential consumers, actual consumers, and other "readers." The meanings, whether intended or incidental, formed by this synthesis of vocabulary and grammar become a higher order feature of this medium's semantics, just as "each of the thousands of languages spoken around the world has its own system and rules, its own subversions, its own quixotic beauty" (Xu, 2010, p. 11). Understanding the workings of a medium's "language" is a precondition that provides the foundation on which effective media literacy must build.

This precondition demands that prevention professionals acknowledge and work with two important facts: (1) an individual mass medium such as magazines or television brings together a wide range of people, contents, practices, and technologies, and (2) mass media technologies and delivery methods are rapidly morphing to gain "mindshare" and influence among their audiences. This development accelerates change in the media landscape, so that even a historically dominant medium such as television holds less general influence—relative to other mass media and relative to its own history as a medium—than it did less than a decade ago.

Media Literacy: An Expanded Working Definition

The concept of media "literacy" is the focus of considerable discussion, study, and controversy (Potter, 2001; Schwarz and Brown, 2005). In general, the definition offered by Hobbs (1998), a leading media educator in the United States, is quite useful. According to Hobbs (1998), media literacy refers to the skills, knowledge, and perspective that form "the process of critically analyzing *and learning to create one's own messages* [emphasis added] in print, audio, video, and multimedia" (p. 16). This definition confirms that, as one form of "critical social consciousness" (Piran, 2001, 2010), "critical viewing skills" are important components of media literacy, particularly as a form of resistance to unhealthy cultural messages about weight and shape.

Hobbs' definition also indicates that experts in media education have a much broader perspective about the meanings of media literacy in the realm of images, bodies, and body image than do most experts in eating disorder prevention and virtually all newcomers to media literacy (Brown, 2001; Hobbs, 1998, 2005; Levine & Smolak, 2006). There are four important assumptions embedded in this broad perspective. First, media literacy is "the ability to access, analyze, evaluate, and communicate messages in a wide variety of forms" (Aufderheide & Firestone, 1993, as quoted in Hobbs, 2005, p. 74). Second, media literacy is neither media cynicism nor blanket condemnation of "other people's pleasures." One prominent meaning of the adjective "critical" is "exercising or involving careful judgment or judicious evaluation." Consequently, "critical" may "imply an effort to see a thing clearly and truly in order to judge it fairly" (*Merriam-Webster Dictionary*, n.d.). This definition, in turn, means that a critical appraisal includes a deeper appreciation of artistic, enjoyable, and other positive elements.

Third, there is the multifaceted assumption that (a) all mass media (including, of course, this chapter) are constructed (re)presentations that both intentionally and unintentionally emphasize certain elements and ignore or distort others; (b) the meanings and implications of mass media use and mass media messages emerge from a transaction between the perceiver, the "text(s)," and the cultural con-texts; and (c) the contexts for transactions between individuals and the media are defined on many levels, including historical, economic, political, peer, and familial (Keery, van den Berg, & Thompson, 2004; Silverstein & Perlick, 1995; Smolak & Levine, 1996).

The fourth implication of Hobbs' expanded conception of media literacy extends the emphasis on person-media transactions and is therefore very important for acknowledging the challenges of understanding and harnessing new media. Most prevention professionals hold a critically proactive stance towards media. However, to be effective, they must also assume and respect that the audiences for their media literacy efforts—students, teachers, parents, coaches, and media professionals—are active, decisive, individual "information processors and consumers," rather than simply naive, gullible, and passive victims of an insidious and/or conspiratorial mass media. This assumption is reinforced by success in the most effective prevention efforts (from the education, mass communication, and critical studies fields), which tend to favour the type of interactive, dialogue-based, and discovery-based learning methods emphasized by Piran (see Chapter 7 in this volume); Steiner-Adair and her colleagues (2002); Jennifer O'Dea (see, e.g., O'Dea & Abraham, 2000; Wade, Davidson, & O'Dea, 2003); and the ATLAS/ATHENA programs (see, e.g., Goldberg et al., 2000; see also Chapter 1 in this volume).

We believe that another increasingly important element of media literacy for prevention professionals and their various audiences is what might be called "marketing awareness" (Kelly, 2002b). Successful marketing is the *raison d'être* and financial lifeblood of most mass media. Regardless of the "channels" through which media are delivered, their creators carefully orchestrate form and content to stir up, reinforce, and extend the desire to purchase products and services, including more consumption of mass media itself. One particularly frequent, salient, and effective marketing strategy is promising that the goods, services, or lifestyles being promoted will reduce, in short and satisfying order, the negative feelings that tend to result from the discrepancy between unreal, "perfect" images common to mass media and the diverse body shapes and weights of normal, healthy individuals (Levine & Harrison, 2009).

The Limits of Literacy

Functioning as influential social constructions, mass media both reflect and generate cultural symbols that are embedded in social values and social institutions of power. These values (e.g., sexism and consumerism) and institutions (e.g., corporate marketing) contribute to—and often benefit from—appearance-related anxiety and dissatisfaction. Therefore, media literacy is embedded in the goal of looking critically at cultural symbols and aiming to transform both media and culture (Piran, 2009, 2010; see also Levine, Piran, & Stoddard, 1999).

The more proximal determinants of risk influenced by mass media, peers, families, and other socio-cultural sources include internalization of the slender or muscular beauty ideal, social comparison tendencies, sexual objectification of the female body, and implicit and explicit prejudice against fat people (Goodman, 2005; Puhl & Latner, 2007; Smolak & Murnen, 2004; Thompson & Stice, 2001; and Chapter 6 in this volume). All of these socio-cultural factors are social constructions (Levine & Smolak, 2006; Piran, 2001; Smolak & Murnen, 2004). Therefore, "a critical social consciousness" is an important first step in deconstructing and changing unhealthy and unfair media influences (Levine & Piran, 2004; Piran, 2001, 2010). But it is only a first step.

The tantalizing belief that media awareness and media analysis inevitably protect young people from the media's negative effects presumes a kind of alchemy. It is expressed in the following syllogism about "media literacy":

- Mass media are bad because they exert a set of very negative influences on our society and, in particular, on impressionable children and youth.
- People who know how to "read" mass media can instantly see right through media's motives and techniques and, thus, are relatively invulnerable to such toxic effects, especially if they are experts in eating disorders and mass communication.

- Therefore, people committed to prevention should do everything they can to understand the construction of seductive and unhealthy media messages and teach others how to shield themselves and embrace healthier values and practices.

Most educators and mental health professionals can easily perform basic analyses of static media communications such as the notorious covers of *Cosmopolitan* magazine and teach others to do the same. They can reveal that the model's flawless, eye-catching, and slender but somehow big-breasted image must have been constructed by technicians and technology, if only because her figural presence and skin tone are impossibly "soft" and there are no more hairs out of place on her head than there are visible pores on her face. However, this kind of deconstruction is only a preliminary step in developing effective media literacy.

Many people committed to eating disorder prevention can recall the thrill of "having the light go on" when they first came to understand the full extent and impact of media tricks such as Photoshopped magazine covers. Perhaps this excitement became energetic optimism when they took the additional step of sharing this critical consciousness in meaningful ways with colleagues and students. It is important to honour these moments of insight and subsequent opportunities for connection through education. At the same time, it is also important to question, as Piran (1995) always did, whether a full understanding of media intentions and media tricks will contribute significantly to prevention and health promotion by inoculating citizens against the insidious effects of media.

The evidence indicates that effective media literacy involves careful content analysis, critical appraisal of the messages' delivery, understanding the interaction between the media creator and the media perceiver, and learning how to create media. In other words, effective media literacy goes beyond knowing how this immense, powerful, and continually evolving socio-cultural influence works—it continues by challenging media's harmful effects by teaching participants to proactively express and assert themselves in and through media.

Media as New, Rapidly Changing Languages
One barrier to effective action is the fact that, in many important ways, the people and institutions that create and embody media (e.g., *Seventeen* magazine, Simon Cowell, Facebook, Lady Gaga, and Google) are exponentially more literate in media than are eating disorder professionals and thus have a greater range of "linguistic" options (e.g., options beyond email, Google, and Facebook). In this regard, as Manuela Ferrari (Chapter 5 in

this volume) explains, the evolution, diversity, and complexity of media (such as Web, cellular, and other communication technologies) will continue to explode and catch on at exponential rates. Therefore, the most effective approaches to media literacy will need to adopt a wider vision that starts from (rather than ends with) the foundation of media analysis and media reaction, continuing on to encompass media creation and media action.

Another related barrier is that adults of a certain age (including the authors of this chapter) tend to privilege a centuries-old technology—the written word printed on paper (e.g., newspapers, detailed journal articles, and books)—as the most organized, thought-filled, analytic, meaningful, · and useful media language. This preference means that people like us, who are versed primarily in older media (including twentieth-century innovations such as broadcasting) will struggle to comprehend the vocabulary, grammar, and semantics of constantly evolving "new media" (such as Wikis, VOIP, webcasts, webinars, podcasts, social networking, and so on) because the latter are built using unfamiliar, rapid, and highly competitive technological innovations. Adding to the difficulty, new media are framed by rapid breakthroughs in the psychology of communications, marketing, and leisure time. These new media privilege a complex blend of images, sounds, text, and interaction that have already made PowerPoint, and perhaps even books, outdated and "quaint" to those individuals we hope to influence with our prevention efforts.

The Ecology of New Media

The new media's vocabulary and grammar are made up of symbols, images, and arrangements that operate on substantially different foundations—including real-time user-to-user interaction and collaboration—than do books, television, radio, or other familiar "one-way" media. Moreover, to the extent that it can be even captured in words, the "normal" media environment of a vast number of young(er) people ages 8 through 30 is a multi-systems ecology of instant messaging, YouTube, texting, online personal revelation, iPads, smart phones, corporate collection of personal data and preferences, DVD players in minivans, "educational" DVDs for infants, flip-cams, Skype, a 500-channel cable-television universe, Web porn, mindshare—the list goes on and grows weekly. If prevention does not keep up with this ecological change, we will be no more successful than if we had tried to use the Latin alphabet to write Chinese. Media multiplicity, novelty, and speed—branching and networking in ways that intentionally, carelessly, and brashly fuse image and substance—constitute a major, complex challenge that we must face personally, professionally, and collaboratively in order to make media literacy an effective prevention tool.

Prevention and Media Literacy: Brief Review and Summary

When thinking about media literacy as a prevention tool, it is useful to recall that prevention programs combine theory, knowledge, and techniques into a systematic attempt to avoid or delay development of a spectrum of disordered eating by decreasing risk factors, increasing the resilience to sources of risk, and otherwise promoting health (see Chapter 1 in this volume). As noted, while it is important to teach media analysis and resistance skills to individuals (as we often do in classrooms), the best "primary" or "universal" prevention strategies seek to change institutions, communities, and cultural practices. To do so, it is necessary to work with and use (i.e., exploit) mass media to change mass media and other important aspects of culture. To paraphrase Lorde (1984), it is impossible to use the media's tools to dismantle the media's house, but there is evidence that the media's tools can be used to mitigate negative impacts of media—especially marketing-driven media.

Attempts to identify "best practice" themes have been only partially successful (Levine & Piran, 2004; Levine & Smolak, 2006). Nevertheless, it appears that the chances of sustained success in prevention are increased when the following components (what we call the "five Cs") are present: Consciousness raising; Competence building; developing strong Connections between participants and between participants and adult mentor-leaders; fostering the experience of Choice in learning and action; and engaging participants in envisioning and pursuing meaningful Changes in their worlds. All of the five Cs are found in the current "best practices" in regard to media literacy as a form of prevention (see, e.g., Neumark-Sztainer, Sherwood, Coller, & Hannan, 2000).

In the 1990s, experts began to propose that media literacy be incorporated into the prevention of disordered eating (see reviews by Irving, 1999; Levine et al., 1999). The resulting programs varied considerably in content and approach, but a compilation of key (and, arguably, ideal) elements is presented in Table 1. Investigations of the effects of media literacy can be categorized into analog laboratory studies, brief interventions, and longer, more intensive programs. Evaluation studies have been reviewed in detail elsewhere (Levine, 2009; Levine & Murnen, 2009; Levine & Smolak, 2006, Chapter 13). This chapter will exemplify and summarize the principal findings, incorporating very recent studies where they are relevant.

Analog Studies

Controlled laboratory experiments demonstrate both the negative effects of mass media (Grabe et al., 2008; Groesz, Levine, & Murnen, 2002) and the ability of pre-exposure inoculations to eliminate or reduce those unde-

TABLE 1: GOALS OF INTENSIVE MEDIA LITERACY PROGRAMS

- Develop critical thinking skills, including an enhanced ability to "read" and "decode" media messages about gender, appearance, weight, and shape.
- Promote healthier body image and eating behaviours by (1) challenging the thinness schema for girls and the idealization of muscularity for boys and (2) considering carefully the benefits and costs of comparing one's own weight and shape to that of peers, fashion models, actors, athletes, and so on.
- Foster a stronger sense of personal self-confidence and autonomy as well as the power of collaboration with peers. In so doing, redefine the body-mind-spirit connection as site of effective action, not self-consciousness and shame about the body.
- Improve communication and other skills necessary for expressing one's self and working with others to change individual behaviour, group norms, and media messages.
- Learn advocacy skills, specifically how to "use" local, mass, "new," and old media (for example, websites, blogs, public-access television, and so on) for social marketing and the promotion of healthy messages.
- Provide participants with peer and adult role "models" who discuss and demonstrate the availability and the benefits of a diversity of roles and identities for females and males as a group.

sirable effects. Very brief written or video interventions can inoculate college-age women, including those who already have a negative body image, against the general tendency to feel worse about their bodies and themselves immediately after viewing slides or video containing images of the slender beauty ideal (Posavac, Posavac, & Weigel, 2001; Yamamiya, Cash, Melnyk, Posavac, & Posavac, 2005). The most effective analog intervention highlights the clash between the artificial, constructed nature of the slender, flawless, "model look" versus two stark realities: (1) human biodiversity—the fact that women's actual shapes and weights naturally and beneficially vary substantially across and within populations, and (2) dieting is risky—the fact that dieting to attain a weight/shape that is unnatural for a given individual has many undesirable long-term effects, including risk for an eating disorder and for increased weight gain. Controlled studies also provide solid evidence that high-school girls are more likely to have their consciousness raised in potentially healthy ways by information about the traps sprung when one begins to make a social comparison of one's body against the images of beauty and sexiness in magazines, movies, and television programs (Levine & Smolak, 2006, Chapter 9).

The limitations of this research include the lack of follow-up evaluations (even short-term reviews) to determine the potency of the effects.

With the exception of foundational work on the negative effects of pro-anorexia websites (e.g., Bardone-Cone & Cass, 2007), there is also a notable absence to date of controlled studies that examine "new" media messages about weight, shape, and beauty, such as the content of advertising and user exchanges on social networking sites such as Twitter and Facebook.

Brief Curricular Programs

Three doctoral dissertations completed in the United States from 1998 to 2000 found that approximately 1 to 2 hours of media literacy training had a number of positive effects, over a couple of months at least, for girls ages 9 through 14 (Levine & Smolak, 2006). Program content varied, but, consistent with the findings of analog research, each intervention emphasized the narrow and constructed nature of beauty ideals as well as the futility of pursuing this artificial "perfection." Several programs for high-school and college-age females used 30-to-90-minute slide presentations or Jean Kilbourne's video *Slim Hopes* to help participants discuss the history of changing, but consistently restrictive, beauty ideals and to address fundamental literacy questions such as: Do real women look like the models? Will I look like the model if I buy the advertised product?[1]

An important feature of these brief curricular programs is information about how various people involved in media creation (e.g., marketing psychologists, corporate executives, fashion models, magazine production staffs, videographers, "cosmetic" surgeons, computer graphics designers, make-up artists, and other technicians and technologies) construct, perfect, and "sell" idealized images. Although the positive effects of these media literacy programs are limited and variable across studies, they do tend to reduce an important risk factor for disordered eating—the internalization of the slender beauty ideal (Thompson & Stice, 2001; see also Chapter 6 in this volume).

Intensive Programs

Multi-lesson, multifaceted media literacy programs create richer opportunities to accomplish many of the goals they share with briefer programs. The intensive programs incorporate the key element of helping students and mentors to translate their critical consciousness into educating peers and into consumer activism (Levine & Smolak, 2006; Piran, 2010). Well-controlled studies of programs that unfold over 1 to 2 months (see, e.g., Neumark-Sztainer et al., 2000; Wilksch & Wade, 2010) have shown that the more intensive media literacy programs help girls and boys ages 10 through 14 to reduce risk factors such as the internalization of the slender or muscular ideal, while increasing the potentially protective factors of self-acceptance, self-confidence in friendships, and confidence in their ability to be activists who challenge narrow and prejudicial social norms concerning weight and shape (Levine & Smolak, 2006).

Implications for Best Practices and Further Developments in Prevention
Media literacy is a promising area for prevention because it has the potential to foster and reinforce potent forms of consciousness raising, connections, competence building, choice, and cultural change (Levine, 2009; Levine & Piran, 2004; Levine & Smolak, 2006; Piran, 2001, 2010). Specifically, these media literacy methods use collaboration, activism, and advocacy to engage students in interactive learning, creating new and healthier group norms, and changing their own efficacy expectations and ecologies. As such, media literacy contains elements considered crucial to preventing problematic youth behaviour such as cigarette smoking and alcohol use/abuse (Botvin, 2000).

Of course, a lot more research is needed. None of these programs are designed specifically to address new media. In addition, we need to follow Piran's (1995, 2001, 2010) and Sarah Stinson's (2010) lead in learning more about the "participatory actions" and "participatory research" strategies necessary to establish, enact, evaluate, and embed media literacy programs in communities, schools, and other social organizations such as Girl Scouts (Neumark-Sztainer et al., 2000), 4-H groups (www.4-h.org), and religious groups.[2]

At present it appears that media literacy programs will work best in the body image and disordered eating field if four conditions are met. First, leaders need to develop skills and invest the time to facilitate respectful dialogues and relationship building within the groups (Piran, 2001). Second, these programs are not "just for kids" and neither are they "just for girls." Adult and boy participation is also essential. Media literacy programs need to be conceived and implemented as part of an integrated ecological approach (see Chapter 1 in this volume). Mass (and targeted) media for health promotion and advocacy require extensive consultation with local stakeholders, along with the education and involvement of adult mentors, businesses, and other community connections (Levine et al., 1999; Piran, 2001; Levine & Smolak, 2006, Chapter 15). Authentic collaboration between adults and youth (inside and outside of schoolrooms) is the foundation for healthier relationships among youth and between youth and their cultures.

Third, serious attention needs to be paid to the possibility that, for reasons that are as yet poorly understood, media literacy training may be most effective for youth ages 9 through 14 and for young adults (see

Levine & Smolak, 2006; Watson & Vaughn, 2006). A recent study by Wilksch, Durbridge, and Wade (2008), conducted with very rigorous methodology, found that eight 50-minute media literacy lessons (with topics such as the analysis of advertising and the methods of consumer activism) had no significant effects on shape and weight concern, media internalization, dieting, and self-esteem of Grade 10 Australian girls (mean age = 15) at a 3-month follow-up, as compared to a control group. In contrast, the same Australian investigators conducted a methodologically rigorous evaluation that found that a version of the same *Media Smart* curriculum produced desirable effects (of small to moderate size) in Grade 8 girls and boys (ages 13-14) on body dissatisfaction, weight and shape concern, dieting, and reports of ineffectiveness and depression (Wilksch & Wade, 2010). Particularly striking is the fact that these effects were observed 2.5 years after the baseline assessment.

Fourth, in keeping with the ethical principles that guide professionals such as psychologists, those individuals committed to prevention need to carefully consider the potential risks of media literacy approaches. Austin, Pinkleton, and Funabiki (2007) documented a "desirability paradox" in which media literacy training regarding tobacco advertising increased adolescents ability to use logic in resisting tobacco advertising while also increasing (not decreasing) the perceived desirability of the tobacco portrayals communicated by media. This important outcome needs to be investigated in the area of body image and disordered eating. It appears to demonstrate that media literacy training is beneficial in large part because it "alters the decision-making process itself, in addition to affecting beliefs" (p. 503) about perceived realism and peer norms. Nevertheless, until long-term effects of any increase in the desirability of media portrayals are shown to be harmless, we need to think carefully about benefit-risk ratios in considering the ethical implications of media literacy research.

Activism

Understanding and accepting the powerful and multi-faceted impact of media in our culture will ultimately help us to resist the temptation to blame any specific cultural influence (such as media) as if it was some detached, nefarious "Other." Although it is critically important to clarify and address cultural risk factors for eating disorders, doing little more than pointing (or wagging) one's fingers at the media will never mitigate those risk factors. We shape the culture and the media with our own behaviour. For over 30 years, eating disorders expert Amy Baker Dennis (personal communication to Levine, October 1987) has told her clients, their families, and her colleagues: "*No one* is responsible for the development of an eating disorder; *everyone* has a responsibility to participate in treatment and prevention."

Personal and collective agency are important and intertwined goals in preventing eating disorders (Piran, 2001). Whether from a feminist, social cognitive, humanistic, or existential perspective, two pillars of agency are the power to choose and the responsibility to take a stance (i.e., make choices, express one's self, and connect with others), despite complexity, doubt, and inevitable mistakes (Funder, 2007; May, Angel, & Ellenberger, 1958). The word "existence" itself is derived from the Latin *ex* (out) and *sistere* or *stare*, which means "to stand" (*Merriam-Webster Dictionary* (n.d.). In other words, to be (and not to be) is to step out and take or make a stance (May et al., 1958). Such a decision includes taking a stand about the individual and collective choices we make as participants in the development of our culture.

The impact of such choices can be seen in the following example. The United Nations Children's Fund (2008) estimates that Africa's under-5 mortality rate would drop by 30% (and its maternal mortality rate by 15%) if a strategy costing less than US$3 per capita—a total of less than $2.8 billion for the entire continent—was implemented. Meanwhile, according to the National Sporting Goods Association (2008), US consumers spent more than six times that amount, or US$17.4 billion, on sport shoes in 2007. Even more startling, the National Restaurant Association (n.d.) estimates that US consumers spent more than 200 times as much—US$558 billion—eating out in 2008. Prevention professionals take stands that can shape our culture by speaking up when we are unhappy with the values, "desired" consumer behaviour, expectations, and so on, that the culture communicates to us, to our families, and to our constituencies. We cannot encourage and reinforce agency in others (especially young people) unless we courageously and consistently engage in the process of acting on our own responsibilities and choices (Irving, 1999; Maine, 2000).

One very important way to improve the cultural environment is through activism and advocacy (Irving, 1999; Levine et al., 1999; Levine & Smolak, 2006; Maine, 2000). Drawing on the media-based prevention work of Wallack, Dorfman, Jernigan, and Themba (1993), Levine has long made a useful distinction between activism and advocacy (Levine et al., 1999; Levine & Smolak, 2006). Activism is better recast as re-activism because the focus is responding negatively to unhealthy messages and positively to healthy messages. Advocacy is pro-active, even though its stimulus may be a re-action to problems. Specifically, advocacy involves using the principles and forms of mass media in order to promote and market positive social changes (Wallack et al., 1993). Kelly (2002a, 2002b), Maine (2000,

TABLE 2: KEY ELEMENTS OF EFFECTIVE MEDIA ACTIVISM

• Work in groups.	• Use humour and satire.
• Find leverage points.	• Let media know what you're doing.
• Find "hidden" ally.	• Welcome and utilize controversy.
• Do honest research.	• Say "thanks."
• Have attitude and fun.	• Be persistent.

2004; Maine & Kelly, 2005), and others have argued that people will get at the roots of risk factors and sow the seeds of real, positive transformations only by becoming active advocates for change in the media and for collaboration with mass media to bring about other important changes in institutions, public policies, and cultural practices (see also Kilbourne, 1999; Lamb & Brown, 2006).

Despite a long and illustrious history of social activism by women and men around the world (see, e.g., Willie, Ridini, & Willard, 2008), prevention initiatives that focus on media and other sociocultural factors continue to be met with questions that illustrate the enormity of the task, such as: "But, really, what can anyone *do*?" or "OK, we have to do something, but *what*, and *how*?" Table 2 identifies some basic steps, based on the experience of media activists, including the authors. The following section provides a concrete example of these principles in action.

Allies in Activism I: Dads and Daughters

In the early 2000s, a US-based non-governmental organization (NGO) called Dads and Daughters (DADs) encouraged its few thousand members to email, write, and/or call corporations that advertise and market in ways that affect girls (Kelly served as president and spokesperson for Dads and Daughters during its 9.5 years of existence). The organization found that a relatively small number of dads could have a marked impact by using "new" media to advocate for their daughters and other girls. Fathers and stepfathers are not the "usual suspects" to become advocates for positive developments in female body image, media messages, and prevention. So, why did this small group of dads have more clout than many people (including the fathers themselves) expected?

The answer to this question reveals the importance of leverage and unexpected allies in creating advocacy (see Table 2). Many dads and stepdads care passionately about, and are fiercely protective of, their daughters. Helping a dad to "connect the dots" between his concern for his daughter's well-being and the cultural dangers she faces from media and marketing can leverage this protective response to create a potential ally in multiple important areas (Kelly, 2002a, 2002b; Maine, 2004). As "first men" in the lives of their daughters, fathers and stepfathers set important familial standards for masculinity in the eyes of their daughters—including what men value and appreciate in girls and women. Leveraging this influence in combination with males' disproportionate positions of influence in a patriarchal culture, Dads and Daughters transformed fathers and stepfathers (a previously untapped, natural resource) into media advocates (Kelly, 2002a, 2002b).

Of course, fathers often inadvertently reinforce the dominant and destructive cultural messages that encourage females to believe that outward appearance is what men value most in girls and women (Maine, 2004). Ironically, a father's "first man" position also gives him a position of leverage in positively shaping and encouraging a daughter's life and self-image—if he becomes media literate about the problematic cultural messages his daughter receives and if he grasps the corrosive impact of any paternal (and paternalistic) responses that strive to seal the daughter off from the larger culture and its dangers. With this sort of feminist consciousness, fathers have the potential to be important prevention resources for daughters—when they use their primary influence to debunk the cultural lie that "how you look is more important than who you are." A father or stepfather can show in words, attitudes, and numerous direct and indirect actions that he values his daughter, and other women, for who they are, what they do, and what they care about—not for their appearance (Kelly, 2002a, 2002b; Levine, 1994; Maine, 2004). Similarly, dads have leverage with sons—who are also damaged by the culture's lie that the size of a woman's cleavage is more important than the size of her heart, brains, or spirit (Brooks, 1995; Kelly, 2004).

Fathers as Leverage: Two Case Examples of Confronting the Negative

A critical social consciousness (Piran, 2001, 2010) of media, gender, and power readily reveals the fact that men head up nearly all of the media, marketing, and advertising companies in North America (Women CEOs, 2010). Approximately, 97% of Fortune 500 chief executive officers (CEOs) are men, fathers, and/or grandfathers. Mass media generators are big businesses that are fuelled by other big businesses and that reflect the unequal distribution of power in society. Power inequity can be considered a risk factor in the development of eating disorders themselves (see Chapter 7 in this volume).

Dads and Daughters advocated against gender inequity in society through active membership in, and/or a partnership with, the National Coalition of Women and Girls in Education, the Women's Sports Foundation, the

Ms. Foundation for Women, the Feminist Majority Foundation, the Save Title IX coalition, the Domestic Violence Hotline, and other advocacy groups. Simultaneously, Dads and Daughters worked to mobilize its predominantly male membership to make tactical use of the gendered power imbalance. Helping less privileged fathers and stepfathers recognize how "dads like us" run Fortune 500 and other influential corporations helped them realize the potential influence of communicating father to father to CEOs about the marketing messages sent to our kids. If a group of men (as fathers) ask a CEO (as a father) to put his daughter's or granddaughter's face into the images and texts of what he's selling and how he's selling it, the recipient CEO may give special legitimacy and weight to that request.

In effect, Dads and Daughters consciously adopted a two-track strategy for working outside and within a patriarchal business system in the United States: (1) team with women advocating against gender disparity in society, and (2) use fathers' position of male privilege to agitate against unhealthy media messages directed at girls and women.

Campbell's Soup

In the autumn of 2000, the Campbell's soup company broadcast a 30-second television commercial during after-school programs, marketing soup to prepubescent girls as a diet aid.[3] The Dads and Daughters system of media activism and advocacy generated father-to-father emails to Campbell's male CEO. Two days later, Campbell's vice-president John Faulkner telephoned DADs to say that the company had pulled the commercial. Faulkner explained that, when creating the commercial, Campbell's had not recognized the dangerous subtext of the message, but its negative connotations became very clear to him and his company after reading the opinions of the fathers who protested.

Thirty-second national television commercials are very expensive to produce and air. Nevertheless, Campbell's was willing to swallow the loss in response to emails from one small organization. Why? In order to succeed, today's marketers must also be agile and respond quickly to what consumers feel and say. The mass of consumers reached by a mass media Campbell's soup advertisement is exponentially greater than the number of men involved in the DADs protest. However, the competition for loyal consumers keeps growing, so businesses and marketers have a big stake in listening closely when even small numbers of consumers speak up. Thus, speaking father to father, a few dozen DADs' members got an important message through to a major corporation. The number of dads involved in this successful piece of activism is roughly the same small size as the number of contributors to this volume.

Dads and Daughters and the Campaign for Commercial-Free Childhood (CCFC)

In 2006, DADs partnered with the Campaign for Commercial-Free Child-hood (CCFC), a coalition of health care professionals, educators, advocacy groups, parents, and individuals devoted to limiting the impact of com-mercial culture on children.[4] The target of their mutual concern was the Hasbro toy company, which had announced plans to launch a line of dolls for girls as young as 6 that were replicas of the Pussycat Dolls, a real-life music group famous (or infamous) for its sexualized lyrics, outfits, and dance routines.[5]

The CCFC and DADs launched an email campaign strongly urging Hasbro not to release the dolls and, further, to end its licensing agreement with the Pussycat Dolls group. Specifically, the messages urged Hasbro's CEO Alfred J. Verrecchia to put his elementary-school-aged granddaugh-ter's face in the picture—and to think and act (i.e., to take a stance) as a grandfather before releasing the new line of dolls. The emails reminded Verrecchia: "You would never encourage your young grandchildren to engage in or aspire to hyper-sexualized behaviours six or seven years before they reach adolescence, and I am sure you did not do the same with your own children when they were very young. But that is exactly what [the "toy"] Pussycat Dolls will do to children." A few weeks later, Verrecchia announced that Hasbro was dropping the Pussycat Doll project altogether.

Fathers as Leverage: A Case Example of Recognizing and Rewarding the Positive

In 1999 and 2000, Chevrolet regularly aired a television commercial depict-ing a lifelong father-daughter relationship in which a dad consistently sup-ports his daughter's dream of being a competitive skier. Eventually, as a young woman, the daughter wins an important race and is immediately surrounded by cheering female coaches and teammates. Through the con-gratulatory hugs, she searches for her dad in the crowd of spectators. Their eyes meet and, as the music swells melodramatically, they give each other an excited thumbs-up. Then the male announcer's basso, macho voice intones: "Year after year, it's good to have someone to depend on. Chevy. The most dependable, longest-lasting trucks on the road."

Just as parents try to "catch" children being good in order to reward positive behaviour, Dads and Daughters also occasionally used the lever-age of concerned, loving fathers to point out examples of positive media messages. To draw attention to Chevrolet, positive portrayal of a father-daughter relationship (a rarity in mass media), DADs mobilized its mem-bers to write emails of thanks and encouragement to both Chevrolet and

Campbell-Ewald, its Michigan ad agency. DADs gave both companies a Father's Day award, which the companies then publicized themselves.

Lessons from the Field

These advocacy success stories are not evidence that groups such as DADs and the CCFC can get what they want every time they take responsibility, take a stance, and speak out. In fact, only about 15% of DADs' member-mobilization campaigns achieved the desired outcome. Sometimes, companies did not respond at all to DADs' well-orchestrated and assertive actions. However, even in the apparently "unsuccessful" cases, there were clear benefits in the enthusiastic fatherly teamwork. Anecdotally, fathers and stepfathers reported that taking responsibility, making a stand, and choosing to act helped them—and their families—feel less overwhelmed by the wide influence of media. Moreover, DADs' advocacy campaigns helped its members set a positive example for their children by showing fathers' willingness to speak up and take a very public advocacy stance.

Allies in Activism II: GO GIRLS! of Red Wing, Minnesota

GO GIRLS! is the acronym for Giving Our Girls Inspiration and Resources for Lasting Self-Esteem! According to Levine et al. (1999), this intensive media literacy program was developed in 1998 by the Seattle-based NGO Eating Disorders Awareness and Prevention, Incorporated, the organization that eventually evolved into the National Eating Disorders Association (NEDA).[6] Its 12 weekly lessons are marketed by NEDA as the GO GIRLS! *Curriculum for High School Girls* (1998). As noted by Levine and Smolak (2006), GO GIRLS! incorporates the five C's of prevention because it is "an organized but flexible set of media-related activities that help adolescent girls understand—through experience, observational learning, and action—that they have a 'voice' as consumers and citizens, and that together they can use that voice and their skills to effect social, corporate, and personal changes" (pp. 319-320).

Beginning in 1999, this vision of media literacy, activism, and advocacy was spectacularly realized in Red Wing, Minnesota, a city of about 16,000 people located on the Mississippi River about 50 miles southeast of the Twin Cities. Veteran eating disorders therapist, educator, and activist Sarah Stinson led and mentored high-school girls participating in the Red Wing GO GIRLS! program. For 12 years, Stinson guided the participating girls—and enabled the girls to guide themselves—to a number of important accomplishments, including: (1) obtaining more than US$70,000 in grants and donations; (2) creating videos, songs, and PowerPoint presentations for educating themselves and peers about mass media, media literacy, and risk factors for negative body image and disordered eating; (3) delivering their messages during broadcast television and radio appearances as well as in-person media literacy and other presentations to over 2,000 people in three states and 11 cities; (4) presenting at several national NEDA conferences; (5) participating in several Washington, DC, congressional lobby days organized by the Eating Disorders Coalition; and (6) making presentations and serving as "big sisters" at the Turn Beauty Inside Out leadership conferences in 2005 (in Los Angeles), 2006 (in Queens, NY), and 2007 (in New York City) (GO GIRLS! 2007).[7]

Their most ambitious project illustrates the extent to which Stinson and the girls encouraged each other to "think big" and "live large" as activists and advocates. Drawing on their own media literacy experience (and after more than a year of planning and fundraising), members of Stinson's GO GIRLS! group travelled in 2009 to Fiji to respond—on location—to the implications of Anne Becker's groundbreaking studies of the negative effects of television's introduction to this developing Pacific island nation (Becker, Burwell, Gilman, Herzog, & Hamburg, 2002). While there, they discussed body acceptance, media's impact on body-esteem and self-esteem, media activism, and media advocacy with 50 Fijian secondary school students, ages 12 to 19 years old. The Minnesota girls found that many of these Fijian students had cellphones and said they watched television an average of 5 hours per day.

The group also made a media literacy presentation to 20 male Fijian soldiers at an army base. One teen GO GIRLS! participant reported: "The men asked us what they should take home with them to tell their wives and daughters. They kept asking, 'How do you know if a [media image] is real or fake?'" (personal communication from Stinson to Kelly, May 9, and May 19, 2010). The transcultural media literacy approach of these small-town girls and their mentor is supported by preliminary evidence in a recent doctoral dissertation by Hennessey (2008) that the GO GIRLS! program can have numerous positive effects on body image and healthy eating among Tanzanian adolescent girls.

Prevention in Larger Contexts: Reality in the Marketing Age
Mass media have had an impact on bodies, body image, gender identity, and eating for more than a century and a quarter (Banner, 1983) and for over 500 years, if we include the first mass medium technology—Gutenberg's fifteenth-century printing press. One phenomenon setting our current age apart from other times in cultural history (for example, the Roaring 1920s) is the exponentially greater ubiquity, frequency, and effectiveness of media as a means of marketing (Silverstein & Perlick, 1995). What constitutes

community today is a culture increasingly saturated with instantaneous electronic connections and profit-imperative marketing.

In his media literacy trainings for parents and professionals who work with families, Kelly (2002a, 2002b; see also Maine, 2000) uses a thought experiment that demonstrates that the average daily time most people spend out of the presence of marketing can be measured in mere minutes. Regardless of his or her age, the rest of the modern person's waking hours are saturated in marketing, whether they are conscious of it or not—a powerful argument for why the era we live in could be called "the market-ing age."

Immersion in this marketing culture has implications that reach beyond ongoing, legitimate concerns over the degree to which marketers willingly sell girls' and women's health and well-being down the river to make a profit (see, e.g., Kasser & Kanner, 2004). According to Maine and Kelly (2005), living in the marketing age means that, to use a key concept in the study of mass communications, media intentionally and incidentally cul-tivate symbolic worlds in which the following principles constitute truth:

- We should never feel uneasy or uncomfortable, except when we "fail" by being without certain socially desirable attributes, goods, and services.
- We should be afraid of the world but fearlessly pursue the goods, the services, and the credit necessary for taking advantage of market commodities, many of which purport to minimize uneasiness and discomfort.
- We should be vigilant about, and afraid of, illness, aging—and espe-cially death—but somehow not think too deeply or care too much about the consequences of overeating, consuming too much alcohol, or smoking cigarettes.
- If we are ever uneasy, uncomfortable, or fearful—including being con-cerned about mass media and other cultural icons—that is a failing on our part as a person—there is something wrong with us. The preferred alternative is for us to "just do it," "have it our way," and get with the larger program of being consumers.

To one degree or another, life in the marketing age leads many people to lose touch with some important realities. For example, life is uncertain and ambiguous, so unease (dis-ease) and discomfort are normal. Over 50 years ago, cultural commentators such as Erich Fromm (1956) and Rollo May and his colleagues (1958) demonstrated that markets, mar-keting, "deals," and consuming will never provide meaningful, peaceful, loving, and authentic solutions to the problems and ambiguities necessarily involved in existing. Real life, the genuine article, provides existential dilemmas revolving around freedom (versus bondage of various sorts), meaning (versus meaninglessness and chaos), love and other connections (versus misunderstanding, hate, alienation, and objectification), and being (versus stagnation, destruction, and death). Facing, accepting, and transcending these inevitable dilemmas requires responses and responsibilities with some type of spiritual dimension. Faith, courage, hope, love, acceptance, competence, and integrity cannot be purchased and obtained—and certainly not by coveting, pursuing, and consuming market commodities such as thinness and sexiness.

Professionals are wise to approach prevention work with a strong awareness of the consequences of living in, and actively responding to, the marketing age. This central contextual step in media literacy must include reflections on how marketing cultures affect one's ability to experience fully the wonders of reality and a genuine life, including creativity, intimacy, and true connection with one another. Hope lies in the knowledge that humans still retain the capacity for connection (to reality and each other) regardless of circumstance. Hope also lies in the examples of how people—even people such as the Red Wing teen girls, who do not hold positions of substantial social power—can use activism and advocacy to transform our marketing age into something better.

Conclusions and Implications

At present, it is fair to conclude that media literacy programs in schools, in other organizations, and perhaps at home hold a great deal of promise for harnessing the key elements of effective prevention. However, it is also important to note that relatively little is known about the key features of these programs, how they work, and what their long-term outcomes are with regard to the actual prevention of body image distress and eating disorders. Moreover, research concerning the impact of media literacy education in other public health arenas (such as the promotion of healthy nutrition and non-violence) yields a mixed, inconclusive picture (Bergsma & Carney, 2008).

One response to the current state of affairs is more focused research on "health-promoting media literacy education" (Bergsma & Carney, 2008, p. 522). Another response is to expand the scope of inquiry and actions. This volume is a testament to the work of Gail McVey, Dianne Neumark-Sztainer, Niva Piran, Linda Smolak, Susan Paxton, and others in demonstrating that eating disorders and related conditions are community problems that must be prevented, treated, and managed by implementing a multiple-systems, public health perspective (see Chapters 1, 3, 6, 7, and

8 in this volume). This perspective follows Bronfenbrenner's (1979) well-known scheme for understanding normal and abnormal development in terms of the independent and interactive influences of families, neighbourhoods, educational settings, athletics, healthcare, and, of course, media. In keeping with this ecological perspective, it is important to expand our focus to the broader (and deeper) social ecology and phenomena in which media systems operate.

The eating disorders prevention field is filled with many examples of education, exercises, and actions that attempt to undo what Maine and Kelly (2005) call "the Body Myth" — the mistaken belief that life's meaning, our self-worth, and our worth to others are (and should be) based on how our body looks, what we weigh, and what we eat. Comprehensive and contextual understanding of media literacy — as awareness, analysis, activism, and advocacy — can give professionals and everyday citizens the power to harness the five C's of prevention in order to create the healthy, equitable, and authentic cultures we want to inhabit (see Chapter 6 in this volume).

Notes

1 Slim Hopes, Media Education Foundation. Retrieved from http://www.mediaed.org/cgi-bin/ commerce.cgi?preadd=action&key=305.
2 4-H groups. Retrieved from http://www.4-h.org.
3 Campbell's Soup Company. Retrieved from http://www.campbellsoup.com.
4 Campaign for Commercial-Free Childhood. Retrieved from http://www.commercial exploitation.org.
5 Hasbro. Retrieved from http://www.hasbro.com; Pussycat Dolls, online: http://www.myspace.com/pussycatdolls.
6 National Eating Disorders Association. Retrieved from http://www.nationaleating disorders.org.
7 Eating Disorders Coalition. Retrieved from http://www.eatingdisorderscoalition.org; and Turn Beauty Inside Out leadership conferences, online: http://www.mindonthe media.org.

References

Arnett, J. J. (1995). Adolescents' uses of the media for self-socialization. *Journal of Youth and Adolescence, 24*, 519-533.

Austin, E. W., Pinkelton, B. E., & Funabiki, R. P. (2007). The desirability paradox in the effects of media literacy training. *Communication Research, 34*, 483-506.

Banner, L. (1983). *American beauty.* New York: Alfred Knopf.

Bardone-Cone, A. M., & Cass, K. M. (2007). What does viewing a pro-anorexia website do? Experimental examination of website exposure and moderating effects. *International Journal of Eating Disorders, 40*, 537-548.

Becker, A. E., Burwell, R. A., Gilman, S. E., Herzog, D. B., & Hamburg, P. (2002). Eating behaviors and attitudes following prolonged exposure to television among ethnic Fijian adolescent girls. *British Journal of Psychiatry, 180*, 509-514.

Bergsma, L. J., & Carney, M. E. (2008). Effectiveness of health-promoting media literacy education: A systematic review. *Health Education Research, 23*, 522-542.

Botvin, G. (2000). Preventing drug abuse in schools: Social and competence enhancement approaches targeting individual-level etiologic factors. *Addictive Behaviors, 25*, 887-897.

Bronfenbrenner, U. (1979). *The ecology of human development: Experiments by nature and design.* Cambridge, MA: Harvard University Press.

Brooks, G. R. (1995). *The centerfold syndrome: How men can overcome objectification and achieve intimacy with women.* Hoboken, NJ: John Wiley.

Brown, J. A. (2001). Media literacy and critical television viewing in education. In D. G. Singer & L. L. Singer (Eds.), *Handbook of children and the media* (pp. 681-697). Thousand Oaks, CA: Sage.

Comstock, G., & Scharrer, E. (2007). *Media and the American child.* Burlington, MA: Academic Press.

Fromm, E. (1956). *The art of loving.* New York: Harper Books.

Funder, D.C. (2007). *The personality puzzle* (4th ed.). New York: Norton.

GO GIRLS! (1998). *Curriculum for High School Girls* (Grades 9-12). Seattle, WA: Eating Disorders Awareness and Prevention.

GO GIRLS! (2007). In Sarah Stinson, *Higher self case statement* (pp. 4-5). Unpublished report [on file with the author].

Goldberg, L., MacKinnon, D. P., Elliot, D. L., Moe, E. L., Clarke, G., & Cheong, J. (2000). The adolescents training and learning to avoid steroids program: Preventing drug use and promoting healthy behaviors. *Archives of Pediatrics and Adolescent Medicine, 154*, 332-338.

Goodman, R. J. (2005). Mapping the sea of eating disorders: A structural equation model of how peers, family, and media influence body image and eating disorders. *Visual Communication Quarterly, 12*, 194-213.

Grabe, S., Ward, L. M., & Hyde, J. S. (2008). The role of the media in body image concerns among women: A meta-analysis of experimental and correlational studies. *Psychological Bulletin, 134*, 460-476.

Groesz, L. M., Levine, M. P., & Murnen, S. K. (2002). The effect of experimental presentation of thin media images on body satisfaction: A meta-analytic review. *International Journal of Eating Disorders, 31*, 1-16.

Hennessey, M. (2008). Body dissatisfaction, eating disorders and a media literacy intervention among Tanzanian females (UMI No. AAI3298643). *Dissertation Abstracts International, 69*(1-B), 679.

Hobbs, R. (1998). The seven great debates in the media literacy movement. *Journal of Communication, 48*(1), 16-32.

Hobbs, R. (2005). Media literacy and the K-12 content areas. In G. Schwarz and P. U. Brown (Eds.), *Media literacy: Transforming curriculum and teaching* (104th yearbook of the National Society for the Study of Education, part I, pp. 74-99). Malden, MA: Blackwell Publishing.

Irving, L. (1999). A bolder model of prevention: Science, practice, and activism. In N. Piran, M. P. Levine, & C. Steiner-Adair (Eds.), *Preventing eating disorders: A handbook of interventions and special challenges* (pp. 63-83). Philadelphia, PA: Brunner/Mazel.

Kasser, T., & Kanner, A. D. (Eds.). (2004). *Psychology and consumer culture: The struggle for a good life in a materialistic world.* Washington, DC: American Psychological Association.

Keery, H., van den Berg, P., & Thompson, J. K. (2004). The Tripartite Influence Model of body dissatisfaction and eating disturbance with adolescent girls. *Body Image, 1,* 237-251.

Kelly, J. (2002a). *Dads and Daughters: How to inspire, understand, and support your daughter.* New York: Broadway Books.

Kelly, J. (2002b). Marketing: Girls in the crosshairs. *Daughters: For Parents of Girls, 7*(2), 4.

Kelly, J. (2004). Dad's influence on his daughter? Just ask her. *Daughters: For Parents of Girls, 9*(6), 12.

Kilbourne, J. (1999). *Deadly persuasion: Why women and girls must fight the addictive power of advertising.* New York: Free Press.

Lamb, S., & Brown, L. M. (2006). *Packaging girlhood: Rescuing our daughters from marketers' schemes.* New York: St. Martin's Press.

Levine, M. P. (1994). "Beauty myth" and the beast: What men can do and be to help prevent eating disorders. *Eating Disorders: Journal of Treatment and Prevention, 2,* 101-113.

Levine, M. P. (2009). Aportaciones desde el campo del la prevención: Implicaciones para la educación en comunición [Lessons from the field of prevention: Implications for Media Literacy Programs]. *Aula de Innovación Educativa* [Educational Innovations for the Classroom], *178,* 14-18.

Levine, M. P., & Harrison, K. (2009). Effects of media on eating disorders and body image. In J. Bryant & M. B. Oliver (Eds.), *Media effects: Advances in theory and research* (3rd ed., pp. 490-515). Mahwah, NJ: Lawrence Erlbaum Associates.

Levine, M. P., & Murnen, S. K. (2009). "Everybody knows that mass media are/are not [*pick one*] a cause of eating disorders": A critical review of evidence for a causal link between media, negative body image, and disordered eating in females. *Journal of Social and Clinical Psychology, 28,* 9-42.

Levine, M. P., & Piran, N. (2004). The role of body image in the prevention of eating disorders. *Body Image, 1,* 57-70.

Levine, M. P., Piran, N., & Stoddard, C. (1999). Mission more probable: Media literacy, activism, and advocacy as primary prevention. In N. Piran, M. P. Levine, & C. Steiner-Adair (Eds.), *Preventing eating disorders: A handbook of interventions and special challenges* (pp. 3-25). Philadelphia, PA: Brunner/Mazel.

Levine, M. P., & Smolak, L. (1996). Media as a context for the development of disordered eating. In L. Smolak, M. P. Levine, & R. Striegel-Moore (Eds.), *The developmental psychopathology of eating disorders* (pp. 235-257). Mahwah, NJ: Erlbaum.

Levine, M. P., & Smolak, L. (2006). *The prevention of eating problems and eating disorders: Theory, research, and practice.* Mahwah, NJ: Erlbaum.

Lorde, A. (1984). *Sister outsider: Essays and speeches.* Trumansburg, NY: Crossing Press.

Maine, M. (2000). *Body wars: Making peace with women's bodies. An activist's guide.* Carlsbad, CA: Gürze Books.

Maine, M. (2004). *Father hunger: Fathers, daughters, and the pursuit of thinness* (2nd ed.). Carlsbad, CA: Gürze Books.

Maine, M., & Kelly, J. (2005). *The body myth: Adult women and the pressure to be perfect.* Hoboken, NJ: John Wiley

Marsh, J. (2006). Emergent media literacy: Digital animation in early childhood. *Language and Education, 20,* 493-506.

May, R., Angel, E., & Ellenberger, H. F. (Eds.). (1958). *Existence: A new dimension in psychiatry and psychology.* New York: Basic Books.

Merriam-Webster Dictionary. (n.d.). The definition of "critical." Online: http://www.merriam-webster.com/dictionary/

National Restaurant Association. (n.d.). Eating out spending for 2008. Online: http://www.restaurant.org/pdfs/research/2008forecast_factbook.pdf

National Sporting Goods Association. (2008). *Sporting goods sales reach $53.5 billion in 2007; NSGA expects flat 2008.* Online: http://www.snewsnet.com/cgi-bin/snews/11987.html

Neumark-Sztainer D., Sherwood N., Coller, T., & Hannan P. J. (2000). Primary prevention of disordered eating among pre-adolescent girls: Feasibility and short-term impact of a community-based intervention. *Journal of the American Dietetic Association, 100,* 1466-1473.

O'Dea, J., & Abraham, S. (2000). Improving the body image, eating attitudes and behaviors of young male and female adolescents: A new educational approach which focuses on self-esteem. *International Journal of Eating Disorders, 28,* 43-57.

Piran, N. (1995). Prevention: Can early lessons lead to a delineation of an alternative model? A critical look at prevention with schoolchildren. *Eating Disorders: The Journal of Treatment and Prevention, 3,* 28-36.

Piran, N. (2001). Re-inhabiting the body from the inside out: Girls transform their school environment. In D. L. Tolman & M. Brydon-Miller (Eds.), *From subjects to subjectivities: A handbook of interpretative and participatory methods* (pp. 218-238). New York: New York University Press.

Piran, N. (2009). El Poder de la imagen: interiorización de los símbolos cultural [The power of the image: The internalization of cultural symbols]. *Journal Aula de Innovación Educativa* [Educational Innovations for the Classroom], *178,* 19-24.

Piran, N. (2010). A feminist perspective on risk factor research and on the prevention of eating disorders. *Eating Disorders: The Journal of Treatment and Prevention, 18,* 183-198.

Posavac, H. D., Posavac, S. S., & Weigel, R. G. (2001). Reducing the impact of media images on women at risk for body image disturbance: Three targeted interventions. *Journal of Social and Clinical Psychology, 20,* 324-340.

Puhl, R. M., & Latner, J. D. (2007). Stigma, obesity, and the health of the nation's children. *Psychological Bulletin, 133,* 557-580.

Potter, W. J. (2001). *Media literacy* (2nd ed.). Thousand Oaks, CA: Sage.

Rentala, L., & Korhonen, V. (2008). New literacies as a challenge for traditional knowledge conceptions in school: A case study from fifth graders digital media production. *SIMILE: Studies in Media and Information Literacy Education, 8,* 1-15.

Schwarz, G., & Brown, P. U. (Eds.). (2005). *Media literacy: Transforming curriculum and teaching* (104th yearbook of the National Society for the Study of Education, part I). Malden, MA: Blackwell Publishing.

Silverstein, B., & Perlick, D. (1995). *The cost of competence: Why inequality causes depression, eating disorders, and illness in women.* New York: Oxford University Press.

Smolak, L., & Levine, M. P. (1996). Adolescents' transitions and the development of eating problems. In L. Smolak, M. P. Levine, & R. Striegel-Moore (Eds.), *The psychopathology of eating disorders: Implications for research, prevention, and treatment* (pp. 207-34). Mahwah, NJ: Lawrence Erlbaum Associates.

Smolak, L., & Murnen, S. K. (2004). A feminist approach to eating disorders. In J. K. Thompson (Ed.), *Handbook of eating disorders and obesity* (pp. 590-605). New York: Wiley.

Steiner-Adair, C., Sjostrom, L., Franko, D. L., Pai, S., Tucker, R., Becker, A. E., & Herzog, D. B. (2002). Primary prevention of eating disorders in adolescent girls: Learning from practice. *International Journal of Eating Disorders, 32,* 401-411.

Thompson, J. K., Heinberg, L., Altabe, M., & Tantleff-Dunn, S. (1999). *Exacting beauty: Theory, assessment, and treatment of body image disturbance.* Washington, DC: American Psychological Association.

Thompson, J. K., & Stice, E. (2001). Thin-ideal internalization: Mounting evidence for a new risk factor for body-image disturbance and eating pathology. *Current Directions in Psychological Science, 10,* 181-183.

United Nations Children's Fund. (2008). *The state of the world's children 2008.* New York: United Nations Children's Fund.

Van Bauwel, S. (2008). Media literacy and audiovisual languages: A case study from Belgium. *Educational Media International, 45,* 119-130.

Wade, T. D., Davidson, S., & O'Dea, J. (2003) A preliminary controlled evaluation of a school-based media literacy and self-esteem program for reducing eating disorder risk factors. *International Journal of Eating Disorders, 33,* 371-383.

Wallack, L., Dorfman, L., Jernigan, D., & Themba, M. (1993). *Media advocacy and public health: Power for prevention*. Thousand Oaks, CA: Sage.

Watson, R., & Vaughn, L. M. (2006). Limiting the effects of the media on body image: Does the length of a media literacy intervention make a difference? *Eating Disorders: The Journal of Treatment and Prevention, 14*, 385-400.

Wilksch, S. M., Durbridge, M. R., & Wade, T. D. (2008). A preliminary controlled comparison of programs designed to reduce risk of eating disorders targeting perfectionism and media literacy. *Journal of the American Academy of Child and Adolescent Psychiatry, 47*, 939-947.

Wilksch, S., & Wade, T. D. (2010). Reduction of shape and weight concern in adolescents: A 30-month controlled evaluation of a media literacy program. *Journal of the American Academy of Child and Adolescent Psychiatry, 48*, 652-661.

Willie, C. V., Ridini, S. P., & Willard, D. A. (Eds.). (2008). *Grassroots social action: Lessons in people power movements*. Lanham, MD: Rowman and Littlefield.

Women CEOs. (2010). *Fortune*. Online: http://money.cnn.com/magazines/fortune/fortune500/2010/womenceos/

Xu, R. (2010). Search engine of the Song Dynasty. *New York Times* (16 May).

Yamamiya, Y., Cash, T. F., Melnuk, S. E., Posavac, H. D., & Posavac, S. S. (2005). Women's exposure to thin-and-beautiful media images: Body image effects of media-ideal internalization and impact-reduction interventions. *Body Image, 2*, 74-80.

CHAPTER FIVE

Mass Media 2: Advocacy, Activism, and Social Change in the Digital Era: The Potential of Cyber-Action

Manuela Ferrari, *University of Toronto*

Never doubt that a small group of thoughtful, committed people can change the world.
Indeed it is the only thing that ever has.

— *Margaret Mead*

I remember what it was like to be a student radical without the help of the Internet, or even a fax machine, to try to drum up some support for a cause. As a teenager in the 1960s, I protested against the war in Vietnam. I defended a doctor who championed women's right to choose whether to have a child when they became pregnant. I criticized the Canadian government, then under Prime Minister Pierre Elliott Trudeau, when it sent troops into Quebec to round up hundreds of innocent people after terrorists kidnapped a British diplomat and a Quebec cabinet minister. I was an activist, '60s style…It was all about getting groups of people who really cared to tell other groups of people about your issues. It was all about word of mouth—but the word traveled at the speed of atoms, not bits.

—*Don Tapscott (2009)*

It might not be the first time for some of you to find Margaret Mead's quote at the beginning of an article or chapter related to advocacy and/or activism. I found this quote several times during my readings. I decided to open this chapter with Mead's words because, first, I truly believe in the power of people, even if just a few, to generate social change and, second,

I also believe that meaningful collaboration between people, enhanced by their ability to overcome differences in culture, status, generation, and/or knowledge, is the key to overcoming social inequity and promoting world changes. As described by Tapscott (2009), the way in which people have engaged in activism and advocacy has changed over time. The tools used by activists in the 1960s and 1970s were different from the ones currently available to people in the digital era. Activists in the present day still fight similar injustices and continue to engage in preserving human rights (e.g., the Vietnam War in the 1960s versus the recent war in Iraq; women's rights to education and to vote versus women's employment rights). However, the methods of organizing, communicating, and sharing the messages and tools used to gain political attention have changed (Fisher, 1998; Myers, 1994; Tapscott, 2009). In the digital era, traditional advocacy tools, such as sit-ins, demonstrations, and lobbying, have been integrated with new Internet-based tools (McNutt & Menon, 2008). The digital era, with the introduction of computers, the Internet, wireless networks, cellphones, and digital audio/video equipment, opened the doors to new forms of activism known as cyber-activism. Cyber-activism, or Internet activism, refers to the use of communication technologies such as email, websites, podcasts, and social networks to enable the faster dissemination of knowledge and resources to the public (McCaughey & Ayers, 2003; McNutt & Menon, 2008). Proper use of these technologies can enhance awareness in citizens and help them to organize, mobilize themselves, and take action or react to things that matter (McNutt & Menon, 2008; Myers, 1994).

The purpose of this chapter is to explore how cyber-activism can help advocacy and activism initiatives within the eating-related disorders field. I aim to answer several questions, such as: What are the new Internet-based tools available for modern activists? How do activists utilize Internet-based communication? How are the new advocacy tools different from traditional ones used to change social systems and policies? And, finally, can Internet activism help eating disorder activists to organize, plan, and take action? While this chapter will answer those questions, the ultimate goal is to provide the reader with a new perspective on cyber-activism. It will define new tools to disseminate information as well as dynamically share insights and viewpoints on an authentic and engaged model for activism and advocacy aimed at broad social change.

In the eating-related disorders field, advocacy can be used to reduce or control the incidence and prevalence of eating-related problems in the whole population, especially within its youngest members. Eating disorder prevention specialists are often engaged in advocacy initiatives, both at the practical and theoretical levels. Levine has identified and stressed the importance of differentiating between advocacy and activism in theory and practice (see Levine & Smolak, 2006). Indeed, he defines advocacy as "pro-active" behaviours, whereas he views activism as a "re-action" to negative and unhealthy messages with the aim of promoting more healthy messages (see Chapter 4 in this volume). Advocacy and activism are only two of the five A's identified by Levine to promote media literacy as a way of engaging the general public in being more critical and active consumers of media (Levin & Smolak, 2006). The other A's are *awareness,* the consciousness of advertising techniques used to promote specific beauty ideals, gender stereotypes, and the objectification and sexualization of women's bodies; *analysis,* the enhancement of critical thinking about media images, especially those that portray women's bodies as objects; and *access,* access to, and use of, the media to share prevention messages with the larger population. As already mentioned, *activism,* the actions taken towards the media, its images, and implicit and explicit messages regarding the objectification of women; and *advocacy,* the pro-active measures that involve using media to shape dominant social messages towards women's bodies, such as developing new generations of magazines capable of promoting a more positive culture of bodily experiences for women (Levine & Smolak, 2006).

Since activism is based on bringing people together to take action, or to react to things that are important to them, this chapter is directed towards multiple audiences including, but not limited to, research practitioners working in the eating disorders field, members of not-for-profit organizations (e.g., parents), and eating disorder activists. I hope that this chapter will inspire them to establish new partnerships and take action together. This chapter works to showcase youth partnerships aimed at both local and global actions (see TakingITGlobal), partnerships between youth and academic/researchers (see YouthVoices) as well as effective collaborations between youth and a not-for-profit organization (see World AIDS Campaign).[1] I intentionally chose to highlight different partnerships developed using new technologies in health-related fields (e.g., smoking, HIV, gambling, street youth, violence, and so on) that are based on collective attempts to take local or global action to promote social change. This chapter is a call to overcome generational and status barriers in the eating disorders field so that practitioners, researchers, parents, and youth will be able to work together to promote many of the initiatives described in this book (see Chapters 1, 3, & 4 in this volume) as well as foster gender body equity in today's society (see Chapters 7 & 8 in this volume).

Over time, technological advancements have created generational differences in peoples' opportunities and experiences with technology that

FIGURE 1: BABY BOOM GENERATION, GENERATION X, AND NET GENERATION

 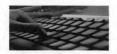 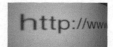

Baby Boom Generation (1946-64)	Generation X (1965-76)	Net Generation (1977-97)
The Baby Generation of children born after World War II (Foot, 1996, 1998) of traditional values (Tapscott, 2009). However, in Europe and North America, Boomers are also associated with traditional materialism as privilege, because many grew up in a time of affluence. This generation saw the diffusion of television in people's live; it is the first to experience war images through television (e.g., the Vietnam War) and, at the same time, to witness – and in same instances witness themselves participating in – street war protests initiated by college students and anti-war groups.	The Generation X (Foot, 1996, 1998) came of age after Vietnam, Generation X observed the end of the Cold War and witnessed the fall of the Berlin Wall; we grew up in times of no major war and relative economic stability. This generation is associated with strong beliefs and values such as the importance of personal relationships, altruism, and community (Tapscott, 2009). Generation X was the first to experience personal computers at home and, later, the Internet, along with new uses of older technologies like radio and television, and was the first to begin using mobile phones.	The Net Generation (Foot, 1996, 1998) experienced a less stable socioeconomic environment compared to Generation X. Indeed, this generation witnessed September 11th, school shootings (e.g., Columbine, Montreal massacre), the war in Iraq, and now the global economical crises. Members of the Net Generation are fully surrounded by digital technology. The majority of them own MP3 players (e.g., iPod), and they can surf the Internet all day, every day – sometimes even with their phone. Indeed, mobile phones are an integral part of their lifestyle. With their phones they not only talk but go online, text-message, and take photos and videos. They are civically aware and engaged in social activism (Tapscott, 1997, 2009).

strongly influence their way of thinking, communicating, and interacting. Many of the therapists and researchers currently working in the field of eating disorders and disordered eating are members of the so-called baby boom generation. However, the majority of the current target "audience" for eating-related disorder interventions belong to the net generation (see Chapter 4 in this volume). Figure 1 provides a short description of the three generations (e.g., the baby boom generation, generation X, and the net generation), along with a description of the different ways in which they grew up interacting with technology. As is evident, the net generation has a unique position and relationship with digital technologies. This generation is highly "connected," and they happily and flexibly utilize several social networking technologies such as Facebook, MySpace, Twitter, and TakeingITGlobal, which I will describe later (Tapscott, 1998, 2009). Members of this generation demand access to free knowledge and resources, they care about justice and freedom, they are civically aware, and, as other generations have done, they engage in social activism but do so in a different way (Tapscott, 1998, 2009).

The expansion of digital technologies has not only influenced the way in which generations live and communicate but also the way in which they share information, organize themselves, and engage in social actions. The net generation is the first real "global generation" that is growing and living with the Internet. Exploring how youth engage in cyber-activism and how they take action on issues that matter to them can help eating disorder researchers/practitioners, parents, and members of not-for-profit eating disorder organizations to see how popular Internet-based tools can be used for activism. And, most importantly, it will help us understand where and how to meet the net generation in order to engage them in meaningful and productive collaborations.

The significance of developing partnerships and collaboration between school staff, community agencies (e.g., public health), researchers, and, most importantly, youth to promote social change is very well established in the eating disorders prevention field (e.g., Girl Talk; Healthy Schools–Healthy Kids program; and the Sorority Body Image Program). Several sections of this book have already showcased these valuable collaborations (see Chapter 1 in this volume). One such example is the valuable collaboration between youth and eating disorder researchers that generated the Sorority Body Image Program (SBIP) (Becker, Bull, Schaumberg, Cauble, & Franco, 2008; Becker, Smith, & Ciao, 2005, 2006; Becker, Stice, Shaw, & Woda, 2009). The spontaneous partnership between Becker and the sorority groups, the largest self-governed female organizations within the Texas university campus, gave life to a new social movement in Texas universities aimed at helping sorority members to feel positive about their bodies, to react to social pressures for a thin body image, and to take a leadership role in this process of change by becoming peer facilitators of the program (Becker et al., 2009). The sororities endorsed Becker's original eating disorder intervention that was developed based on the Cognitive Dissonance Model (Stice, Chase, Stormer, & Appel, 2001) and decided to adapt it to meet the sororities' values and aims. One of the changes made by the sorority president was to emphasize the ability of sorority members to change social systems: "As the largest body of organized women on this campus, you have the power to create change" (Becker et al., 2009, p. 268). The SBIP was first implemented at Trinity University. It quickly gained national attention from other sororities and, since 2007-08, has expanded to a number of universities across the United States. This example illustrates the importance and benefit of meaningful partnerships between youth and researchers. Furthermore, it proves how the net generation has the ability to rapidly promote activism and produce social innovation. This chapter will provide more examples of the importance of overcoming silos of status, generation, and knowledge and of developing valuable collaborations to promote social change.

This chapter next addresses the rationale for using Web-based technologies as advocacy and activism tools within the eating-related disorders field. Subsequently, it provides a short overview of Internet-based applications for advocacy and activism to help readers familiarize themselves with terms and tools. As mentioned earlier, three different models of partnerships will be presented as examples of Internet-based activism—all of these collaborations draw from the work of the pedagogist and activist Paulo Freire (2000) and his self-reflective spiral of action. The first example is from TakingItGlobal, which showcases a youth global partnership that uses social networks to promote local and global social change. The second example is YouthVoice, a former TeenNet project, which portrays a partnership between youth and researchers from the University of Toronto though a participatory research project. They utilized different digital technologies (e.g., Internet, photo, video, and so on) to help youth participate in health promotion and community action. Finally, the World Aids Campaign, which showcased partnerships between not-for-profit organizations and youth through an e-course, was implemented to help youth use new technologies for social action. The chapter concludes with an examination of the implications and recommendations for future use of this type of advocacy.

The Cassandra Paradox: Are We Missing Something?

As mentioned in the beginning of this chapter, the development and expansion of the digital era has profoundly influenced the way in which practitioners and researchers working in the field of eating-related disorders are providing treatment, conducting research, sharing knowledge, maintaining relationships, and taking actions on issues that influence this field. In 2003, the *European Eating Disorders Review* dedicated a full edition to exploring the use of new technologies to prevent and treat eating disorders. This edition collected examples of experts in the field from all around the world who used computer technology as a treatment tool or support tool to work with eating disorder patients. The examples of technologies used ranged from email communications (Yager, 2003) and palm-top computers (Norton, Wonderlich, Myers, Mitchell, & Crosby, 2003) to telemedicine (Mitchell, Myers, Swan-Kremeier, & Wonderlich, 2003) and text messaging (Bauer, Percevic, Okon, Meermann, & Kordy, 2003). This special edition of the *European Eating Disorders Review* summarized the current knowledge on the use of new technologies for the treatment of eating disorders, by saying: "Granted, a good computer program may be more helpful for patients than a bad therapist. However, a good therapist may facilitate the use of a technology-based treatment in such a way that it enables patients to explore previously uncharted territories" (Schmidt, 2003, p. 152). Thus, presently in the eating-related disorders field, attention has been devoted to exploring the efficacy and effectiveness of new technologies in addressing treatment (Mitchell et al., 2003; Yager, 2003) and prevention (Bruning-Brown, Winzelberg, Abascal, & Taylor, 2004; Low et al., 2006; McVey, Gusella, Tweed, & Ferrari, 2009; Taylor, Bryson, Luce, Cunning, & Celio, 2006; Zabinski, Celio, Jacobs, Manwaring, & Wilfley, 2003). However, not enough attention has been paid to exploring the potential of new technologies and its effect on advocacy, activism, and social change. Could it be that new technologies can not only open the doors to new treatment models by better helping clients to explore new territories but also help to promote activist and advocacy initiatives in this area?

In the *Iliad*, Cassandra, the daughter of the king of Troy, advised her fellow Trojans that the Greeks were hiding inside the wooden horse. No one trusted her or believed her warning. The huge wooden horse was right there in front of the Trojans. It was very visible to them and, as such, the attack by the Greeks' was predictable, but the Trojans ignored the warning and what their eyes could see. Hence, a Cassandra paradox occurs when the most obvious possibilities may be ignored or dismissed precisely because they are so obvious. Are we experiencing the Cassandra paradox by ignoring the potential of Internet advocacy?

Many of us use the Internet regularly for both personal and/or work-related reasons. Many people spend several hours of the day surfing the World Wide Web, attending Web conferences/meetings, emailing, watching videos/television, and even shopping online. For the first time in human history, people are able to share knowledge and interact with each other across the world in a rapid and often, but not always, effective manner. Time and space boundaries are beginning to seem antiquated. At the

TABLE 1: CHARACTERISTICS OF INDIVIDUALS USING THE INTERNET

	Any location[a]		
	2005	2007	2009
	Percentage of individuals[b]		
All Internet users	67.9	73.2	80.3
Age			
34 years and under	88.9	93.1	96.5
35-54 years	75.0	79.8	87.8
55-64 years	53.8	60.8	71.1
65 years and over	23.8	28.8	40.7

Notes:

a Internet access from any location includes use from home, school, work, public library, or other and counts an individual only once, regardless of use from multiple locations.

b Percentage of individuals who have used the Internet for personal, non-business reasons in the past twelve months. The target population for the Canadian Internet Use Survey has changed from individuals eighteen years of age and older in 2005 to sixteen years of age and older in 2007.

Source: Statistics Canada (2010).

beginning of the nineteenth century, an optical telegraph could wirelessly transmit a short message from Amsterdam to Venice (1,345 kilometres) in an hour's time. During the second half of the twentieth century, the availability of computers and the Internet has allowed the general public to transmit texts and images around the globe in only a few seconds.

The Internet has entered the life of approximately 29% of the world's population. At the end of 2010, 77.4% of people in North America were using the Internet, along with 61.3% of the population in Oceania/Australia, 58.4% in Europe, and 34.5% in South America/Caribbean (Internet World Stats, 2009). The explosive growth in the number of Internet users is evident in the rapid development of the Internet between 2000 and 2010 in new areas such as Africa (2,357%) and the Middle East (1,825%) — 444% worldwide (Internet World Stats, 2010). Table 1 shows Canadian Internet usage broken down by age. Even after controlling for factors such as educational attainment and household income, age remains a significant and substantive predictor of Internet use.

I argue that there are two main reasons for using new technologies for advocacy and activism within the field of eating disorder and eating-related disorders: (1) the Internet, as a new media, can contribute to the development of eating disorder problems (see Bardone-Cone & Cass, 2007; Tiggemann, 2010), and (2) eating disorders and disordered eating are fast becoming global issues and a more active global collaboration among researchers and practitioner is needed (Treasure, Schmidt, & van Furth, 2003). We need to remind ourselves that our "target" population—or, as I prefer to think, our partners in social change—is "living" online. The Internet can be a beneficial as well as a harmful medium to them, and this is something that we cannot afford to ignore.

Expanding on my first point, the Internet and other digital technologies are a new form of media that, together with traditional media such as magazines and television, are identified as risk factors for the development of body dissatisfaction and disordered eating (see Chapters 4 & 6 in this volume). Exposure to images on the Internet can help promote body dissatisfaction in young women. This subject is still understudied at the moment (Tiggemann, 2008), but preliminary work conducted by Tiggemann (2010) shows how Internet exposure (as well as fashion magazines) among high-school girls was found to correlate with the internalization of the ideal of being thin and a drive for thinness.

In more extreme cases, the Internet can encourage unhealthy weight-control behaviours and strategies through various websites, such as pro-ana/pro-mia websites, which promote anorexia nervosa and bulimia nervosa as lifestyle choices rather than eating disorders. Empirical knowledge is now available to show how exposure to pro-anorexia websites has a negative effect on female viewers. Undergraduate students who were experimentally exposed to the pro-anorexia websites over time found themselves concerned about their weight, perceived themselves as being heavier, and engaged in more body image comparison (Bardone-Cone & Cass, 2007). Still, although the Internet can have a negative impact, it can also help to promote awareness of disordered eating issues within the public and enable social action.

As a follow-up to my second argument, eating disorders and eating-related disorders are assuming global characteristics. Clinicians and practitioners are seeing eating disorder cases all around the world, especially in non-Western countries (Becker, 2004; Becker, Fay, Gilman, & Striegel-Moore, 2007; Treasure, Schmidt, & van Furth, 2003). As a result, it has become critical for clinicians and researchers to share technical and experiential knowledge. At the clinical level, therapists are now seeking recommendations on "best practices" in treatment by participating in list-serve discussions via special Internet-based networks formed by the Academy for Eating Disorders' Special Interest Groups on Assessment and Diagnosis and Inpatient/Residential Treatment. Furthermore, therapists are looking for follow-up care for clients after treatment by contacting the Academy for Eating Disorders' members via its email list. At the research level, the number of international research collaborations is rapidly increasing, and digital technologies are now a vital way for eating disorder research teams to communicate effectively and rapidly, despite the vast distances between them. The value of new technologies, such as email, in media literacy and activism campaigns is well described in Chapter 4 of this book. Digital technologies can help members of the eating-related disorder field to share information and organize themselves over a wider geographic range, often engaging with people who cannot physically attend meetings or be reached through a door-to-door campaign.

As mentioned, digital technologies are now integral parts of our private, interpersonal/social, and work-related lives. The Internet is rapidly growing as a result of the increased number of users populating and constantly recreating this cyber-environment. The Internet is also helping create new forms of social community. By its nature, the Internet is a communication network. It is an ideal environment for social movements, as it allows for the development of groups of similar or diverse individuals to share common ideology and social goals.

Overview of New Internet-Based Advocacy Tools

Social movement activists have long engaged with, and depended on, the successful use of technology, such as mass media, to disseminate their message to potential members of the movement (Myers, 1994). As McCaughey and Ayers (2003) state: "Technology is hardly new to activists. Social-movement groups have historically incorporated new technologies into their social change struggle. Whether newspaper, radio, TV, or film, activists have embraced new communications media to circulate information, make statements, raise consciousness, raise hell" (p. 4).

Often activists have to resort to radical behaviours to get media attention and then, with little or no control over it, need to rely on television networks and other media (e.g., newspapers) to disseminate the message (McNutt & Menon, 2008; Myers, 1994). Indeed, the mass media involve one-way communication, whereas the Internet provides individuals with great communicative power and much more control (McNutt & Menon, 2008; Myers, 1994). Social networks, including MySpace, Facebook, Twitter, Blogger, YouTube, Yahoo, and Flicker have the ability to reach people located in different geographical areas, and they also allow people to retrieve, return, react to, and share communications. In summary, Internet-based tools offer opportunities for clarification and solicitation of an agreement on the plans of action. Furthermore, activists can access and use Internet-based tools with minimal technical skills when compared to other technologies, such as television or radio broadcasting (McNutt & Menon, 2008; Myers, 1994).

Before the advent of the Internet, especially since Web 2.0, citizens were generally limited, in terms of their access to news, by what was available through their local/national media news. In order to express themselves politically, people used to call or write directly to local officials and to the offices of politicians and/or send letters to newspapers with no guarantee that the letter(s) would be published or shared with the public (Myers, 1994). Now, not only can people search online for information from mainstream sources related to social and political issues,[2] but they can also use the Internet to find out what other citizens think and to correspond with them (Schellenberg, 2004; Veenhof, Wellman, Quell, & Hogan, 2008).[3] Indeed, the Internet is both an alternative source of mainstream information as well as a place where people outside of the mainstream institutions can share and discuss political ideas. Once again, members of the net generation have tended to be most active in terms of reading and discussing political issues with others (Veenhof et al., 2008).

Without a doubt, the growth of Web 2.0, defined as the use of Web-based collaborative technologies, has had a powerful influence on the use of technology for advocacy. The "old Web" was about reading and sharing content/information, whereas Web 2.0 is about creating and contributing to information. Internet users have moved from a position of observer to a position of active user and content creator. Furthermore, Web 2.0 is democratic and transparent by nature; all users potentially have a voice on the Internet. Activists, or simply the general public, who desire to express their opinions, simply need to post it; other online users are able to find, read, and respond to it when desired. Figure 2 provides a description of three categories of different Internet-based tools: those that enhance awareness; those that promote discussion, planning, and mobilization for action; and those that allow action and reaction to social issues. As illustrated in Figure 3, although new technologies have been used for advocacy and activist purposes within the eating disorders field, they do not always fall so clearly into one of these three categories. It is important to realize that the categories are not rigid and that tools can be used for multiple purposes (e.g., an email can be used to share knowledge and to take action). Let us now explore how youth have used Web 2.0, particularly for the purpose of social networking to promote activism.

FIGURE 2: INTERNET-BASED TOOLS

Internet-based tools that enhance awareness and reflection: Information sharing and distribution is the first major step in promoting citizen awareness of special issues. Information, from general knowledge to advanced research data, is important to activate passion and motivation, encourage critical thinking, influence public health policy, and mobilize social groups. Internet technologies allow fast and easy access to information for both general users (e.g., email, newsgroups, Google, Wikipedia, etc.), practitioners, and researchers (e.g., listserv, discussion group, electronic peer-reviewed journals).

- Email and newsgroups, and related technologies such as discussion groups and groupware, constituted the first and easiest use of technology in activism (McNutt & Menon, 2008).
- Websites are useful for educational and informational purposes, but less useful for recruiting because users have to actively decide to visit the website (McNutt & Menon, 2008), even if it "pops up" first or second on a search engine.
- Electronic journals and research engines have dramatically changed how students, researchers, and policy-makers are able to access and disseminate information. Electronic journals are scholarly periodicals available via the Internet and on computers, rather than in paper format. The majority of electronic journals are subscription-based or require pay-per-view access. However, "open access journals," a new form of electronic journal accessible via the Internet without making a payment, are rapidly developing. Many students and faculty are able to access electronic journals through university subscriptions, but it is also possible for individuals to subscribe.

Internet-based tools that promote discussion and planning actions (e.g., social organization mobilization): Digital technologies can help mobilization in three different ways: (1) help coordinate meetings, lobbies, and other offline activities via emails or Web postings; (2) assist in initiating online meetings and actions as a substitute for the offline activities— as mentioned earlier, the Internet can help maximize an organization's time and resources; (3) facilitate organization and mobilizations possible only online, as in the case of large geographical separations or the dissemination of sensitive information that needs to be shared with a large group in a very short period of time.

- A Wiki is a web page or collection of pages designed to enable users to contribute to or modify the content in a simple way, without requiring specific knowledge of Internet coding. Wikipedia is probably the best-known example of a wiki. Wikis are often used to create collaborative websites and to power community websites. Wikis can be incorporated into a larger website to enhance its interactivity and the quality of the content. Examples of these groups include email, calendaring, text chat and wiki and social software such as social networks like MySpace, Second Life, and Facebook. These tools are very successful bringing people together and maintaining a community, as well as planning and coordinating action.
- Blogs, or weblogs, are websites, usually maintained by an individual or organization, that provide users with commentary, descriptions of events, or other material such as graphics or video. Blogs are another example of "one-to-many communication" tools because they allow the blog visitors to respond and/or comment to the blog.
- Podcasting, the downloading of audio or visual information, is also a product of Web 2.0 technology.

Internet-based tools that allow action and reaction to social issues: The word "activism" is based on action (or re-action) toward something that concerns a group of people. Traditional activist behaviors, such as door-to-door campaigns, sit-ins, demonstrations, and lobbying can, as mentioned, be coordinated online, but can also take place entirely online. Other online actions, such as hacking, can be considered extreme activism, straddling the line between legal and illegal action.

- Internet petitions, such as those on www.petition.com, are a form of petition posted on a website. Visitors to the petition website can add their email addresses or names, and after enough "signatures" have been collected, the resulting letter may be delivered to the subject of the petition, usually via email. The use of Internet petitions is not without controversy. Internet petitions are easy to set up and can generate many signatures in very little time. However, Web petitions cannot fully control the legitimacy of the people who electronically sign it; as a result, invalid signatures can jeopardize the petition. Furthermore, the efficacy of Web petitions directed to a government agency has not been fully explored

- Hacktivism, defined as activism through hack action, is "the nonviolent use of illegal or legally ambiguous digital tools in pursuit of political ends. These tools include website defacements, redirects, denial-of-service attacks, information theft, website parodies, virtual sit-ins, virtual sabotage, and software development (Samuel, 2004, p. iii)." It is often understood as the writing of code to promote political ideology: such as expressive politics, free speech, human rights, or information ethics. Acts of hacktivism are carried out in the belief that proper use of code will have leveraged effects similar to regular activism or civil disobedience. Fewer people can write code, but code on the Internet affects many. Internet hacking is at best controversial, as it is often an illegal, malicious, and destructive act that jeopardizes the security of the Internet. However, for those belonging to the hacktivist movement, cyber-attacks, even illegal ones, are an acceptable form of direct action. By its nature, hacktivism seems more relevant and visible within Web-based, political, or economic topics (e.g., privacy, Internet issues, human-rights issues) and less within the eating-related issues community.

- A virtual sit-in is a form of "electronic civil disobedience." Virtual sit-ins are considered a form of legal hacktivism that interferes with normal functioning or accessibility of a targeted website. During a virtual sit-in, hundreds of activists concurrently and continually try to access a target website. If the virtual sit-in action is run properly, this action will cause the website to run slowly or even collapse entirely, preventing anyone else from accessing it. Many of you may be familiar with the shutdown of a grant agency website on the last day of the grant submission period – without knowing it, by logging on all at once, you have helped to create the same outcome as a virtual sit-in! Virtual sit-ins are considered legal because users are simply visiting a website; it is the least controversial form of hacktivism.

FIGURE 3: ADVOCACY AND ACTIVIST IN THE EATING DISORDERS FIELD

Activism

- Email: The ease of forwarding messages and sending the same message to multiple sites can result in a tremendous diffusion of information in an extremely short period of time. In late 1992, Mattel released a new Barbie doll called Teen Talk Barbie. These dolls were programmed to say different things that were related to being a teenage woman. One sentence spouted by the teen Barbie was "Math class is tough." Recognizing that this message reinforced the prevailing socialization of young women to fear math and to feel unable to perform mathematical tasks, an association of women scholars mounted a campaign to get Barbie to stop saying "Math class is tough." Part of this attempt was an email message sent to female academics explaining the situation, urging action, and providing names and addresses of the Mattel headquarters. The result of the Barbie campaign was a promise by Mattel to replace dolls that spoke the words and to volunteer Barbie for pro-math advertising. Similarly, as mentioned in Levine and Kelly's chapter, an email was sent by Dads & Daughters to the CEO of Sun-In, a hair-bleaching product, to protest the use of disturbing advertising. A simple email with powerful and insightful content was enough to persuade the CEO to discontinue the advertising.
- Websites are useful for educational purposes as well as to provide users with action orinted tools. For example, the Eating Disorders Coalition for Research, Policy, and Action (http://www.eatingdisorderscoalition.org/index.htm) aims "to advance the federal recognition of eating disorders as a public health priority." One of their goals is to "mobilize concerned citizens to advocate on behalf of people with eating disorders, their families, and professionals working with these populations." To do so, they make effective use of the Internet and its technology. The Eating Disorders Coalition's website provides information on how to contact a member on the House of Representatives and how to write a letter to the editor (www.eatingdisorderscoalition. org/take-action.htm). Also, the site provides information on upcoming events such as "Lobby Day". Furthermore, websites can also be used to conduct online petition drives (e.g., www.petition.com) to collect data through Web surveys (e.g., www.surveymonkey.com), and to organize demonstrations and other political actions.
- Internet petitions are a form of petition posted on a website. In Oct. 16, 2009, Quebec Minister Christine St-Pierre, the minister responsible for culture, communications and the status of women, introduced to *La charte québécoise pour une image corporelle saine et diversifiée,* or Quebec charter for an healthy and diverse body image, a first agreement between the government body and the Quebec's fashion industry to promote a healthier image of women within campaign and initiatives. The charter was developed by fashion and media industries and the government; it calls for a change in mentality about the image portrayed in the media. The charter includes seven avenues for action, with pledges to promote a healthy diversity of body images, including different heights, proportions and ages; discourage excessive weight-control practices or appearance modification; and act as agents of change to promote healthy eating and weight-control practices and realistic body images. The province of Quebec invites everyone in Quebec to sign an online petition to support the charter (http://www.jesigneenligne.com). People can also share and/or sign the petition using Facebook and Twitter.

Advocacy

- Web 2.0 technology allows the development of wiki, a web page or collection of pages designed to enable users to contribute to or modify the content in a simple way, without requiring specific knowledge of Internet coding. For example, About-Face is an organization that is based in San Francisco but active all around the world via the Internet; it aims to provide "women and girls with tools to understand and resist harmful media messages that affect their self-esteem and body image." About-Face offers "action media-literacy workshops" but also, thanks to Web 2.0 technology, enables women and girls to act on media images via the Internet. The About-Face website shows the top 10 most recent ads that promote positive images of women, as well as the top 10 that sexualize or objectify women's bodies; this is called the "gallery of offenders." Within the "gallery of offenders," viewers are provided with information on how to critically analyze the ads and are given easy access to the company's email to send a complaint. Also, the About-Face website helps support off-site actions and protests. For example, disgusted by a new Fox show called "The Swan," which "depicts normal-looking women entering a beauty pageant against each other, after having extensive cosmetic surgery, doing brutal workouts, and going on very restrictive diets," About-Face decided to send collected signatures to Fox Television's chairwoman, Gail Berman; more than 500 letters were signed by women, girls, fathers, boyfriends, husbands, and brothers.

Social Network for Social Change: TakingITGlobal

Many of you may be familiar with social networks such as Facebook and MySpace, but you may be less familiar with TakingITGlobal. In 1999, Michael Furdyk and Jennifer Corriero, who were 17 and 19 at the time, envisioned an online space where youth could work together with other youth around the word to promote social innovation. This idea soon became known as TakingITGlobal.[4] TakingITGlobal provides youth between the ages of 13 and 30 with a global online social network and hub for civic participation; content and tools for educators to facilitate rich, interactive learning experiences; outreach and collaboration tools for events, networks, campaigns, and causes; and research, development, and sharing of best practices on youth engagement. TakingITGlobal aims to be a Web platform to provide youth with access to global opportunities, cross-cultural connections, and meaningful participation in decision-making.

To date, TakingITGlobal has more than 290,000 members. Four million young people were reached in 2008, and over 14 million since its launch in 2000. Knowledge and discourses are shared across 12 languages and across more than 200 countries. Over time, TakingITGlobal has developed partnerships with UN agencies, dozens of international civil society organizations, several top-tier technology companies (Google, Microsoft,

Adobe, Cisco, Hewlett Packard), and leading-edge foundations in North America (e.g., the Trillium Foundation, the Walter and Duncan Gordon Foundation, and the UN Foundation). TakingITGlobal is supported by a board of directors and advisory committees composed of community and academic institutions.

TakingITGlobal has seven defined areas for youth engagement: media (sub-issues include creative commons and freedom of expression); peace and conflict (sub-issues include arms control, genocide, and youth violence); health diseases (sub-issues include HIV/AIDS, maternal health and child mortality, mental health, sexuality, sports, and substance abuse); environment (sub-issues include animal rights, climate change, natural disasters, and sustainable development); human rights (sub-issues include child and youth rights, gender equality, lesbian, gay, bisexual, and transgender rights, and refugee rights); technology (sub-issues include digital citizenship, digital divide, and digital literacy); education (sub-issues include educational technology, global education, informal/experiential learning, and literacy), globalization (sub-issues include child labour, corporate social responsibility, food security, labour rights, migration, and poverty); and culture (sub-issues include global citizenship and language).

TakingITGlobal broadly connects people to the issues that matter to them by providing them with online resources, tools, and opportunities for collaboration that can be used to make a positive and stable impact in communities all over the world. The global issue pages provide an interactive opportunity for TakingITGlobal's members to generate their own content through the group blogs, discussion boards, petitions, and online events. Members can also share their commitments with others. Furthermore, the global issue pages are all wiki pages, which allow members to contribute their knowledge on specific issues.

For example, to learn more about women's rights, members can "virtually visit" the Women's Art Gallery.[5] This gallery explores women's issues as well as showcases female artists' work from all around the world. Women's rights issues are organized into six themes: language, bodies, global inequalities, feminism, work, and resisting violence. Every theme contains artwork, photographs, and other objects revealing information on the subject. The Women's Art Gallery celebrates women who devote their lives to what they are passionate about—whether it is art, labour rights, sustainable development, violence awareness, or feminism. The following quotation is a sample of the content provided in the theme about "bodies":

> Women's bodies are frequently the site of controversial discussions regarding sexuality and autonomy. Women's bodies are at once sexualized, used to sell goods (advertising, fashion pornography), or they are "protected" to

maintain honour and duty to a belief system. Through their bodies, women are usually reduced to simple equations—good girls and bad girls—both impossible stereotypes.

The virtual visitor can admire the artwork of Georgia O'Keefe, the Venus of Willendorf, and Pan Yuliang's self-portrait. They can read a poem by Adrienne Rich and learn more about her poetry and how over the years her work has become one of the most "provocative voices" on the politics of sexuality, race, language, power, and women's culture. Finally, they can also admire a photo of Simone de Beauvoir, a French philosopher and novelist, who was concerned with women's right to abortion and the broad social status of women. Visitors also have access to supplementary resources (e.g., books, articles, websites, and so on). After visiting the gallery, TakingITGlobal's members are invited to take action by joining the discussion boards on the topics of women and violence, language, work, health and sexuality, global inequalities, and feminism, and they are also encouraged to start their own thread on the discussion boards. Members can also express themselves by submitting their artwork (e.g., pictures, drawings, videos, paintings, and so on) to the Welcome to the TakingIT-Global Global Gallery, which showcases youth perspectives on human rights and environmental issues through art. Global Gallery is an excellent example of youth advocacy, where youth actively generate new media images that better represent their value, vision, and hope.

TakingITGlobal's members base their social action initiative on the following steps: (1) reflect and get inspired, (2) identify and get informed, (3) lead and get others involved, (4) get connected, (5) plan and get moving, and (6) have a lasting impact. They have access to action tools to help them create a petition, make a commitment for a better world, or use one of TakingITGlobal's action guides to learn how to start a community project on a global issue of their choice. TakingITGlobal's action guide is available in six languages (English, French, Portuguese, Russian, Chinese, and Arabic).

Among the several initiatives and social actions promoted by TakingIT-Global's members, this active social community was able to inspire its teachers to work together to promote social change. In 2006, the TakingITGlobal for Educators (TIGed) was launched. This new section of TakingITGlobal allows teachers to bring global perspectives into the classroom in ways that meet the needs of their learning environments. The ultimate goal is to empower students to think and act as world citizens. TIGed uses technology, especially Web 2.0 tools (e.g., blogs, podcasts, maps, digital image galleries, discussion boards, live video chat, online file space, and so on), to make it easier for teachers to connect, share ideas, and work together. At the same time, it allows students to use collaborative technology in order to connect with other youths from around the world and learn about global issues.

In order to join the TIGed community, TakingITGlobal members who are actively engaged as educators in their community need to apply for an "educator badge." This badge allows users to search the member database for educators so they can identify potential colleagues, partners, and "allies." Teachers also have access to a collaboration database to develop partnerships with other classrooms around the world. The TIGed blogs and newsletters help teachers to stay up to date on developments and events related to the TIGed community. The discussion forum allows educators to share successes, challenges, strategies, and ideas with respect to integrating technology and global perspectives into education. In order to help the teacher get familiarized with TIGed environment and enhance both digital literacy and global citizenship literacy, teachers are provided with a guide to "best practices in global education and collaborative technologies," which showcases the different ways in which teachers around the world are utilizing TIGed.[6] Furthermore, teachers can link their TIGed course to curriculum benchmarks, using the *Mid-Continent Research for Education and Learning Compendium* of kindergarten to Grade 12 standards. TakingITGlobal recognizes both the power and the danger inherent in social and collaborative uses of the Internet, as a result TIGed offers teachers the ability to create and manage private, advertising-free virtual classrooms, through which students can take advantage of the benefits of Web 2.0 tools without sacrificing their security.

TakingITGlobal has many more rich, engaging, and interactive examples than what I have described so far. After a few minutes on their site, readers will find many inspiring works by youth. According to Westley, Zimmerman, and Patton (2006), social innovation and changes are like a "flow." Sometimes you may be the one to initiate the process and at other times "the flow is taking you": "Social innovation is as much about letting go as it is about taking control. Effective social innovators know how to let it find them—how to recognize and ride social flow, trusting that the world will provide if we are open to it" (p. 155). To be open to social change, we need to remind ourselves to listen and reflect—listen to youth voices and reflect together to find new directions, learn from each other, and plan new action together.

YouthVoices

YouthVoices, a former TeenNet Research Program, was developed through the collaboration between the Department of Public Health Sciences at the University of Toronto, presently known as Dalla Lana School of Public

Health, 57 young people, and five community partners (e.g., the Canada International Scientific Exchange Program, the St. Stephan's Community House, the Davenport Perth Neighbourhood Centre, the Young Men's Christian Association's [YMCA] Youth Gambling Awareness Program) (see Chen, Poland, & Skinner, 2007; Ridgley, Maley, & Skinner, 2004; Skinner, 2002). Founded by Dr. Harvey Skinner in 1995, TeenNet has pioneered the use of Internet-based technology to engage youth in health promotion and community action. The TeenNet team collaborates locally and internationally to involve young people from diverse backgrounds in community health issue identification (e.g., smoking, gambling, poverty, homelessness, betrayal, racism, and so on), community action (e.g., developing a website, video, and interactive workshop on the globalization of tobacco), and learning resource development that includes websites, videos, songs, photo exhibitions, and youth activism manuals (Morrision, Lombardo, Biscope, & Skinner, 2005; Ridgley et al., 2005; Skinner & Biscope, 2005).[7]

Several e-Health promotion projects and applications have been developed without an explicit model to guide the design, evaluation, and ongoing improvement of the program. To overcome this lack of knowledge in the field and generate new theoretical knowledge, the YouthVoice team has developed the Spiral Technology Action Research (STAR) Model (see Skinner, Maley, & Norman, 2006). This model was developed based on the team's practical experiences with creating a youth health promotion website called CyberIsle, which was the result of a series of collaborations between TeenNet's community partners and youth.[8] The model comprises five principles (participatory, relevance, active learning, autonomy supporting, and access) that bring together continuous awareness, community involvement, and technological development (Skinner et al., 2006).[9] The STAR model not only incorporates behaviour change strategies (e.g., self-determination theory, social cognitive theory, and the Trans-Theoretical Model), but it also emphasizes the need to organize and build capacity for community well-being and action. Indeed, community organization and action research methods are used to continuously build knowledge and provide feedback to encourage improvement, learning, and capacity building.

Launched in 1996, when there were only 11,000 websites across the world, CyberIsle is a teens-only island that takes a holistic approach to teen health. Ongoing dialogue and collaboration between the TeenNet's community partners generated the idea of establishing a smoking-specific website using CyberIsle called the Smoking Zine, which aims to prevent youth non-smokers from starting to smoke (i.e., to increase resistance self-efficacy) and assist youth smokers to stop or cut down their cigarette use (action self-efficacy). The program offers information, self-assessment tools, and guided self-change. Furthermore, youth have the opportunity to connect with other youth as well, which yields the opportunity to receive social support around smoking and/or coping skills and action planning for resisting cigarette use. A series of interactive games and quizzes and an online bulletin board are used within five distinct, tailored stages to deliver the intervention to the youth.

As mentioned earlier, the YouthVoice team's practical knowledge generated a theoretical framework that serves to inform future programs (e.g., the STAR Model) and the E-Health Literacy Model (see Norman & Skinner, 2006). Furthermore, the team has carefully assessed their work though outcome evaluation (e.g., Norman, Maley, Li, & Skinner, 2008) and process evaluation (e.g., Norman & Skinner, 2007), using both qualitative and quantitative methodologies. For example, once the first prototype of the Smoking Zine site was launched, pilot evaluation determined the appropriateness and feasibility of conducting a future systematic evaluation. A small, randomized trial was conducted (n = 118) at 15 diverse settings (e.g., shopping malls, youth centres, public libraries, and youth employment centres in urban, suburban, and rural settings) throughout the province of Ontario (Norman, Maley, Li, & Skinner, 2008). Youth (ages 12 to 19 years) were randomly assigned to complete the Smoking Zine or a guided Web-surfing task. Data were compared to determine the effects of any short-term shifts in the measured variables on tobacco use. Additional data were collected from youth who completed the Smoking Zine through a short, one-page qualitative feedback form.

The promising results of the pilot trial encouraged the development of a larger-scale randomized trial conducted in 14 Toronto-area high schools. This randomized trial was done in partnership with Toronto Public Health. A total of 1,402 students in Grades 9, 10, and 11 were randomly assigned to complete either the Smoking Zine or a control website program. Results of the study indicated that the Smoking Zine had more influence in terms of reducing smoking-related intentions and smoking behaviour with boys than girls and among students in Grade 10 versus the other grades—data were collected following the intervention and at 3-month and 6-month follow-ups. The findings from the randomized trial suggest that the Smoking Zine significantly influenced students' behavioural intentions to smoke and consume cigarettes. In 2003, the Smoking Zine was simplified and adapted into the traditional Chinese language in collaboration with the Shanghai Center for Disease Control. This was then used for smoking prevention with youth in China as well as with recent immigrants to Canada. Similar work is under way in the Portuguese and Spanish languages, where the Smoking Zine is being adapted for youth smoking prevention in South

America (Brazil, Argentina, and Chile), and in Arabic/Hebrew/Farsi languages for use in the Middle East.

The STAR Model was also used to develop YouthBet.net, a multimedia website based on public health theories, such as health promotion, harm reduction, and problem prevention, aimed at preventing gambling problems among youth (Korn, Murray, Morrison, Reynolds, & Skinner, 2006).[10] Similar to the Smoking Zine, YouthBet.net is part of CyberIsle and features games, information, and help resources to protect youth from gambling-related harm. YouthBet.net was designed by youth for youth! A youth working group worked for several months to design the look and feel of the site to ensure that it would appeal to youth ages 10 though 19.

The site provides information on the gambling industry and gambling statistics. This information was intended to help youth gain a better understanding of gambling phenomena and related issues. Furthermore, the site's "tool kit" provides games and interactive activities for youth on time management, money management, general risk perception, decision-making skills, odds/randomness and probability, gambling self-assessment, and minimizing negative consequences. Mirroring the YouthBet.net content, a website for parents was developed to increase parents' awareness on youth gambling.

Usability testing of the site was implemented with 34 youths. Participants had no difficulties navigating the site, finding content, and playing games. Youth participants indicated that they liked the interactive manner in which gambling information was presented via realistic games and quizzes. The youth also commented that they would return to the site and would recommend it to a friend if they were having a problem with gambling. Additionally, the youth indicated that YouthBet.net would be a fun and educational tool to be used by teachers in the classroom. YouthBet.net is, at present, one of the most comprehensive websites designed for youth gambling.

The YouthVoice team's work has been disseminated through traditional academic channels (e.g., conferences, books, and peer-review journals) as well as through new academic frontiers, such as open access journals and online documentary videos. The members of the YouthVoice team strongly believe that open access, which is defined as digital/online literature free of charge and free of most copyright and licensing restrictions, is a more effective medium to reach a large audience, especially policy-makers. A few theoretical papers, such as the E-Health Literacy Model, were published in the *Journal of Medical Internet Research*, which is a leading open-access peer-reviewed trans-disciplinary journal on health and health care in the Internet age (Norman & Skinner, 2006). This principle of access to knowledge is supported by evidence from literature showing that open-access publishing can reach more readers than subscription-access publishing (Davis, Lewenstein, Simon, Booth, & Connolly, 2008; Douw, Vondeling, Eskildsen, Simpson, 2003; Eysenbach, 2006a, 2006b).

In a randomized controlled trial of 11 published journals (a total of 1,619 research articles and reviews) aimed at assessing article readership (measured as downloads of full text, PDFs, and abstracts) and a number of unique visitors (Internet protocol addresses), it was found that open access was associated with 89% more full-text downloads, 42% more PDF downloads (32% to 52%), and 23% more unique visitors (16% to 30%) (Davis et al., 2008). However, open-access articles were no more likely to be cited than subscription-access articles in the first year after publication. In total, 59% of open-access articles were cited 9 to 12 months after publication in comparison to 63% of subscription-access articles (Davis et al., 2008).

On the other hand, other media for knowledge sharing, such as Youth-Voice video/documentary, may be more suitable in capturing the attention of youth. "Deal Me In" is a documentary developed entirely by youth to show how gambling behaviours can impact people at multiple levels. The idea of using a documentary generated by youth to increase awareness on gambling was conceived during an "anon conference," a non-structured gathering between researchers, members of community organizations, and youth to freely and openly discuss a topic. The youth who attended the meeting brought forward the idea of developing a documentary that could be disseminated though YouTube. YouthVoice researcher team members and community members from the YMCA's Youth Gambling Awareness Program developed a proposal for the Ministry of Health Promotion and were able to ensure funding for a 2-year project. A working group of six youth, called "youth directors," developed the content/script, shot the documentary, and edited the material to produce "Deal Me In," which is now available on YouTube.[11]

As this section shows, many interesting and powerful projects can be generated when researchers, members of community organizations, and youth start to work together. I would like to highlight three key aspects of this meaningful collaboration. First, it is the need to adopt and/or develop a theoretical model/framework to guide the partnership/collaborations between members. YouthVoices used the STAR Model as well as the TakingITGlobal's members' guide. Their social action initiative used similar steps (reflect/listening, dialogue, and action). It is extremely important that researches take time to meet and collaborate with youth and, most importantly, listen and understand their perspectives and needs. The outcomes of these discussions are then clarified and negotiated through ongoing and open dialogue before any specific action plans are initiated. This framework is not unknown within the eating disorder prevention field. Using critical social/feminist theories, the Healthy School Model, and Freire's (2000) dialogism, Piran (1998, 1999a, 1999b, 2001) helped students to engage in ongoing dialogue to "create system changes" within Canada's National Ballet School and then to establish a school environment where children, especially girls, can feel safe and good about their own body shape, including a positive experience of the body changes that occur during puberty.

Second, it is important to continue evaluating the work done through initiatives in order to inform future directions. Within social action and innovation initiatives, ongoing evaluation helps to ensure meaningful sustainability of actions, to identify new directions, and to prevent possible harm. Sustained evaluation also means that the end of one social action initiative can lead to the beginning of another, as in the case of the Youth-Bet.net project, which led to the development of the "Deal Me In" documentary. New forms of knowledge dissemination, such as documentaries and/or open-access journals, should be considered to increase the awareness of both the general public and policy-makers on eating disorder issues.

World AIDS Campaign

Sometimes, eating disorder prevention practitioners refer to the smoking-prevention literature to understand how policy changes can be implemented to better prevent eating disorder problems (Levine & Smolak, 2006). The smoking-prevention literature can certainly influence our knowledge around more effective prevention policy interventions, but I would argue that the AIDS movement can better inspire us to promote broader social changes and provide us with a new philosophy on youth engagement. Within the HIV/AIDS movement, there is a long history of people and communities affected by HIV mobilizing themselves to create responses to overcome the stigma of the disease. The HIV/AIDS movement emphasized that people living with HIV must be involved in any initiative that directly or indirectly affects their life—people with HIV embraced the motto: "Nothing for us, about us, without us!"

The youth AIDS/HIV movement started during 1993 at the South Africa HIV/AIDS conference. At that time, only twenty youth attended the conference. However, youth soon recognized that although they were one of the largest groups affected by HIV, they were not present at the decision-making table. Thus, their need to organize themselves found an outlet in 1994 when the Paris AIDS Summit took place and 42 countries declared the *Greater Involvement of People Living with HIV and AIDS (GIPA)* to be critical to the ethical and effective national responses to the epidemic.[12] Today, the *GIPA* principle is the backbone of many worldwide interventions emphasizing youth engagement. People living with, or affected by, HIV (e.g., parents, siblings, friends, and so on) are involved in a wide variety of activities at all levels of the fight against AIDS, from simple tasks to participating in major decision-making and policy-making activities. As reported in the Paris AIDS Declaration,

> The participation and contribution of people living with HIV is one of the best examples of global progress in public health. We have come from a place where people openly living with HIV were stoned to death, to a place where we have been invited to stand among the leaders of the world to shape international policies. There is still a long way to walk but we have made historical changes and gains of which we can be proud.[13]

In 2010, the World AIDS Campaign Youth Constituency Programme decided to implement an e-course entitled Towards Universal Access: Young People in Action.[14] The course's purpose was to help youth change how HIV affected their communities and the world though advocacy and activism (De Pauw & McCelland, 2010). In harmony with "young people's rights," the program felt that youth needed the opportunity to receive training to fight for their rights and for issues that mattered to them. The e-course was designed to help youth "to build or strengthen many leadership skills necessary for addressing global issues." It was based on six pillars: *global awareness*, including how to understand and address global issues and to work with people from different cultures, religions, and backgrounds; *civic literacy*, including how to understand policy-making, how to use human rights to influence decision-makers, and how to engage in advocacy at the local, national, and global level; *health literacy*, including how to understand and address public health issues; *creative thinking*, including how to brainstorm innovative ways to mobilize youth and gain public attention; *critical thinking*, including how to use a question-posing stance to explore health issues and to identify solutions addressing the root causes; *group skills*, such as communication and collaboration; and *information and communication technology literacy*, including how to access and use social media for social change (De Pauw & McCelland, 2010, p. 2).

Students from 15 different countries around the world were invited to take the e-course to improve their general knowledge and their advocacy skills and to take direct action. Using social media, such as Facebook, Blogger and YouTube, students had the opportunity to meet online, communicate, discuss relevant topics, learn from others, and implement their own global HIV responses (De Pauw & McCelland, 2010). The 8-week e-course asked youth to read policy documents and reports and to watch videos on the topic. Using an ongoing online discussion, participants were able to better understand these materials and had the opportunity to think critically about the content and issues. Many participants' way of understanding how HIV affects their community changed after taking this course. They were able to share their new understanding and thoughts with other members of their community within their personal blog. They also had the ability to create their own "evidence" by using Fotovoice and implement their own advocacy campaign. After the completion of the course, participants who demonstrated exceptional leadership skills had the opportunity to apply for one of the five leadership projects, which included up to $500 and ongoing coaching. The World AIDS Campaign Youth Constituency Programme thought that through the leadership projects, youth leaders could be supported on their ongoing advocacy work (De Pauw & McCelland, 2010).

Participants' feedback about the e-course provided useful lessons for the development of similar and/or new projects. First, the design phase of any e-course should clearly explore and expand youth access to the Internet. Second, the Internet provides a large variety of content (e.g., research data, policy reports, videos, and so on) that can be easily incorporated in an e-course. Third, e-learning does not need to be fancy or expensive. This e-course used free Web-based tools that youth were already using (e.g., YouTube, Facebook groups, Blogger.com, and Skype) as well as existing videos, articles, and websites that were easily accessible as learning material. Fourth, it is important to include not only content-area learning outcomes but also technology-related learning outcomes. And, finally, it is necessary to build capacity for ongoing use of social media for awareness raising and mobilization.

To conclude this section, not-for-profit organizations or coalitions, such as the World AIDS Campaign, are in a perfect position to build capacity for advocacy and activism for youth, parents, and practitioners. As illustrated in the development of this *Young People in Action* e-course, the end of one social innovation can lead to the beginning of another. After taking the e-course, youth were able to open new doors for social change and expand their own social actions.

Discussion: Limitations and Recommendations for Future Directions

I have presented different case studies to demonstrate how Internet-based tools can be used for advocacy and activism and, most importantly, how they can lead to powerful and meaningful collaborations between people, particularly youth. However, "there are no simple formulas—serious and significant social changes necessarily involve recognizing and dealing with complex systems, which seem to operate with a logic and life of their own, are far from inert, and battle for their own preservation" (Westley et al., 2006, p. ix).

To truly understand activism and social change, we need to embrace the idea that activism cannot be explained by exploring each of its elements (e.g., a visionary leader, motivated and skilful people, resources, communication tools, or a process of pre-defined steps) and then assuming that when all of these elements come together one can attain the whole product: advocacy or activism. The key to understanding social change is in exploring how all of these elements work together as a whole and in exploring the relationship between them. Complex science embraces the idea that social change is unpredictable, even when an alignment of circumstances makes actions possible. This will help us to make the impossible possible! As a result, this chapter "goes beyond" exploring cyber-activism by unpacking its elements, tools, and process to stress the importance of building new collaborations, overcome existing generational gaps, and learning from each other.

New technologies and Internet-based tools have the potential to influence advocacy and activism within the eating-related disorders field, but, most importantly, these tools will provide the ability to work together for social change in the eating disorders field. The time for "action" is here and now, and the following simple but important steps need to be taken to overcome possible barriers:

- If you are member of the baby boomer generation or if you are simply unskilled with, or skeptical about, new technologies try to overcome your anxiety and prejudices so that you can explore new Internet tools and be humble, open, and curious about them and take the time to explore their potential!
- If you are unfamiliar with Internet tools, especially Web 2.0 technologies such as YouTube, take some time to explore this world. You will soon discover that there is an eating disorder cyber-world that needs your support and action (e.g., pro-ana/pro-mia websites) as well as youth willing to work and help you (e.g., TakingITGlobal).
- If you are dissatisfied with Internet content, images, and video, remember that you can change it yourself by publishing new public content and helping Internet users enhance their critical thinking.
- If you are publishing with an electronic peer-reviewed journal or publisher, you should consider publishing in open-access or hybrid

open-access journals, knowing that open-access journals are effective knowledge sharing and dissemination tools to reach policy-makers and the general public.

- If you are a professor or researcher working in the field (e.g., faculty advisor of graduate students), you could encourage and support your students in developing and evaluating advocacy and activism efforts using the tools described in this chapter.
- If you are member of a not-for-profit organization or a researcher interested in advocacy and activism, you should consider alternative ways to build capacity in our community around advocacy and activism for eating-related disorders using new technology. An e-course on the topic can be an effective way to start.
- If you are involved in advocacy and activism regarding eating-related disorders, explore how new technologies can facilitate your work and actions. Remember to combine off-line and online initiatives and remember that all tools can facilitate social change.
- If you are already involved in cyber-activism, remember that we need to continually engage in reflection and evaluation to assess the efficacy, effectiveness, and usefulness of our online actions.
- Remember to take the time to develop meaningful collaborations before starting your advocacy journey. Remember to ask and involve youth in your work and action—they will be powerful resources to you.

Conclusions

The digital era offers activists working in the eating-related disorders field a new and potentially very effective set of tools to promote awareness, mobilize social groups, and co-ordinate actions to promote social change. The added value to using Web-based technologies as advocacy and activism tools include, but are not limited to, accessibility, time and cost effectiveness, more effective information gathering, and dissemination. Many of the tools described in this chapter have already been used to build capacity within the eating disorders community to promote social cohesion and change, but there are still many possibilities yet to be explored. Current eating disorder advocacy and activism initiatives have been able to achieve important results, but the future could hold much promise for newer and more exciting efforts, thanks to Internet-based applications and tools. There is still much to be learned about the positive or negative influences of the Internet in terms of its role in the prevention of weight-related disorders. There is more to gain by meeting at the crossroads and joining youth online to collectively advocate for social change.

Notes

1 TakingITGlobal, retrieved from http://www.tigweb.org; YouthVoices, retrieved from http://www.youthvoices.ca; World AIDS Campaign, retrieved from http://www.worldaidscampaign.org.

2 In 2003, as reported in the General Social Survey (GSS) on social engagement, approximately one-third (33.2%) of Canadians ages 15 to 29 searched for information on political issues (online or offline) while only one-quarter of those ages 30 to 49 (25.3%) and 50 to 64 (24.5%) searched for such information (Schellenberg, 2004).

3 Nearly one-third (29.2%) of Canadian home Internet users read other Canadians' comments and posts concerning political and social issues in 2005, and 13.8% said they used the Internet to correspond with Canadians about specific political or social issues (Veenhof, Wellman, Quell, & Hogan, 2008).

4 TakingITGlobal is funded by a range of sources, including government and UN agencies, foundations, corporations, and non-profit organizations. The funding they receive is either associated with specific projects that have deadlines and deliverables or it goes towards core operational costs. As a registered charity, it also accepts individual donations. TakingITGlobal's office is located in Toronto (main location) and New York.

5 Women's Art Gallery. Retrieved from http://www.tigweb.org/themes/women/.

6 For more information, see http://tig.phpwebhosting.com/tiged/TIGed-MTC.pdf.

7 For more information, see http://www.youthvoices.ca/.

8 CyberIsle. Retrieved from http://www.teennetproject.org./node?page=5.

9 Participatory: key involvement (ownership) at all stages by youth. Relevance: focus on personal, health, and social issue identified by youth. Active learning: fun, engaging, flexible, and highly interactive, stimulates self-directed learning. Autonomy supporting: respects individual choice and exploration of options regarding health behaviour. Access: designed and adapted to be accessible and relevant to diverse groups and settings, especially marginalized populations.

10 YouthBet.net. Retrieved from http://www.youthbet.net.

11 To view this documentary, see YouTube, http://www.youtube.com/watch?v=ta0A IFaW0Z4andfeature=PlayListandp=188BE1941E2E9F97andindex=4.

12 *Greater Involvement of People Living with HIV and AIDS.* Retrieved from http://data.unaids.org/pub/Report/2007/JC1299-PolicyBrief-GIPA_en.pdf.

13 Ross, Gracia Violeta, National Chair, Bolivian Network of People Living with HIV/AIDS, Paris AIDS Declaration (1994).

14 The World AIDS Campaign is a global coalition of national, regional, and international civil society groups, basically a coalition of AIDS/HIV not-for-profit organization, united by the call for governments to honour their AIDS commitments under the slogan "Stop AIDS. Keep the Promise" (McCelland and De Pauw, 2010). Inside the World AIDS Campaign, the Youth Constituency Programme aims to strengthen campaigning of young people around universal access to prevention, treatment, care, and support (McCelland and De Pauw, 2010).

References

Bardone-Cone, A. M. & Cass, K. M. (2007). What does viewing a pro-anorexia website do? An experimental examination of website exposure and moderating effects. *International Journal of Eating Disorders, 40*, 537-548.

Bauer, S., Percevic, R., Okon, E., Meermann, R., & Kordy, H. (2003). Use of text messaging in the aftercare of patients with bulimia nervosa. *European Eating Disorders Review, 11*, 279-290.

Becker, A. E. (2004). Television, disordered eating, and young women in Fiji: Negotiating body image and identity during rapid social change. *Culture, Medicine and Psychiatry, 28*, 533-559.

Becker, A. E., Fay, K., Gilman, S. E., & Striegel-Moore, R. (2007). Facets of acculturation and their diverse relations to body shape concern in Fiji. *International Journal of Eating Disorders, 40*, 42-50.

Becker, C. B., Bull, S., Schaumberg, K., Cauble, A., & Franco, A. (2008). Effectiveness of peer-led eating disorders prevention: A replication trial. *Journal of Consulting and Clinical Psychology, 76*, 347-354.

Becker, C. B., Smith, L. M., & Ciao, A. C. (2005). Reducing eating disorder risk factors in sorority members: A randomized trial. *Behavior Therapy, 36*, 245-254.

Becker, C. B., Smith, L. M., & Ciao, A. C. (2006). Peer facilitated eating disorder prevention: A randomized effectiveness trial of cognitive dissonance and media advocacy. *Journal of Counseling Psychology, 53*, 550-555.

Becker, C. B., Stice, E., Shaw, H., & Woda, S. (2009). Use of empirically supported interventions for psychopathology: Can the participatory approach move us beyond the research-to-practice gap? *Behaviour Research and Therapy, 47*, 265-274.

Bruning-Brown, J. B., Winzelberg, A. J., Abascal, L. B., & Taylor, C. B. (2004). An evaluation of an Internet-delivered eating disorder prevention program for adolescents and their parents. *Journal of Adolescent Health, 35*, 290-296.

Chen, S., Poland, B., & Skinner, H. (2007). Youth voices: Evaluations of participatory action research. *Canadian Journal of Program Evaluation, 22*, 125-150.

Davis, P. M., Lewenstein, B. V., Simon, D. H., Booth, J. G., & Connolly, M. J. L. (2008). Open access publishing, article downloads and citations: Randomized trial. *British Medical Journal, 337*, a586.

De Pauw, L. & McCelland, A. (2010). Towards universal access: Young people in action e-course outline. World AIDS Campaign. Retrieved from http://www.worldaidscampaign.org/en/Constituencies/Youth/Youth-ecourse.

Douw, K., Vondeling H., Eskildsen, D., & Simpson, S. (2003). Use of the Internet in scanning the horizon for new and emerging health technologies: A survey of agencies involved in horizon scanning. *Journal of Medical Internet Research, 31*, Article e6. Retrieved from http://www.jmir.org/2003/1/e6

Eysenbach, G. (2006a). Citation advantage of open access articles. *PLoS Biology, 4*(5), Article e157. Retrieved from http://dx.doi.org/10.1371/journal.pbio.0040157

Eysenbach, G. (2006b). The open access advantage. *Journal of Medical Internet Research, 8*, 2-6.

Fisher, D. R. (1998). Rumoring theory and the Internet: A framework for analyzing the grass roots. *Social Science Computer Review, 16*, 158-168.

Foot, D. K. (1996). *Boom, bust and echo: How to profit from the coming demographic shift.* Toronto: Macfarlane Walter and Ross.

Foot, D. K. (1998). *Boom, bust and echo 2000: Profiting from the demographic shift in the new millennium.* Toronto: Macfarlane Walter and Ross.

Freire, P. (2000). *Pedagogy of the oppressed* (30th anniversary edition). New York: Continuum.

Internet World Stats. (2009). Retrieved from http://www.internetworldstats.com/

Internet World Stats. (2010). Retrieved from http://www.internetworldstats.com/

Korn D., Murray M., Morrison M., Reynolds J., & Skinner H. A. (2006). Engaging youth about gambling using the Internet: The YouthBet.Net Website. *Canadian Journal of Public Health, 97*, 448-453.

Levine, M. P., & Smolak, L. (2006). *The prevention of eating problems and eating disorders: Theory, research, and practice.* Mahwah, NJ: Lawrence Erlbaum Associates.

Low, K. G., Charanasomboon, S., Lesser, J., Reinhalter, K., Martin, R., & Jones, H., Winzelberg, A., Abascal, L., & Taylor, C. B. (2006). Effectiveness of a computer-based interactive eating disorders prevention program at long-term follow-up. *Eating Disorders, 14*, 17-30.

McCelland, A., & De Pauw, L. (2010). *Towards universal access: Young people in action e-course lessons learned report.* World AIDS Campaign (Unpublished manuscript) [on file with the author].

McCaughey, M., & Ayers, M. D. (2003). *Cyberactivism: Online activism in theory and practice.* New York, NY: Routledge.

McNutt, J. G., & Menon, G. M. (2008). The rise of cyberactivism: Implications for the future of advocacy in the human services. *Families in Society, 89*, 33-38.

McVey, G., Gusella, J., Tweed, S., & Ferrari, M. (2009). A controlled evaluation of web-based training for teachers and public health practitioners on the prevention of eating disorders. *Eating Disorders, 17*, 1-26.

Mitchell, J. E., Myers, T., Swan-Kremeier, L., & Wonderlich, S. (2003). Psychotherapy for bulimia nervosa delivered via telemedicine. *European Eating Disorders Review, 11*, 222-230.

Morrison, M., Lombardo, C., Biscope, S., & Skinner, H. (2005). *Youth action guide: Community-based smoking prevention.* TeenNet Research: University of Toronto. Retrieved from https://www.box.com/s/etuasidldtml3xhvn85c

Myers, D. J. (1994). Networks to activism communication technology and social movements: Contributions of the computer. *Social Science Computer Review, 12*, 250-260.

Norman C. D., Maley, O., Li, X., & Skinner, H. A. (2008). Using the Internet to assist smoking prevention and cessation in schools: A randomized controlled trial. *Health Psychology, 27*, 799-810.

Norman, C. D. & Skinner, H. A. (2006). eHEALS: The eHealth Literacy Scale. *Journal of Medical Internet Research, 8*, 47-52.

Norman, C. D. & Skinner, H. A. (2007). Engaging youth in eHealth promotion: Lessons learned from a decade of TeenNet Research. *Academic Medicine: State of the Art Review, 18*, 357-369.

Norton, M., Wonderlich, S. A., Myers, T., Mitchell, J. E., & Crosby, R. D. (2003). The use of palmtop computers in the treatment of bulimia nervosa. *European Eating Disorders Review, 11*, 231-242.

Piran, N. (1998). A participatory approach to the prevention of eating disorders. In G. Noordenbos & W. Vandereycken (Eds.), *Prevention of eating disorders* (pp. 173-186). London: Athelone Press.

Piran, N. (1999a). The reduction of preoccupation with body weight and shape in schools: A feminist approach. In N. Piran, M. P. Levine, & C. Steiner-Adair (Eds.), *Preventing eating disorders: A handbook of interventions and special challenges* (pp. 194-206). Philadelphia, PA: Brunner/Mazel.

Piran, N. (1999b). Eating disorders: A trial of prevention in a high risk school settings. *Journal of Primary Prevention, 20*, 75-90.

Piran, N. (2001). Re-inhabiting the body from the inside out: Girls transform their school environment. In D. L. Tolman & M. Brydon-Miller (Eds.), *From subjects to subjectivities: A handbook of interpretive and participatory methods* (pp. 218-238). New York: New York University Press.

Ridgley, A., Maley, O., & Skinner, H. A. (Fall 2004). Youth voices: Engaging youth in health promotion using media technologies. *Canadian Issues: Association for Canadian Studies* 21-24.

Samuel, A. W. (2004). *Hacktivism and the future of political participation* (Ph.D. dissertation, Department of Political Science, Harvard University, Cambridge, MA) [Unpublished].

Schmidt, U. (2003). Getting technical. *European Eating Disorders Review, 11*, 147-154.

Schellenberg, G. 2004. 2003 General social survey on social engagement, Cycle 17: An overview of findings. Statistics Canada Catalogue no. 89-598-XIE, July. Retrieved from http://www.statcan.ca/bsolc/english/bsolc?catno=89-598-X

Skinner, H. A. (2002). *Promoting health through organizational change*. San Francisco, CA: Benjamin Cummings.

Skinner, H. A., & Biscope, S. (2005). Making change work in youth centres. TeenNet Research, University of Toronto. Retrieved from http://www.thcu.ca/yetp/pubs/pdf/making_change_work_YETP.pdf

Skinner, H. A., Maley, O. & Norman, C. D. (2006). Developing eHealth promotion Internet-based programs: The spiral technology action research (STAR) model. *Health Promotion Practice, 7*, 1-12.

Statistics Canada. (2010). CANSIM, Tables (for fee) 358-0123, 358-0124, 358-0125 & 358-0126. Retrieved from http://www.statcan.gc.ca/tables-tableaux/sum-som/l01/cst01/comm35a-eng.htm

Stice, E., Chase, A., Stormer, S., & Appel, A. (2001). A randomized trial of a dissonance-based eating disorder prevention program. *International Journal of Eating Disorders, 29*, 247-262.

Tapscott, D. (1998). *Growing up digital: The rise of the net generation*. Montreal: McGraw-Hill.

Tapscott, D. (2009). *Grown up digital: How the net generation is changing your world*. New York: McGraw-Hill.

Taylor, C. B., Bryson, S., Luce, K. H., Cunning, D., & Celio, A. (2006). Prevention of eating disorders in at-risk college-age women. *Archives of General Psychiatry, 63*, 881-888.

Tiggemann, M. (2008, May). *Media and body image: Research findings and implication*. Paper presented at the meeting of the Academy of Eating Disorders International Conference, Seattle, WA.

Tiggemann, M. (2010, June). *The Internet and adolescent girls' drive for thinness*. Paper presented at the meeting of the Academy of Eating Disorders International Conference, Salzburg, Austria.

Treasure, J., Schmidt, U., & van Furth, E. (2003). *Handbook of eating disorders* (2nd ed.). Southern Gate, Chichester: John Wiley and Sons.

Veenhof, B., Wellman, B., Quell, C., & Hogan, B. (2008). *How Canadians' use of the internet affects social life and civic participation*. Statistics Canada Catalogue no. 56F0004M — no. 016. Retrieved from http://www.statcan.gc.ca/pub/56f0004m/56f0004m2008016-eng.pdf

Westley, F., Zimmerman, B. D., & Patton, M. Q. (2006). *Getting to maybe: How the world is changed*. Toronto: Random House Canada.

Yager, J. (2003). E-mail therapy for anorexia nervosa: Prospects and limitations. *European Eating Disorders Review, 11*, 198-209.

Zabinski, M. F., Celio, A. A., Jacobs, M. J., Manwaring, J., & Wilfley, D. E. (2003). Internet-based prevention of eating disorders. *European Eating Disorders Review, 11*, 183-197.

PART TWO

Risk, Resilience, and Prevention

CHAPTER SIX

Risk and Protective Factors in Body Image Problems: Implications for Prevention

Linda Smolak, *Kenyon College*

Causal models of the development of body image and eating problems, supported by empirical data, are an important element in designing prevention programs. Indeed, along with an assessment of the needs, strengths, and weaknesses of the target community, such models are arguably the most crucial component for program designers to consider. Knowledge of risk and protective factors in the development of body image problems will aid program designers in identifying the most appropriate audiences; the most mutable behaviours, attitudes, and environmental characteristics; and the best matches between audiences and target behaviours.

Risk factors are typically defined as variables that increase the likelihood of problematic or even pathological outcomes. The definitions of risk factors suggested by Kraemer and colleagues (1997) have been particularly influential in body image and eating disorder research, especially work rooted in the bio-psycho-social approach (e.g., Jacobi, Hayward, deZwaan, Kraemer, & Agras, 2004; Shisslak & Crago, 2001; Stice, 2002). Kraemer and her colleagues (1997) made two major contributions in defining risk factors. First, they distinguished between "fixed" and "variable" risk factors. As the names imply, "fixed" risk factors may mark risk and may even be causative, but they cannot be changed and are, therefore, often of limited interest to prevention researchers. Gender and ethnicity are often treated as fixed risk factors (e.g., Jacobi et al., 2004). The variable risk factors, whose levels or influence can be altered, such as media images or peer teasing, tend to receive greater attention. Not surprisingly, variable risk factors are often the focus of prevention programs.

Second, Kraemer et al. (1997) delineated the requirements for establishing a risk factor as causal. First, it must show temporal precedence to the outcome variable, which requires prospective, longitudinal data. This specification is the minimal requirement for establishing a causal relationship. Second, following in the tradition of empiricism, one has to demonstrate, preferably through experimental manipulation, that altering the level of the risk factor changes the level of the outcome variable in some predictable fashion. Such action might be accomplished in studies that look directly at a particular putative risk factor (e.g., Calogero, 2004) or as part of a prevention study (see, e.g., Levine & Smolak, 2006, for a review).

There are also factors that reduce the likelihood that problem behaviours will develop, even in the face of substantial risk. Such variables are termed protective factors. Hypothetically, increasing the frequency and intensity of protective factors could be at least as powerful an approach as lowering risk factors in reducing body image problems. However, compared to risk factors, protective factors have been more difficult to identify. Hence, protective factors have played a less central role in prevention programs, although there has been some attention to empowerment and embodiment (Piran, 1999, 2001; Chapter 7 in this volume), self-esteem (O'Dea & Abraham, 2000), family relationships (Archibald, Graber, & Brooks-Gunn, 1999), and feminist identity (Peterson, Tantleff-Dunn, & Bedwell, 2006).

There are numerous reviews of risk and protective factors in the development of body image and eating disturbances, ranging from general reviews (e.g., Smolak, 2009; Stice, 2002) to analyses of specific variables such as media (Bartlett, Vowels, & Saucier, 2008; Grabe, Ward, & Hyde, 2008), ethnicity (Grabe & Hyde, 2006; Roberts, Cash, Feingold, & Johnson, 2006), social comparison (Myers & Crowther, 2009), and feminist identity (Murnen & Smolak, 2009). Rather than repeat these analyses, the primary goal of this chapter is to describe how major risk and protective factors in the development of body image and eating problems might be incorporated into prevention programs. Risk and protective factors are not monoliths. They will vary with age, gender, ethnicity, social class, and other broad culturally defined factors. Some factors will be associated with the onset of problems, others with the maintenance. Thus, this undertaking is complex and will, of necessity, be selective. There are five sections in the chapter. Four of these sections will focus on different categories of risk factors: biological factors, socio-cultural factors, individual factors, and cultural influences. The fifth will examine protective factors. Within each section, developmental issues will be raised.

Biological Risk Factors

There are at least four "biological" risk factors that have been related to body image issues and eating problems: body mass index (BMI), puberty, neurochemistry, and genetics. Biological factors are frequently treated as "fixed" risk factors. They are viewed as being intrinsic features of the individual. It is frequently, assumed, then, that these features can be treated as "moderators" in the relationship between socio-cultural variables and body image or as direct causal influences on body image. They are variables that identify "groups" of people—for example, underweight versus obese, early versus on-time puberty, or specific serotonin imbalances, which might identify individuals who are differentially susceptible to other risk factors for the development of eating disorders. If "at-risk" levels of these variables can be identified, they can be used to select participants for targeted prevention programs.

BMI

BMI has been related to body image. Researchers routinely find that even among the thinnest group of girls (the tenth percentile of BMI), there are those who wish to be thinner (which is not the case with boys). Nonetheless, heavier weights are typically associated with greater body dissatisfaction, even in childhood (Field et al., 2001; Ohring, Graber, & Brooks-Gunn, 2002). However, except perhaps in situations where weight interferes with physical well-being or functioning, the weight status per se is not what typically creates the body dissatisfaction. Rather, it is the prejudice and discrimination against "fat" as well as the cultural emphasis on the thin ideal for girls and women and the lean ideal for both genders (Smolak & Murnen, 2008) that likely creates the link between BMI and body dissatisfaction (Puhl & Latner, 2007). Relatedly, research has not consistently documented a relationship between BMI and a drive for muscularity among boys (Holt & Ricciardelli, 2002; McCabe & Ricciardelli, 2005). BMI might be a useful tool in designing prevention programs for at least two reasons. First, it may help to identify children who are at particular risk for body image problems. Second, understanding the negative psycho-social effects of BMI may help to identify cultural forces in body image development. However, BMI is not a truly "biological" influence on body dissatisfaction.

Puberty

There is a possibility of hormonal involvement in the development of eating problems (Kaye, Frank, Bailer, & Henry, 2005; Klump, Keel, Sisk, & Burt, 2010), an argument spurred by the gender difference in anorexia nervosa that appears to increase from about 5 girls for every boy to 9 girls for each boy during adolescence (Watkins & Lask, 2009). Furthermore, body image, eating disorders, and depression are interrelated, and depression has been related to pubertal hormonal levels (Graber, Archibald, & Brooks-Gunn, 1999). Nonetheless, evidence for a substantial role for pubertal hormones in the development of body image and eating problems is currently limited (e.g., Klump et al., 2010). Nor is this the main focus of research linking puberty to body image. Most research has instead examined the relationship of pubertal timing to body image.

Early puberty is associated with a variety of behavioural problems in girls, including body dissatisfaction (Hayward et al., 1997). This is not true for boys, perhaps reflecting the negative social aspects of having an adult woman's body but the positive value of an adult man's body. During early adolescence, girls who are early developers (often defined as girls who reach menarche by age 11 or as the highest quintile of the Pubertal Developmental Scale) appear to have lower body esteem and higher body dissatisfaction (Hayward, 2003; Wertheim, Paxton, & Blaney, 2009). However, this effect seems to wash out over time such that by middle adolescence there is not a consistent difference between early and on-time maturers. The on-time and late maturers seem to catch up to the early-maturing girls in terms of body image problems. Some research indicates that mediators such as weight gain, which tend to be associated with early puberty, may be related to increases in body and eating concerns (Wertheim, Martin, Prior, Sanson, & Smart, 2002). Nonetheless, in general, researchers agree that pubertal timing does not have long-term implications for body image and eating dysfunction (Wertheim et al., 2009). Yet, for prevention programs aimed at pre-adolescents or early adolescents (approximately the ages of 9 to 12), pubertal timing might be considered to be a selection factor for targeted prevention. Discussion of pubertal changes and pubertal timing, including the facilitation of the acceptance of the pubertal weight gain, with students of this age group might also reduce the increases in body dissatisfaction and dieting.

Neurobiology and Neurochemistry

There is substantial evidence of neurochemical abnormalities during episodes of anorexia nervosa and bulimia nervosa (e.g., Jimerson & Wolfe, 2006; Kaye, Fudge, & Paulus, 2009; Kaye et al., 2005). Given the starvation and purging involved in eating disorders, this finding is not surprising. These findings almost certainly have implications for the pharmacological treatment of eating disorders. The larger question involves the role of neurobiology as a risk factor for the development of anorexia nervosa and bulimia nervosa. Reviewers frequently suggest that the serotonin system is a likely risk factor for the development of anorexia nervosa (e.g., Kaye et al., 2009). Steiger (2004) has hypothesized that genetics might create a serotonin system that is vulnerable to trauma, hence increasing the likelihood of developing bulimia nervosa. However, there are no prospective studies establishing serotonin disturbances as a causal factor in the development of anorexia nervosa and bulimia nervosa. Instead, the arguments that serotonin dysfunction or imbalances may be a risk factor are based on studies of people who have recovered from anorexia nervosa or bulimia nervosa. Beyond the difficulties in agreeing on what constitutes "recovery," this theory is problematic because the disorders themselves may have long-term, and perhaps permanent, effects on brain functioning (Streigel-Moore & Smolak, 2001). Such lingering marks of eating disorders are sometimes called "scar effects" (Lilenfeld, Wonderlich, Riso, Crosby, & Mitchell, 2006). Neuroscience has clearly established that even the adult brain is susceptible to environmental influences. Environmental events of various sorts may result in reorganizations of the brain's anatomic, chemical, or metabolic systems (see Cicchetti & Curtis, 2006, for a review). Furthermore, some of the serotonin system changes that have been observed in women who have recovered from eating disorders, including increased levels of some forms of serotonin and hypersensitivity to acute tryptophan depletion are consistent with the effects of early malnutrition seen in animal experiments (Jimerson & Wolfe, 2006; Schmidt & Georgieff, 2006).

Perhaps early nutrition deficits, associated with maternal dieting or even maternal anorexia nervosa during pregnancy or childhood dieting, actually create a vulnerable serotonin system that "overreacts" to later tryptophan reductions associated with dieting, thereby creating an increased risk for eating disorders (Cowen, Clifford, Walsh, Williams, & Fairburn, 1996). The average female brain may be more susceptible than the typical male brain to dieting induced changes in tryptophan (Walsh, Oldman, Franklin, Fairburn, & Cowan, 1995). Interestingly, animal research has shown that early malnutrition is also linked to reductions in the GABA transmitter (Schmidt & Georgieff, 2006). Topiramate, a drug that has recently shown some effectiveness in treating bulimia nervosa (Nickel et al., 2005), appears to work in part by increasing GABA levels (e.g., White, 2005).

Early malnutrition is not the only environmental event that might alter neurobiology. Animal studies have clearly demonstrated, and human studies have suggested, that stress alters serotonin levels (Cichetti & Curtis, 2006; Steiger, 2004). The prospective animal data indicate that the effects of social stress may be permanent. Behavioural research with Romanian orphans indicates that the permanence of the effects of social stress depends on the timing of the interventions (Rutter & the English and

Romanian Adoptees Study Team, 1998). Furthermore, even gender differences in brain functioning that might be associated with reactions to
stress may be attributable to social experiences rather than prenatal brain
organization (Dedovic, Wadiwalla, Engert, & Pruessner, 2009). In a similar vein, Bohon and Stice (2010) have suggested that differences between
women suffering from bulimia nervosa and women in the control group in
neurological food intake reward systems (e.g., in the insula) may be attributable to a history of binge eating highly palatable food. The point here is
that the brain is a self-organizing system that is constantly reorganizing
itself in response to experience and to the environment (Cichetti & Curtis,
2006). Genes may help to probabilistically determine how an individual's
brain will react to the environment (Gottlieb, 1995).

Unfortunately, we do not yet have the data necessary to explain how
these processes work during childhood and adolescence to contribute
to the development of body image and eating problems. Such research,
while time-consuming and expensive, is desperately needed to illuminate
whether and how neurochemical systems increase the risk for eating disorders. Perhaps the best way to use the currently available information is
to design prevention programs that appear to reduce factors that might
negatively impact serotonin or GABA systems. These might include child
sexual abuse, early social stress/deprivation, and early nutritional patterns
(perhaps particularly those that are associated with maternal dieting or
eating disorders during pregnancy).

Genetics

There has been considerable enthusiasm recently for genetic explanations
of various eating disorders—anorexia nervosa, bulimia nervosa, and binge
eating disorder—and their symptoms, including body dissatisfaction.
There have been several reviews of the recent explosion of research in this
area (e.g., Mazzeo, Landt, van Furth, & Bulik, 2006; Suisman & Klump,
2011). In general, these reviews suggest family aggregation of eating disorders and moderate to high heritability estimates (50-85%) (Klump, Suisman, Burt, McGue, & Iacono, 2009). While there are some clues about
specific chromosomal or autosomal loci for the disorders or the symptoms,
there have not been consistent findings.

There are a variety of general critiques of the behavioural genetics
approach that also apply to eating disorder studies (e.g., Gottlieb, 1995).
For example, the model used in most of the eating disorder research
reflects three components: genetics, unique environment, and shared
environment. There is no component explicitly representing the interactions between genes and the environment. These genetic models tend to

assume that genetics influence environment more than the environment influences genetics and so include genetic-environment interactions under the genetic components of the model (Klump et al., 2009). This procedure tends to overestimate genetic and underestimate shared environment influences. These models also do not recognize what Gottlieb (1995) refers to as the probabilistic effect of genes, which will depend heavily on the timing and availability of environmental factors. Thus, for example, evidence suggests that there are interactions between genetics and prenatal exposure to cigarettes in affecting self-regulation but that the expressions of these interactions are different in infants than in preschoolers (Wiebe et al., 2009). One implication of this probabilistic approach is that some of the influence of the genes will be fully moderated by environmental factors. If such environmental factors could be identified, they would become important targets of interventions (including prevention programs), particularly those aimed at high-risk children (Rutter, 2003).

Most of the genetic studies have been performed with adult samples. It is not clear that these studies are applicable to children and adolescents since there are important differences between eating disorders of children and adults (see Watkins & Lask, 2009). For example, bulimia nervosa is more common than anorexia nervosa in adults, but the reverse is true in children. The gender difference in eating disorders is more pronounced in adults than in children. Indeed, the limited research suggests different levels of heritability in prepubertal girls compared to pubertal (defined as being mid-pubertal according to the Pubertal Development Scale) or older adolescents and women (Culbert, Burt, McGue, Iacono, & Klump, 2009; Klump et al., 2010; Klump, McGue, & Iacono, 2000, 2003). In prepubertal twins, genetic influences seem to be negligible, while shared environment is a significant contributor to the Minnesota Eating Disorders Inventory scores. The correlations for monozygotic and dizygotic twins were virtually identical for this age group. In pubertal and 17-year-old twins as well as adult women (ages 20 to 41), however, genetic influences were significant, while shared environment effects were negligible. These studies certainly require replication.

It is unclear how genes might be involved in the development of body image and eating problems. Thus, while it continues to be reasonable to consider children with parents or siblings who suffer from eating disorders at "high risk" and, hence, as an appropriate target of prevention programs, it is not likely that they will be a sizeable focus of prevention efforts. While research on genetics may ultimately yield important clues concerning body image and eating disturbances, extant data have limited implications for current prevention efforts.

Socio-Cultural Risk Factors

Much research has focused on socio-cultural factors in the development of body image and eating problems. Indeed, the dominant theories of body image development, such as the Tripartite Influence Model, focus on socio-cultural factors mediated by individual characteristics (Thompson, Heinberg, Altabe, & Tantleff-Dunn, 1999). The three influences that have received the most attention are the media, parents, and peers.

Media

Media have probably received more research attention than any other risk factor. Indeed, the emphasis on media has resulted in the development of a number of media literacy prevention programs (Levine & Smolak, 2006). Experimental, correlational, longitudinal, and meta-analytic data all demonstrate relationships between various forms of media (e.g., television and magazines) and the development and intensification of body dissatisfaction in girls (e.g., Grabe et al., 2008; Groesz, Levine, & Murnen, 2002; Want, 2009). Boys are similarly affected, although the effects may be somewhat weaker (Bartlett et al., 2008).

Various forms of media affect body image. For example, Grabe, Ward, & Hyde (2008) found that magazines and television seemed to have comparable effects. Recent experimental research indicates that both male and female undergraduates experience lower body esteem after playing "body emphasizing" video games (Bartlett & Harris, 2008). While more research is needed to explicate the nature of these relationships at various ages and in different ethnic groups, it is evident that media influence is an important factor to consider in prevention programs. Multi-level intervention is preferable with activism to actually change the media images and individual rejection and criticism of the extant images among the potential components of prevention programs. Such issues are discussed in detail by Michael Levine and Joe Kelly in Chapter 4 in this volume.

Parents

Parents clearly impact their children's body image, although there are differences according to the age of the child as well as the gender of the child and the gender of the parent (Field et al., 2001; Santfer, Crowthers, Crawford, & Watts, 1996; Smolak, Levine, & Schermer, 1999; Wertheim et al., 2002). Generally speaking, mothers are more influential than fathers for both boy and girl children (McCabe & Ricciardelli, 2005). Girls may be more affected than boys.

Parents might influence children's body image either through modelling body dissatisfaction or by making direct comments about the child's body (Smolak et al., 1999; Stice, 1994). While some studies indicate that maternal weight loss behaviours increase daughters' body dissatisfaction, others find no such relationship. Findings concerning parental comments and pressures on children to be thin are more consistent. Research, including longitudinal work, indicates that parental comments show a small to moderate relationship to daughters' body image (e.g., Smolak et al., 1999; Stice, Shaw, & Nemeroff, 1998).

In addition, parents may attempt to control their children's eating. They might, for example, withhold desserts from the child until more nutritious foods are eaten. Or they may control when and how much children can eat. Such rules may be attempts to increase the nutritional content of the child's diet, or it may represent an attempt to control a child's weight from an early age (Costanzo & Woody, 1985). Studies indicate that parental attempts to control children's eating in these intrusive ways is associated with increased risk for obesity, lower levels of ability to self-regulate eating, and lower self-esteem (Addessi, Galloway, Visalberghi, & Birch, 2005; Fisher & Birch, 2000; Galloway, Fiorito, Francis, & Birch, 2006). These negative effects on body image and eating begin to appear during the preschool years.

Thus, there are a variety of ways in which parents might affect a child's body image and eating patterns. It is clear that parents should be included in prevention efforts. Given busy parental schedules and, perhaps, parents' own body issues, including them can be challenging (Graber et al., 1999). Gathering information from parents prior to instituting a prevention program may help to identify ways to involve them.

Peers
As with parents, peer influences on body image may take various forms. Peers may model body dissatisfaction and dieting. Girls and boys may compare themselves to their peers in order to assess how well they meet cultural criteria for attractiveness. Peers may also discuss weight and shape, especially among girl friends. Such discussions may include "fat talk" in which girls disparage their bodies in order to be more socially acceptable and to motivate themselves regarding appearance (Nichter, 2000). Peers may also comment on each other's weight and shape. Teasing might be included among these direct comments.

All of these forms of peer influence have been associated with girls' body dissatisfaction. So, for example, appearance conversations with friends, appearance social comparison to friends, dieting by friends, and peer teasing have all been prospectively related to body dissatisfaction among adolescent girls (e.g., Jones, 2004; Paxton, Eisenberg, & Neumark-Sztainer,

2006). Such direct relationships have not always been found for younger girls (Clark & Tiggemann, 2008) although appearance related peer inter-actions have been associated with the development of appearance schemas in pre-adolescent girls (Sinton & Birch, 2006). Appearance schemas, in turn, have been related to body dissatisfaction in this age group (Clark & Tiggemann, 2008; Sinton & Birch, 2006). Thus, the specific nature of peer effects may show developmental variation. These age differences will be important to consider in designing prevention programs.

Peer sexual harassment may also affect body image and disordered eating. Even among elementary-school children, cross-gender sexual harassment is related to negative weight-shape esteem in girls but not boys (Murnen & Smolak, 2000). By high school, the substantial major-ity of girls have experienced sexual harassment, with unwanted romantic attention, demeaning comments about gender, teasing about appearance, and unwanted physical contact being the most common forms (Leaper & Brown, 2008). Researchers have used both qualitative (e.g., Larkin, 1994) and quantitative (Harned, 2000; Piran & Thompson, 2008) techniques to relate sexual harassment to body dissatisfaction and disordered eating among adolescent girls and adult women. Prospective data are, however, desperately needed to better understand the extent and nature of these relationships, including the gendered context within which sexual harass-ment is interpreted (Smolak, 2010).

Peer teasing about appearance and weight and shape is also a powerful influence on girls' body image and disordered eating (Menzel, Schaefer, Burke, Mayhew, Brannick, & Thompson, 2010). For example, in a study of Swedish girls that began when they were 10 years old, those girls who were teased and bullied by their friends had lower weight esteem at age 13 and more body shame at age 18 (Lunde, Frisén, & Hwang, 2007; Lunde & Frisén, 2011). Furthermore, BMI is not related to the strength of the rela-tionship between teasing and body dissatisfaction, although heavier girls are more likely to be teased (Wertheim et al., 2009).

Boys, too, are certainly affected by peer influences. So, for example, social comparisons to peers are related to body dissatisfaction among ado-lescent boys (Jones, 2001). Peer teasing is related to higher body dissatisfac-tion (Phares, Steinberg, & Thompson, 2004). Although the link between weight-related teasing and body dissatisfaction is stronger in girls, the link between appearance-related teasing and body dissatisfaction is similar for both genders (Menzel et al., 2010). However, boys are somewhat less likely than girls to engage in peer social comparisons or appearance conversa-tions (Jones, 2001, 2004). These peer influences on body dissatisfaction and eating problems have several implications for prevention programs. First, they suggest particular behaviours to target in prevention programs.

Programs can encourage children to not engage in weight-related teasing or can teach children how to cope with such teasing, for example. Second, these findings provide a rationale for universal prevention. By including all children in a program, the actual peer context may be altered.

It is noteworthy that in addition to friends, children often have siblings who are close to their age. Very limited research suggests that sisters might influence one another's body dissatisfaction and disordered eating. This influence may come through modelling or through being targets for social comparison. Such effects may be mediated by social comparison or thin ideal internalization tendencies (Coomber & King, 2008). While research on sisters' influences is very limited and has not yet examined developmental differences, this does raise another site for prevention, particularly for prevention aimed at families.

Individual Psychological Factors

Individual psychological factors may have a direct effect on the development of body image and eating problems. For example, Bearman, Presnell, Martinez, and Stice (2006) reported that negative affectivity was prospectively related to increases in body dissatisfaction among adolescents. This was true for both boys and girls. Martin and colleagues (2000) also reported that childhood negative emotionality was related to the later development of eating and body image problems, especially among girls.

However, individual psychological characteristics are often examined within the context of complex moderating and mediating relationships. Socio-cultural and biological factors may sometimes have direct effects on body image. More commonly, they are filtered through mediating or moderating variables. In many cases, such variables represent characteristics of the individual. Such mediators or moderators include appearance schema, internalization of the thin ideal, and social comparison.

For example, one popular socio-cultural model is the Tripartite Influence Model (Thompson et al., 1999). This model suggests that the effects of peers, parents, and media are mediated by thin ideal internalization and social comparison. There is research with boys and girls as well as with college-age women that supports this model (e.g., Coomber & King, 2008; Keery, van den Berg, & Thompson, 2004; Smolak & Stein, 2006). Jones (2004) reported that appearance social comparisons predicted body dissatisfaction among adolescent girls, while commitment to muscular ideals predicted body dissatisfaction in boys. Research also supports a direct influence of thin ideal internalization and appearance schema on body dissatisfaction (Clark & Tiggemann, 2008).

The treatment of these factors as mediators of the relationship between socio-cultural influences and body dissatisfaction means that the theorists and researchers are arguing that the socio-cultural factors actually create the individual characteristics. For example, media and parent comments about weight and shape might be seen as actually shaping appearance schemas (Sinton & Birch, 2006) or thin ideal internalization (Groesz et al., 2002). Thus, prevention programs might try to target socio-cultural factors in order to decrease the likelihood that the mediators will develop. If, however, the mediating characteristics are already in place, as is likely among adolescents and adults, then attempts to reduce the mediators themselves might be a more effective approach.

Moderators, on the other hand, are variables that define groups that are assumed to be differentially affected by risk or protective variables. Gender and ethnicity are commonly treated as moderators. Particular genomes may also be treated as moderators. Gender and ethnicity are often treated as fixed risk or protective variables, although this tendency may not appropriately represent the complexity of these constructs (see Chapter 8 in this volume). If moderators are identified, they may be useful in tailoring prevention programs to various audiences.

Cultural Factors

Prevention programs generally focus on giving girls tools to critique and resist media, parent, and peer influences. This process reflects the bias of many psychologists that body image and disordered eating are the problems of individuals. Thus, this review has emphasized individual problem behaviours. Alternatively, ecological theorists argue that the context within which problems develop is important. This is the distinction between "causes of cases" and "causes of incidence" (see Piran, 2010, for a discussion of how this distinction applies to eating disorders). While "causes of cases" focus on what leads an individual to develop a disorder, "causes of incidence" seek to explain why certain groups may be more susceptible to a particular disorder. Shared life experiences of groups may increase or decrease their risk for problem behaviours. Given the consistent gender differences in body image and disordered eating as well as the common finding that Black girls and women are more body satisfied than other ethnic groups (Grabe & Hyde, 2006), gender and ethnicity may both hold important implications for prevention programs.

Gender

Gender and ethnicity represent broad cultural values and experiences. It is a mistake to think of these "macro-factors" as being uniform, fixed factors. For example, gender roles are socially defined and constructed. A variety of aspects of these roles, including investment in romance, emphasis on appearance, sexual harassment and sexual violence experiences, and career opportunities are culturally defined. All of these aspects are potentially related to body image and disordered eating (see Piran, 2010; Smolak & Murnen, 2010; Chapter 8 in this volume). Even individual level variables are best understood within the context of macro-level variables. Thus, for example, both sexual harassment and self-silencing appear to occur among both men and women. However, the meaning and implications of both of these experiences differ considerably with women being substantially more negatively affected than men are (Smolak, 2010). Long-term change and prevention of these problems will require societal-level modifications in how gender roles are constructed (Piran, 2010; Chapter 8 in this volume).

Ethnicity

Black girls and women have better body image and lower rates of dieting-related disordered eating than girls and women from other American ethnic groups (Grabe & Hyde, 2006; Levine & Smolak, 2010). No other ethnic group appears similarly protected. This may reflect the definition of attractiveness among Black communities. This definition endorses a wider range of body types as attractive and emphasizes attitude over physical characteristics in determining attractiveness. Thus, one lesson from studying ethnic group differences in body image and eating concerns is that changing the prevailing definition of attractiveness may be important in prevention programs. It also means that prevention aimed at Black girls and women will need to acknowledge the different definitions of attractiveness.

Prevention programs also need to consider other ethnic group differences in influences on body image and disordered eating. For example, in a study of South Asian-American college women, Iyer & Haslam (2003) reported that a history of being teased about ethnic issues (including, but not limited to, appearance) was indeed positively correlated with body image disturbance, even after controlling for self-esteem and BMI. Thus, experiences of discrimination should be considered in programs working with girls from ethnic minority groups. As with gender, then, ethnicity is actually a term that summarizes shared experiences. Those experiences need to be examined in order to both understand risk and protective factors and to appropriately tailor prevention programs to different ethnic minority groups.

Protective Factors

The research on factors that might reduce the likelihood of body image problems is limited. At least two potential factors have been identified: participation in certain sports and feminist identity. Smolak, Murnen, &

Ruble (2000) reported that participation in non-elite high-school sports was associated with more positive body image. Murnen & Smolak (2009) have recently documented weak relationships between feminist identity (particularly the "synthesis" stage in which feminist identity becomes integrated and women move away from thinking of men as the "enemy") and positive body image. Internalization of the thin ideal, in particular, was positively impacted by feminist identity. In a similar vein, empowering girls by giving them control to identify and resolve some of the gendered discrimination and sexist experiences they face is also associated with decreases in body dissatisfaction and disordered eating (see Chapter 8 in this volume).

Two other factors may protect against body dissatisfaction during childhood. Autonomy—the ability to resist social pressures—may protect against declining body satisfaction during childhood (Clark & Tiggemann, 2008). Second, the actual rejection of thin, sexy media images may be associated with better body image among elementary-school girls (Murnen, Smolak, Mills, & Good, 2003).

These findings underscore the importance of designing prevention programs that emphasize that girls and women are more than just attractive bodies. Investing in roles that emphasize competence and control for girls may increase the success of prevention programs. This approach may also suggest other variables that might be included in prevention efforts. The burgeoning field of positive psychology, particularly research that focuses on the development of positive body image, may also offer suggestions for protective factors (Tylka, 2011).

Conclusions

Research has established that there are a variety of biological, socio-cultural, and individual psychological risk factors for the development of body image and eating disturbances. These factors work interactively and reciprocally to create problems, although protective factors may decrease the risk of negative outcomes. Both individual and contextual factors should be considered. Prevention programs can build on this empirical information to create universal and targeted prevention programs that are at least age and gender appropriate, reflecting differences in cognitive development, self-system development, and gender role investment. The more explicit program developers are about the empirical and theoretical bases for their programs, the greater the chance that appropriate measures will be selected to evaluate programs and the more likely the programs will be successful (Levine & Smolak, 2006).

On the other hand, it is not imperative that causal models of body image or eating problems be fully explicated before successful prevention programs can be developed (Levine & Smolak, 2008). Indeed, prevention programs can provide experimental evidence of the effects of certain variables. This possibility enhances the importance and value of prevention efforts.

References

Addessi, E., Galloway, A. T., Visalberghi, E., & Birch, L. L. (2005). Specific social influences on the acceptance of novel foods in two five-year-old children. *Appetite, 45*, 264-271.

Archibald, A., Graber, J., & Brooks-Gunn, J. (1999). Associations among parent-adolescent relationships, pubertal growth, dieting, and body image among young adolescent girls. *Journal of Research on Adolescence, 9*, 395-415.

Bartlett, C. P., & Harris, R. (2008). The impact of body emphasizing video games on body image concerns in men and women. *Sex Roles, 59*, 586-601.

Bartlett, C. P., Vowels, C., & Saucier, D. (2008). Meta-analyses of the effects of media images on men's body image concerns. *Journal of Social and Clinical Psychology, 27*, 279-310.

Bearman, S. K., Presnell, K., Martinez, E., & Stice, E. (2006). The skinny on body dissatisfaction: A longitudinal study of adolescent girls and boys. *Journal of Youth and Adolescence, 35*, 229-241.

Bohon, C., & Stice, E. (2011). Reward abnormalities among women with bulimia nervosa: A functional magnetic resonance imaging study. *International Journal of Eating Disorders, 11*, 585-595.

Calogero, R. M. (2004). A test of objectification theory: The effect of the male gaze on appearance concerns in college women. *Psychology of Women Quarterly, 28*, 16-21.

Cichetti, D., & Curtis, W. J. (2006). The developing brain and neural plasticity: Implications for normality, psychopathology, and resilience. In D. Cicchetti & D. Cohen (Eds.), *Developmental psychopathology*, Volume 2: *Developmental Neuroscience* (2nd ed.; pp. 1-64). New York: Wiley.

Clark, L., & Tiggemann, M. (2008). Sociocultural and individual psychological predictors of body image in young girls: A prospective study. *Developmental Psychology, 44*, 1124-1134.

Coomber, K., & King, R. (2008). The role of sisters in body image dissatisfaction and disordered eating. *Sex Roles, 59*, 81-93.

Costanzo, P. R., & Woody, E. Z. (1985). Domain-specific parenting styles and their impact on the child's development of particular deviance: The example of obesity proneness. *Journal of Social and Clinical Psychology, 3*, 425-445.

Culbert, K., Burt, S. A., McGue, M., Iacono, W., & Klump, K. (2009). Puberty and the genetic diathesis of disordered eating attitudes and behaviors. *Journal of Abnormal Psychology, 118*, 788-796.

Cowen, P., Clifford, E., Walsh, A., Williams, C., & Fairburn, C. (1996). Moderate dieting causes 5-HT2C receptor supersensitivity. *Psychological Medicine, 26*, 1155-1159.

Dedovic, K., Wadiwalla, M., Engert, V., & Pruessner, J. (2009). The role of sex and gender socialization in stress reactivity. *Developmental Psychology, 45*, 45-55.

Field, A. E., Camargo, C. A., Jr., Taylor, C. B., Berkey, C. S., Roberts, S. B., & Colditz, G. A. (2001). Peer, parent, and media influences on the development of weight concerns and frequent dieting among preadolescent and adolescent girls and boys. *Pediatrics, 107*, 54-60.

Fisher, J., & Birch, L. (2000). Parents' restrictive feeling practices are associated with young girls' negative self-evaluation of eating. *Journal of the American Dietetic Association, 100*, 1341-1346.

Galloway, A., Fiortio, L., Francis, L., & Birch, L. (2006). "Finish your soup": Counterproductive effects of pressuring children to eat on intake and affect. *Appetite, 46*, 318-323.

Gottlieb, G. (1995). Some conceptual deficiencies in "developmental" behavioural genetics. *Human Development, 38*, 131-141.

Grabe, S., & Hyde, J. S. (2006). Ethnicity and body dissatisfaction among women in the United States: A meta-analysis. *Psychological Bulletin, 132*, 622-640.

Grabe, S., Ward, L. M., & Hyde, J. S. (2008). The role of the media in body image concerns among women: A meta-analysis of experimental and correlational studies. *Psychological Bulletin, 134*, 460-476.

Graber, J., Archibald, A. B., & Brooks-Gunn, J. (1999). The role of parents in the emergence, maintenance, and prevention of eating problems and disorders. In N. Piran, M. P. Levine, & C. Steiner-Adair (Eds.), *Preventing eating disorders: A handbook of interventions and special challenges* (pp. 44-62). Philadelphia, PA: Brunner/Mazel.

Groesz, L., Levine, M. P., & Murnen, S. K. (2002). The effect of experimental presentation of thin media images on body satisfaction. *International Journal of Eating Disorders, 31*, 1-16.

Harned, M. S. (2000). Harassed bodies: An examination of the relationships among women's experiences of sexual harassment, body image, and eating disturbances. *Psychology of Women Quarterly, 24*, 336-348.

Hayward, C. (2003). Methodological concerns in puberty-related research. In C. Hayward, K. Hurrlemann, C. Currie, & V. Rasmussen (Eds.), *Gender differences in puberty* (pp. 1-14). New York: Cambridge University Press.

Hayward, C., Killen, J., Wilson, D., Hammer, L., Litt, I., Kraemer, H., Haydel, F., Varady, A., & Taylor, C. (1997). Psychiatric risk associated with early puberty in adolescent girls. *Journal of the American Academy of Child and Adolescent Psychiatry, 36*, 255-262.

Holt, K., & Ricciardelli, L. A. (2002). Social comparisons and negative affect as indicators of problem eating and muscle preoccupation among children. *Journal of Applied Developmental Psychology, 23*, 285-304.

Iyer, D., & Haslam, N. (2003). Body image and eating disturbance among south Asian-American women: The role of racial teasing. *International Journal of Eating Disorders, 34*, 142-147.

Jacobi, C., Hayward, C., deZwaan, M., Kraemer, H., & Agras, W.S. (2004). Coming to terms with risk factors for eating disorders: Application of risk terminology and suggestions for a general taxonomy. *Psychological Bulletin, 130*, 19-65.

Jimerson, D., & Wolfe, B. (2006). Psychobiology of eating disorders. In S. Wonderlich, J. Mitchell, M. de Zwaan, & H. Steiger (Eds.), *Annual review of eating
disorders* (Part 2; pp. 1-15). Oxford: Radcliffe Publishing.

Jones, D. C. (2001). Social comparison and body image: Attractiveness comparison to models and peers among adolescent girls and boys. *Sex Roles, 45,*
645-664.

Jones, D. C. (2004). Body image among adolescent girls and boys: A longitudinal
study. *Developmental Psychology, 40,* 823-835.

Kaye, W., Frank, G., Bailer, U., & Henry, S. (2005). Neurobiology of anorexia
nervosa: Clinical implications of alterations of the function of serotonin and
other neuronal systems. *International Journal of Eating Disorders, 37,* S15-S19.

Kaye, W., Fudge, J., & Paulus, M. (2009). New insights into symptoms and neu-
rocircuit function of anorexia nervosa. *Nature Reviews of Neuroscience, 10,*
573-584,

Keery, H., van den Berg, P., & Thompson, J. K. (2004). An evaluation of the tripartite influence model of body dissatisfaction and eating disturbance with
adolescent girls. *Body Image, 1,* 237-251.

Klump, K., Burt, S. A., Spanos, A., McGue, M., Iacono, W., & Wade, T. (2010).
Age differences in genetic and environmental influences on weight and shape
concerns. *International Journal of Eating Disorders, 43,* 679-688.

Klump, K. L., Keel, P. K., Sisk, C. L., & Burt, S. A. (2010). Preliminary evidence
that estradiol moderates genetic influences on disordered eating attitudes and
behaviors during puberty. *Psychological Medicine, 40,* 1745-1753.

Klump, K., McGue, M., & Iacono, W. (2000). Age differences in genetic and environmental influences on eating attitudes and behaviors in preadolescent and
adolescent female twins. *Journal of Abnormal Psychology, 109,* 239-251.

Klump, K., McGue, M., & Iacono, W. (2003). Differential heritability of eating
attitudes and behaviors in prepubertal versus pubertal twins. *International
Journal of Eating Disorders, 33,* 287-292.

Klump, K., Susiman, J., Burt, S.A., McGue, M., & Iacono, W. (2009). Genetic and
cnvironmental influences on disordered eating: An adoption study. *Journal of
Abnormal Psychology, 118,* 797-805.

Kraemer, H., Kazdin, A., Offord, D., Kessler R., Jensen, P., & Kupler D. (1997). Coming to terms with the terms of risk. *Archives of General Psychiatry 54,* 337-343.

Larkin, J. (1994). *Sexual harassment: High school girls speak out.* Kensington, MD:
Second Story Press.

Leaper, C., & Brown, C. (2008). Perceived experiences with sexism among adolescent girls. *Child Development 79,* 685-704.

Levine, M. P., & Smolak, L. (2006). *The prevention of eating problems and eating disorders: Theory, research, and practice.* Mahwah, NJ: Lawrence Erlbaum
Associates.

Levine, M. P., & Smolak, L. (2008). "What exactly are we waiting for?": The case
for universal-selective eating disorders prevention programs. *International
Journal of Child and Adolescent Health, 1,* 295-304.

Levine, M. P., & Smolak, L. (2010) Cultural influences on body image and the eating disorders. In W. S. Agras (Ed.), *The Oxford handbook of eating disorders* (pp. 223-246). New York: Oxford University Press.

Lilenfeld, L., Wonderlich, S., Riso, L., Crosby, R., & Mitchell, J. (2006). Eating disorders and personality: A methodological and empirical review. *Clinical Psychology Review, 26,* 299-320.

Martin, C., Wertheim, E., Prior, M., Sanson, A., & Oberklaid, F. (2000). A longitudinal study of the role of childhood temperament in the later development of eating concerns. *International Journal of Eating Disorders, 27,* 150-162.

Mazzeo, S., Landt, M., van Furth, E., & Bulik, C. (2006). Genetics of eating disorders. In S. Wonderlich, J. Mitchell, M. de Zwaan, & H. Steiger (Eds.), *Annual review of eating disorders* (Part 2; pp. 17-33). Oxford: Radcliffe Publishing.

McCabe, M. P., & Ricciardelli, L. A. (2005). A longitudinal study of body image and strategies to lose weight and increase muscles among children. *Journal of Applied Developmental Psychology, 26,* 559-577.

Murnen, S. K., & Smolak, L. (2000). The experience of sexual harassment among grade-school students: Early socialization of female subordination? *Sex Roles, 43,* 1-17.

Murnen, S. K., & Smolak, L. (2009). Are feminist women protected from body image problems? A meta-analytic review of relevant research. *Sex Roles, 60,* 186-197.

Murnen, S. K., Smolak, L., Mills, J., & Good, L. (2003). Thin, sexy women and strong, muscular men: Grade-school children's responses to objectified images of women and men. *Sex Roles, 49,* 427-437.

Myers, T., & Crowther, J. (2009). Social comparison as a predictor of body dissatisfaction: A meta-analytic review. *Journal of Abnormal Psychology, 118,* 683-698.

Nichter, M. (2000). *Fat talk: What girls and their parents say about dieting.* Cambridge, MA: Harvard University Press.

Nickel, C., Tritt, K., Muehlbacher, M., Pedrosa, F., Mitterlehner, F. O., Kaplan, P., … Nickel, M. (2005). Topiramate treatment in bulimia nervosa patients: A randomized, double-blind, placebo-controlled trial. *International Journal of Eating Disorders, 38,* 295-300.

O'Dea, J., & Abraham, S. (2000). Improving the body image, eating attitudes and behaviors of young male and female adolescents: A new educational approach which focuses on self-esteem. *International Journal of Eating Disorders, 28,* 43-57.

Ohring, R., Graber, J. A., & Brooks-Gunn, J. (2002). Girls' recurrent and concurrent body dissatisfaction: Correlates and consequences over eight years. *International Journal of Eating Disorders, 31,* 404-415.

Paxton, S., Eisenberg, M., & Neumark-Sztainer, D. (2006). Prospective predictors of body dissatisfaction in adolescent girls and boys: A five-year longitudinal study. *Developmental Psychology, 42,* 888-899.

Peterson, R., Tantleff-Dunn, S., & Bedwell, J. (2006). The effects of exposure to feminist ideology on women's body image. *Body Image, 3,* 237-246.

Phares, V., Steinberg, A. R., & Thompson, J. K. (2004). Gender differences in peer and parental influences: Body image disturbance, self-worth, and psychological functioning in preadolescent children. *Journal of Youth and Adolescence, 33,* 421-429.

Piran, N. (1999). The reduction of preoccupation with body weight and shape in schools: A feminist approach. In N. Piran, M. P. Levine, & C. Steiner-Adair (Eds.), *Preventing eating disorders: A handbook of interventions and special challenges* (pp. 148-159). Philadelphia, PA: Brunner/Mazel.

Piran, N. (2001). Re-inhabiting the body from the inside out: Girls transform their school environment. In D. Tolman & M. Brydon-Miller (Eds.), *From subjects to subjectivities: A handbook of interpretive and participatory methods* (pp. 218-238). New York: New York University Press.

Piran, N. (2010). A feminist perspective on risk factor research and on the prevention of eating disorders. *Eating Disorders: Journal of Treatment and Prevention, 18,* 183-198.

Piran, N., & Thompson, S. (2008). A study of the adverse social experiences model to the development of eating disorders. *International Journal of Health Promotion and Education, 46,* 65-71.

Puhl, R., & Latner, J. (2007). Sigma, obesity, and the health of the nation's children. *Psychological Bulletin, 133,* 557-580.

Roberts, A., Cash, T. F., Feingold, A., & Johnson, B. T. (2006). Are black-white differences in females' body dissatisfaction decreasing? A meta-analytic review. *Journal of Consulting and Clinical Psychology, 74,* 1121-1131.

Rutter, M. (2003). Genetic influences on risk and protection: Implications for understanding resilience. In S. S. Luthar (Ed.), *Resilience and vulnerability: Adaptation in the context of childhood adversities* (pp. 489-509). New York: Cambridge University Press.

Rutter, M., & the English and Romanian Adoptees Study Team (1998). Developmental catch-up and deficit, following adoption after severe global early privation. *Journal of Child Psychology and Psychiatry, 39,* 465-476.

Sanftner, J. L., Crowther, J. H., Crawford, P. A., & Watts, D. D. (1996). Maternal influences (or lack thereof) on daughters' eating attitudes and behaviors. *Eating Disorders: Journal of Treatment and Prevention, 4,* 147-159.

Schmidt, A., & Georgieff, M. (2006). Early nutritional deficiencies in brain development: Implications for psychopathology. In D. Cicchetti & D. Cohen (Eds.), *Developmental psychopathology,* Volume 2: *Developmental Neuroscience* (pp. 1-64). New York: Wiley.

Shisslak, C., & Crago, M. (2001). Risk and protective factors in the development of eating disorders. In J. K. Thompson & L. Smolak (Eds.), *Body image, eating disorders, and obesity in youth: Assessment, prevention, and treatment* (pp. 103-126). Washington, DC: American Psychological Association.

Sinton, M. M., & Birch, L.L. (2006). Individual and sociocultural influences on pre-adolescent girls' appearance schemas and body dissatisfaction. *Journal of Youth and Adolescence, 35,* 165-175.

Smolak, L. (2009). Risk factors in the development of body image, eating disorders, and obesity. In L. Smolak & J. K. Thompson (Eds.), *Body image, eating disorders and obesity in youth: Assessment, prevention, and treatment* (2nd ed., pp. 135-156). Washington, DC: American Psychological Association.

Smolak, L. (2010). Gender and self-silencing. In D. C. Jack & A. Ali (Eds.), *Cultural perspectives on women's depression: Self-silencing, psychological distress, and recovery* (pp. 129-146). New York: Oxford.

Smolak, L., Levine, M. P., & Schermer, F. (1999). Parental input and weight concerns among elementary school children. *International Journal of Eating Disorders, 25,* 263-271.

Smolak, L., & Murnen, S. K. (2008). Drive for leanness: Assessment and relationship to gender, gender role and objectification. *Body Image: International Journal of Research, 5,* 251-260.

Smolak, L., & Murnen, S. K. (2011). The sexualization of girls and women as antecedents of self-objectification. In R. Calogero, S. Tantleff-Dunn, & J. K. Thompson (Eds.), *Self-Objectification in women: Causes, consequences, and directions for research and practice* (pp. 53-76). Washington, DC: American Psychological Association.

Smolak, L., Murnen, S. K., & Ruble, A. (2000). Female athletes and eating disorders: A meta-analysis. *International Journal of Eating Disorders, 27,* 371-381.

Smolak, L., & Stein, J.A. (2006). The relationship of drive for muscularity to sociocultural actors, self-esteem, physical attributes gender role, and social comparison in middle school boys. *Body Image, 3,* 121-129.

Steiger, H. (2004). Eating disorders and the serotonin connection: State, trait and developmental effects. *Journal of Psychiatry Neuroscience, 29,* 20-29.

Stice, E. (1994). Review of the evidence for a socio-cultural model of bulimia nervosa and an exploration of the mechanisms of action. *Clinical Psychology Review, 14,* 633-661.

Stice, E. (2002). Risk and maintenance factors for eating pathology: A meta-analytic review. *Psychological Bulletin, 128,* 825-848.

Stice, E., Shaw, H., & Nemeroff, C. (1998). A longitudinal test of the dual pathway model of bulimia nervosa. *Journal of Social and Clinical Psychology, 17,* 129-149.

Suisman, J., & Klump, K. (2011). Genetic and neuroscientific perspectives on body image. In T. F. Cash & L. Smolak (Eds.), *Body Image: A handbook of science, practice, and prevention* (2nd ed., pp. 29-38). New York: Guilford.

Thompson, J. K., Heinberg, L., Altabe, M., & Tantleff-Dunn, S. (1999) *Exacting beauty: Theory, assessment, and treatment of body image disturbance.* Washington, DC: American Psychological Association.

Tylka, T. (2011). Positive psychology perspectives on body image. In T. Cash & L. Smolak (Eds.), *Body image: A handbook of science, practice, and prevention* (2nd ed., pp. 56-66). New York: Guilford Press.

Walsh, A., Oldman, A., Franklin, M., Fairburn, C., & Cowan, P. (1995). Dieting decreases plasma tryptophan and increases the prolactin response to *d*-fenfluramine in women but not men. *Journal of Affective Disorders, 33,* 89-97.

Want, S. (2009). Meta-analytic moderators of experimental exposure to media portrayals of women on female appearance satisfaction: Social comparisons as automatic processes. *Body Image: International Journal of Research, 6,* 257-269.

Watkins, B., & Lask, B. (2009). Defining eating disorders in children. In L. Smolak & J. K. Thompson (Eds.), *Body image, eating disorders, and obesity in youth: Assessment, prevention, and treatment* (2nd ed., pp. 35-46). Washington, DC: American Psychological Association.

Weibe, S., Espy, K., Stopp, C., Respass, J., Stewart P., Jameson, T., Gilbert, D., & Huggenvik, J. (2009). Gene-environment interactions across development: Exploring DRD2 genotype and prenatal smoking effects on self-regulation. *Developmental Psychology, 45,* 31-44.

Wertheim, E. H., Martin, G., Prior, M., Sanson, A., & Smart, D. (2002). Parent influences in the transmission of eating and weight related values and behaviors. *Eating Disorders: Journal of Treatment and Prevention, 10,* 321-334.

Wertheim, E., Paxton, S., & Blaney, S. (2009). Body image in girls. In L. Smolak & J. K. Thompson (Eds.), *Body image, eating disorders, and obesity in youth: Assessment, prevention, and treatment* (2nd ed., pp. 47-76). Washington, DC: American Psychological Association.

White, H. S. (2005). Molecular pharmacology of topiramate: Managing seizures and preventing migraine. *Headache, 45,* S48-S56.

CHAPTER SEVEN

The Developmental Theory of Embodiment

Niva Piran, *Ontario Institute for Studies in Education, University of Toronto*
Tanya Teall, *Ontario Institute for Studies in Education, University of Toronto*

Embodiment has been a construct developed and discussed mostly in the disciplines of philosophy and critical sociology. A definition of the construct, rooted in the writings of Merleau-Ponty (1962) and his students, that is in line with this chapter is the "experience of engagement of the body with the world" (Allan, 2005, p. 177). This definition reflects not only the breadth of possible subjectively perceived embodied experiences but also their inextricable connection to social contexts and structures. This chapter aims to describe the potential contribution of the theoretical construct of Embodiment in understanding disordered eating and body weight and shape preoccupation. It also aims to delineate the innovative Developmental Theory of Embodiment (DTE) by Piran and her associates (Piran, Carter, Thompson, & Pajouhandeh, 2002; Piran et al., 2007; Piran, Thompson, Legge, Nagasawa, & Teall, 2009), which is located at the intersection of the disciplines of psychology and sociology. This theory proposes that social experiences shape individuals' body experiences through three core pathways: experiences in the physical domain, experiences in the mental domain involving exposure to dominant social labels and expectations, and experiences related to social power. The theory further contends that both protective and risk factors are organized along these three pathways, and, hence, in addition to its etiological significance, the theory could guide both therapy and prevention of eating disorders.

The chapter is divided into two central parts. The first part, entitled the Embodiment Construct and Its Relevance to Eating Disorders, begins with current delineations of the construct of embodiment within the disciplines of philosophy and critical sociology where it has originated. It then continues with a discussion of the relevance of this construct to mental health generally and to eating disorders specifically. The second part, entitled The Developmental Theory of Embodiment, describes the research program leading to the emergence and validation of the theory as well as key constructs of the theory. The conclusion section addresses implications of this theory to treatment and prevention.

The Embodiment Construct and Its Relevance to Eating Disorders

The Embodiment Construct in the Disciplines of Philosophy and Critical Sociology

Current descriptions of the construct of embodiment are anchored in the writings of the French phenomenological philosopher Merleau-Ponty. Merleau-Ponty (1962, p. 281) advanced the understanding of the construct of embodiment by giving rise to the notion of the "lived body" and asserted that consciousness, or human subjectivity, resides in the body. Thus, in contrast with the conceptualization of the mind-body relationship presented by the French philosopher René Descartes in the seventeenth century, who considered mind and body to be distinct from one another and the mind as being superior to the body (Bordo, 1993), Merleau-Ponty's phenomenological position suggested that the mind and body were equivalent, intertwined, and inseparable (Csordas, 1994; Howe, 2003). Furthermore, Merleau-Ponty argued that the body should be considered not only a physical object in the world that is seen and touched by others but also a subjective site that senses and experiences the world meaningfully (Crossley, 1995). As elaborated by Crossley (1995, p. 47), "the body's being-in-the-world is at once mediated through physical presence and perceptual meaning." The term of embodiment therefore became a common term for referring to a state of connection between the mind and the body. For example, Young (1992, p. 90) has described embodiment as the way in which the self "is experienced in and through the body." Morse and Mitcham (1998, p. 668) also considered embodiment to be a "summary term for all aspects of human subjectivity."

In addition to considering the body as the site of human subjectivity, and to seeing the mind and body as inseparable, Merleau-Ponty considered the body to be in a continual dialectical relationship with the social context. As Allan (2005, p. 176) elaborates, Merleau-Ponty's view was that "the body is neither objective nor subjective because it is continually, mutually constructed through perception in each particular social and cultural context." For example, the "body" of a girl who just immigrated to a country where she would be classified as a member of a specific visible minority, an appearance associated with negative social projections by the dominant social group as well as one that exposes her to prejudicial treatment, is different from her pre-immigration "body." This view has been supported by others (Butler, 1988; Rehorick, 1986). Considering this dialectical relationship between body and culture, Allan (2005, p. 177) defined embodiment as the "perceptual experience of engagement of the body in the world."

Embodied experiences at the intersection of body and culture have been a focus of discussion in social critical theory, which has seen the body as a site that both reproduces culture and holds the promise for its transformation. In particular, Foucault (1979), a student of Merleau-Ponty, has added to the construct of embodiment through his discussion of power in modern societies and his description of the "docile body." While, traditionally, "power was embodied in the person of the monarch and exercised upon a largely anonymous body of subjects" (Bartky, 1997, p. 147) in modern society power is anonymous, acting from the "bottom up" through widely disseminated and accepted social expectations with which individual citizens are expected to comply in order to avoid adverse social processes, such as rules regarding gender or social class. In this way, for example, girls post-puberty are encouraged to act "nice" (Brown, 1998; Piran et al., 2009) and are discouraged from looking muscular through social labeling such as "butch" or from expressing agency in sexual desire through social labelling such as "slut" (Piran et al., 2007, 2009). As individual citizens discipline their own bodies to conform to the expectations of their social institutions—for example, girls acting "nice," seeking a smaller body size, or restricting sexual behaviour that responds to their own desire, they produce "docile bodies." Feminist writers, therefore, have emphasized "those disciplines that produce a modality of embodiment that is peculiarly feminine" (Bartky, 1997, p. 132) related to gender oppression. Foucault's discussion of power in modern societies helps explain the willingness with which women engage in objectifying activities and subject themselves to social control (Bordo, 1997). Moreover, the "blind" nature of this disciplinary power makes it difficult to resist and challenge, as Bartky (1997, p. 142) states, "the disciplinary power that inscribes femininity in the female body is everywhere and it is nowhere; the disciplinarian is everyone and yet it is no one in particular." Bordo (1997, p. 91) has warned that it is these disciplining practices that continually make women feel the "conviction of lack, of insufficiency, of never being good enough. At the farthest extremes, the practices of femininity may lead us to utter demoralization, debilitation, and death."

Objectification Theory (Fredrickson & Roberts, 1997) is a more recently articulated theory that is in line with several of the key constructs of Foucault's theory. According to the Objectification Theory, women learn to appraise their body from an outsider's, typically male, gaze, and they internalize this dominant gaze. Fredrickson and Roberts (1997, p. 175) explained that "always present in contexts of sexualized gazing is the potential for sexual objectification...when objectified, women are treated as bodies—and in particular, as bodies that exist for the use and pleasure of others." Consequently, due to their awareness of gaze, women learn to practice self-surveillance as a way of monitoring one's appearance so that one presents in a way that is acceptable to the outsider that observes and evaluates their appearance. The concept of self-surveillance is akin to that described by Foucault previously, as a powerful force where previous experiences of gaze, and the knowledge of the possibility of gaze, teaches the individual to self-monitor, thereby leading to strict body control. Furthermore, Objectification Theory acknowledges that women focus on their appearance, not due to superficiality but, rather, as a learned strategy to cope with and achieve more social power in an objectifying culture that heavily emphasizes feminine beauty and comportment (Fredrickson & Roberts, 1997; Roberts & Waters, 2004).

The Constructs of Embodiment and Body Image in Relation to Disordered Eating and Other Indicators of Mental Well-Being

The authors of this chapter suggest that the construct of "embodiment" may expand the understanding of eating disorders and related mental health issues beyond the construct of body image. In her extensive review of the development of the body image construct, Dionne (2002) describes the perceptual and attitudinal components of body image. The perceptual component refers to "the awareness or knowledge about the shape, size or form of the body" (p. 13). The attitudinal component of body image, or affective/emotional component, refers to "the view of the body as being pleasing or displeasing" (Dionne, 2002, p. 13). The construct of embodiment, defined in this chapter as the "experience of engagement of the body with the world" (Allan, 2005, p. 177) differs from body image in several important ways: its breadth, its inner focus, and the nature of the dialectical relationship with the social context. In terms of breadth, the embodiment construct represents a range of experiences from positive experiences of embodied agency, self-care, joy, attunement with the body, and functionality (Piran, Carter, Thompson, & Pajouhandeh, 2002), to multiple disruptions in embodiment, such as negative body image (Blood, 2005), dissociation (Briere, Kaltman, & Green, 2008), or alexithymia (Taylor, Bagby, & Parker, 1991), which is a range not addressed by the body image construct. Further, the construct of embodiment can address the range of co-existing behavioural disruptions that seem to occur more commonly in girls and women, such as a reduced experience of competence and involvement in physical activities (Biddle, 1993; Richman & Shaffer, 2000; Bradley, McMurray, Harrell, & Deng, 2000; Falgairette, Deflandre, & Gavarry, 2004), sexual involvement without negotiating for protection and without desire (e.g., Tolman, 1994), higher rates of self-harm (Rohde, Lewinson, & Seeley, 1991), or the association of disordered eating patterns with the consumption of substances that are unrelated to obtaining a thin body shape (Gadalla & Piran, 2007; Piran & Gadalla, 2006). The construct of embodiment can therefore address a larger range of issues related to women's health and well-being.

Second, the embodiment construct as a site of human subjectivity anchored in sensory perception and awareness reflects an inside-out perspective in contrast to the construct of body image, which entails an evaluation of oneself from the outside and therefore reflects the internalization of the external gaze towards one's body. That is, while there are varied definitions for the construct of body image, including those that address a perceptual component (awareness or knowledge of body shape), a focus of body image literature is on the attitudinal component (one's view towards the body, which implies an evaluative gaze) (Dionne, 2002). This internalization of the external gaze may be considered a disruptive experience to one's positive embodiment (even when body image is positive) as it implies an objectified perspective of the body. For example, Blood (2005) critiqued research that aimed to provide a quantitative measurement of one's body image as a way of better understanding women's relationships to their bodies and urged more work to be done in the area of embodiment. She explained that "an alternative approach to knowing and experiencing one's body emphasizes the cultivation of 'inner' bodily awareness. Developing an awareness of feeling states and physiological states is crucial in learning to 'live in' or fully inhabit one's body" (Blood, 2005, p. 125). Example of scales that emphasize an awareness of internal states, rather than scales that evaluate the body, are the Toronto Alexithymia Scale (Taylor et al., 1991), which evaluates the capacity to identify internal experiences and feelings and communicate them to other people, and the Body Awareness Scale (Shields, Mallory, & Simon, 1989), which assesses body awareness and responsiveness to bodily sensations. These scales assess the attunement to internal body experiences described by Blood as an aspect of embodiment.

Further, the construct of body image cannot explain the multiple phenomena in the field of eating disorders that would indicate disruption in the experience of engagement of the body with the world, which is our working definition of embodiment. For example, Katzman and Lee (1997) discussed both case studies and larger clinical group studies where women presenting with anorexic patterns discussed how their self-starvation was not motivated by the pursuit of thinness or any disruption with body image. In other words, self-starvation was not in any way related to body image but, instead, related to a lived experience of restricted agency. Similarly, disruption in the experience of engagement of the body with the world, and not negative body image, may explain the development of disordered eating patterns following body violation. For example, Legge (in press) described the case of an adolescent girl sexually harassed by a gang of adolescent boys who starved herself every school year in order to "disappear" from the eyes of her tormentors. This girl did not exhibit a distorted body image; rather she hoped to "disengage" her body from the world in the context of uncontrolled violations. Further, both clinical observations and research document a range of behavioural disruptions, unrelated to negative body image, associated with eating disorders, such as self-harm (Favazza, DeRosear, & Conterio, 1989; Sansone & Levitt, 2004) or the consumption of multiple substances not associated with obtaining particular body shapes or starvation (Gadalla & Piran, 2007). An example would be a survivor of sexual abuse whose body becomes an inhabitable site and who engages in multiple self-harm behaviours, including disordered eating (Young, 1992). Young described disembodiment as an understandable, highly probable, result from experiences of sexual trauma. Young (1992, p. 90) explains:

> The dilemma of the survivor of severe sexual abuse could be formulated this way: How do I live with (but not in?) a dangerous, damaged or dead body? In addition, how do I continue to live in "the body" of a family or a world that is equally dangerous, damaged, or dead? So a child experiencing severe sexual abuse, seemingly faced with physical and psychological annihilation, may abandon the body, make it "outside me," pretend it doesn't exist or turn on it in anger and confusion.

Young (1992) noted that, following abuse, multiple self-harm behaviours, such as substance abuse, eating disorders, dissociative disorders, and depression, relate to a disembodied state of being, whereby the disembodiment allows the victim a degree of control and protection. However, she also acknowledges how this coping mechanism entails a high cost, as "such a solution entails an enormous sacrifice, since it also makes problematic experiencing the everyday pleasures, sensations and comforts of human embodiment" (p. 93). Interestingly, the academic and clinical study of eating disorders since the mid-1900s, spearheaded by Hilde Bruch (1962), started with an emphasis on the disruption of body awareness rather than on body image. For example, Bruch speculated that anorexia could occur due to a severe "falsification of body awareness," such that the individual feels "that he does not own his body, and that he is not in control of its functions" (p. 193).

Third, while body image is considered to emanate from external appraisals of the body by others, the construct of embodiment reflects the complexity of the body culture relation. In particular, embodiment entails an ongoing construction of the experience of the embodied self through meaningful interactions with complex social structures, such as patriarchy (Bordo, 1993). The construct of embodiment, therefore, may reflect disruptions at the intersection of body and culture where the construct of body image may be less relevant. For example, Katzman and Lee (1997), who hold a cross-cultural perspective to eating disorders, were critical of an exclusive body image perspective as it relates to disordered eating. In summarizing and discussing their results, the authors claim that "by construing anorexia nervosa as a body image disorder or Western culturebound syndrome, extant models miss the broader contexts and varied meanings of food refusal. The implications of cross-disciplinary perspectives for theory building and treatment are discussed, acknowledging not only the gendered nature of eating disorders but their embodiment of power differentials as well" (p. 385).

Katzman and Lee (1997, p. 385) further claim that "such conceptualizations have been criticized for overvaluing sexism at the exclusion of other societal systems of oppression such as poverty, immigration, and heterosexism and for academic myopia as the focus of theorizing is often white, Western, middle-class women." They have discussed the clinical presentation of disordered eating in a group of rural Chinese women and highlighted how "feelings of powerlessness, oppression, and experience of sexual abuse are reported, but fat phobia is not" (p. 390) and argue that such women were as distressed as those who have negative body image who meet the full criteria for an eating disorder. Therefore, these authors consider the construct of embodiment to be more inclusive of the multiple and diverse disruptions that individuals may have in the body domain in relation to varied social conditions. Such a perspective is advantageous as societies become increasingly diverse and culturally integrated.

The Developmental Theory of Embodiment: Program of Research and Key Constructs

To date, there is no research-based developmental theory of embodiment that bridges between the "body" as seen through the lens of social critical theory and the embodied experiences of individuals in the process of development, hence linking the domains of sociology and psychology. In particular, while the past 20 years have seen a surge in qualitative studies examining the domain of the "self" in pre- and post-pubertal girls of varied social locations, documenting both the observed appropriations of, and the resistances to, dominant social ideologies and structures (e.g., Brown, 1998; Gilligan, 1991; Taylor, Gilligan, & Sullivan, 1995), the domain of the developing experience of the "body" has not been similarly explored or integrated with inquiries of the "self," likely due to Western dualistic thinking (Bordo, 1993). The Developomental Theory of Embodiment is a developmental theory that has relied on multiple methodologies in its development and validation (Piran et al., 2002, 2009).

Program of Research
To date, the Developmental Theory of Embodiment is based on a mixed-method research program (Jick, 1979) spanning the past 20 years, utilizing the strengths of qualitative approaches in the emergence of innovative constructs and in the detailed consideration of complex contexts within which phenomena occur as well as the strengths of quantitative approaches, such as structural equation models, in validating emergent models. The research program completed to date can be divided into two broad phases with separate stages within each phase.

Phase 1: The Emergence and Validation of a Three-Pathway Risk Factor Model: The Adverse Social Experiences Model (ASEM) for the Development of Eating Disorders
This mixed methodology program of research (see Stages I-V), which has used both a qualitative participatory action research approach as well as quantitative survey data, has led to the emergence and cross-validation of ASEM in the development of eating disorders (Piran, 2001; Piran & Thompson, 2008; Piran & Cormier, 2005). This model suggests that adverse social experiences occur along three pathways in the physical (Violation of Body Ownership), mental (Internalization of Constraining Social Labels), and social power (Exposure to Prejudicial Treatment) domains (see Figure 1).

Stage I: Participatory action research project   This 15-year-long project involved the analysis of themes (Miles & Huberman, 1994) collected from over 300 focus groups with students conducted as part of a prevention program conducted at a competitive residential ballet school (Piran, 2001). Separating into gender-cohesive and age-cohesive groups, these focus groups explored factors in the school environment that students found to adversely affect their body experiences at the school. Similarly, all actions

FIGURE 1: ADVERSE SOCIAL EXPERIENCES MODEL (ASEM)

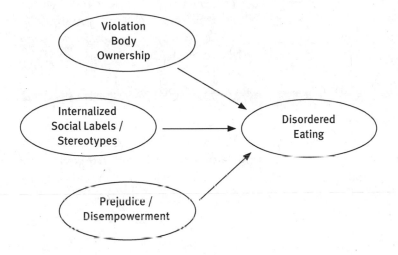

Adapted from Piran 2001; Piran & Cormier, 2005; Piran & Thompson, 2008.

that the students pursued in their school environment were analyzed for themes. The hierarchical thematic analysis of the focus groups' content led to the emergence of three main content categories of adverse social experiences: Violation of Body Ownership (physical domain), Internalization of Constraining Social Labels (mental or social construction domain), and Exposure to Prejudicial Treatment (social power domain) (Piran, 2001). This innovative three-pathway model, ASEM (Piran, 2001; Piran & Cormier; Piran & Thompson, 2008) was based on the content of the focus groups and on transformative actions by the students, and it included a broader range of social experiences than typically addressed in existing social models of eating disorders. The participatory action research project was associated with significant changes in the prevalence of disordered eating patterns at the school (Piran, 1999).

Stage II: Testing ASEM—a structural equation modelling study in a university sample   This study aimed to test the model in which the latent variables Violation of Body Ownership and Exposure to Prejudicial Treatment were hypothesized to exert a direct influence on the development of disordered eating patterns (Piran & Thompson, 2008). In total, 436 university students, ages 18 to 25 (56% European, 27% Asian, and 17% other heritages), completed the Sexual Victimization of Children Survey (Finkelhore, 1979), the conflict Tactics Scale (Strauss, 1979), the Sexual Experiences

Questionnaire (Fitzgerald, Gelfand, & Drasgow, 1995), the Weight Harassment Scale (Piran & Thompson, 2008), the Eating Attitude Test (Garner, Olmsted, Bohr, & Garfinkel, 1982), and behavioural items pertaining to dieting, bingeing, vomiting, the use of laxatives and diet pills derived from the Diagnostic Survey for Eating Disorders (Johnson, 1985). The Violation of Body Ownership was assessed using measures of childhood sexual abuse, childhood physical abuse, adult sexual coercion, and adult exposure to unwanted sexual attention. The Exposure to Prejudicial Treatment was assessed using the measures of gender harassment and weight harassment. Using structural equation modelling (Lisrel 8.51 program) (Jöreskog & Sörbom, 1993) to derive the estimated model, standardized parameters indicated that all paths were significant and the modification indices indicated no need to consider additional paths and all fit indices indicated an excellent fit for the model.

Stage III: Testing ASEM—a structural equation modelling study in a community sample   This study aimed to cross-validate the results of the survey with university students, using the same methodology (Piran & Thompson, 2008). The community sample consisted of 341 women, ages 18 to 25 living in the same city. Of these women, 67.2% self-identified as European and 15.8% self-identified as Asian. The university and community samples differed significantly in terms of ethnic group membership, age, paternal education, and percentage living with parents or with partners. Using the full sample to derive the estimated model, standardized parameters indicated that all paths were significant and modification indices indicated no need to consider additional paths. The fit indices indicated an excellent fit for the model.

Stage IV: Testing ASEM—a multiple-sample analysis comparing the university and community models   A structural model was estimated for multiple-sample analyses to determine model comparability across samples, using the same fit indexes (Piran & Thompson, 2008). In multiple-sample comparisons, the equivalence of the factor structure in both the university and community samples was tested first by allowing parameters to be freely estimated for each sample. Next, model fit was assessed after constraining all parameter estimates to be invariant across samples, thus testing for equality of factor loadings and structural paths in the two groups. Fit statistics for the multiple-sample models indicated an excellent fit for the single model across both samples. Further, the similarity in factor structure and factor loadings in two different samples indicates the stability of the model.

Stage V: Studying the "internalization of constraining social labels" pathway of ASEM—a multiple regression study of the relationship between the internalization by young women of discourses of femininity and disordered eating patterns   In this survey, 394 women from the community completed the Silencing the Self Scale (Jack & Dill, 1992), the State-Trait Anger Expression Inventory (Spielberger, 1996), and the Objectified Body Consciousness Scale (McKinley & Hyde, 1996). Self-silencing of needs and voice, the suppression of the outward expression of anger, and the internalization of the objectified gaze towards one's own body were found, in multiple regression analyses, to significantly predict scores on eating disorder measures (Piran & Cormier, 2005). Together, they explain between 27% and 46% of the variance on these measures. This study supported the need to consider the development of disordered eating within the context of multiple gender-based social constructions.

Phase 2: The Emergence and Validation a Three-Pathway Risk and Protective Developmental Model: The Developmental Theory of Embodiment
The second phase of this program of research aimed to address limitations in Phase 1, specifically the need to further understand the relationship between eating disorders and other disruptions in the body domain, the lack of developmental data, and the exclusive emphasis on risk factors (see, e.g., Piran et al., 2002, 2007, 2009; Piran & Gadalla, 2006). This phase has led to the emergence of the Developmental Theory of Embodiment, which

FIGURE 2: THE DEVELOPMENTAL THEORY OF EMBODIMENT (DTE)

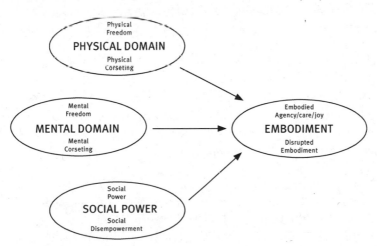

Source: Adapted from Piran et al., 2002, 2007, 2009.

incorporates both risk and protective factors and has led to the emergence of the key research constructs of Embodiment, Body Journey, Physical Freedom (versus Physical Corseting), Mental Freedom (versus Mental Corseting), and Social Power (versus Social Disempowerment) (see Figure 2) (Piran et al., 2002, 2007, 2009). While the specific research projects, and related methodologies, leading to the second phase of the emergence and validation of this theory are described in this section, the theory and its key constructs are described in the next section of this chapter. Importantly, the three pathways of risk factors in the physical, mental, and social power domains, which emerged in Phase 1 were found to emerge as well in the three research projects of Phase 2, suggesting important theoretical convergence (Jick, 1979) (see Figures 1 and 2).

Stage VI: Emergence of the Developmental Theory of Embodiment—a life history qualitative study with young women   The life history approach to qualitative methodology emphasizes the exploration of social-contextual factors in the telling and understanding of life stories as well as the engagement of participants as active co-creators of emergent understandings through a series of dialogical interviews (Piran et al., 2002, 2007, 2009). The life history study involved a total of 30 interviews with eleven women, ages 18 to 27 (three interviews with most women), of diverse backgrounds recruited through community-based advertisements. The inquiry focused on these women's body, self, and related social experiences throughout their lives. The first interview tended to centre on early childhood, childhood, and adolescence, while the second interview continued with this chronological exploration to the present. Detailed hierarchical theme analysis by a team of four researchers led to the emergence of key constructs and structures of the Developmental Theory of Embodiment (Piran et al., 2002) (see next section of this chapter). In order to validate the emergent theory with the participants, a detailed delineation of the general emergent theory, as well as a detailed developmental life story of each participant organized according to the theoretical constructs, were composed and sent to participants prior to the third interview in order to check the validity of the emergent theory. This process of member checking strongly supported the relevance of the theory to their lives (Piran, 2006).

Stage VII: Towards a quantitative validation of the Developmental Theory of Embodiment—the development and validation of the Embodiment Scale for Women: A psychometric study   This project aimed at deriving a quantitative measure of the key constructs of the Developmental Theory of Embodiment, entitled the Embodiment Scale for Women (ESW) (Teall,

2006; Piran & Teall, 2006). Similar to other studies that have developed quantitative scales from qualitative narratives (see, for example, the development of the Silencing the Self Scale from a qualitative study with depressed women Jack & Dill, 1992), subscale items were derived from lower-level themes that were included under the higher-level core constructs in the hierarchical thematic analysis. Wording of items was matched as closely as possible to participants' expressions. The first psychometric study of the scale with one hundred women yielded information regarding its reliability and validity and provided initial quantitative support for the key constructs that emerged in the life history study with young women. The ESW has four subscales, corresponding with four key constructs of the Developmental Theory of Embodiment. The first subscale is entitled the "Experience of Embodiment," reflecting the "experience of engagement of the body with the world" (Allan, 2005, p. 177). Examples of the items included in this scale are: "I have cared more about how my body feels than about how it looks," "I feel at one with my body," or "My body has made me feel depressed/anxious." The "Experience of Embodiment" Subscale has 48 items, was found to have a Cronbach's alpha of .93, and, as predicted, was significantly correlated with the Toronto Alexithymia Scale (r = −.55) (Bagby et al., 1994), the Body Esteem Scale (r = .78) (Mendelson, Mendelson, & White, 2001), and the EAT-26 (r = −.45) (Garner, Olmsted, Bohr, & Garfinkel, 1982). A second subscale of the ESW, entitled "Physical Freedom," addresses the experiences in the physical domain that have enhanced individuals' sense of physical competence and ownership over the body, such as: "I have a strong sense of ownership over my body," "I have engaged in body-based practices (such as yoga, karate, massage, meditation) that have helped me connect with my body in a more positive way"), or "There has been physical violence in my home." This scale has 56 items and was found to have a Cronbach's alpha of .84. As hypothesized, the scale had a strong negative correlation with the Self-Surveillance Scale of the Objectified Body Consciousness Scale (r = −.57). The third subscale of the ESW, entitled "Mental Freedom," includes items that assess the impact of social expectations and labels on one's embodied experience, such as "I have felt that being physically strong conflicts with being a girl/woman," "Different stereotypes about the female gender (e.g., tomboygirlie girl, slut-prude, bitchy-nice) have been a source of stress for me," or "I have been encouraged to think critically about different social pressures that I have experienced." This scale has 37 items and was found to have a Cronbach's alpha of .93 and, as predicted, to be correlated significantly with the Self-Acceptance Subscale of the How I See Myself Scale (r = .50) (Ryff, 1989). The fourth subscale of the ESW, entitled "Social Power," addresses experiences of social empowerment and disempowerment and includes items such as "People who have shared important characteristics with me, such as race, ethnic group membership or gender, have taken pride in our shared group membership," "Learning that society assigns more social power to boys/men than girls/women has had a negative effect on how I have viewed myself," or "I haven't experienced much teasing/harassment/discrimination." The Social Power Subscale has 34 items and was found to have a Cronbach's alpha of .88 and, as predicted, to be correlated significantly with the Autonomy subscale of the How I See Myself scale (Ryff, 1989). Another feature of the ESW is that the same items can be completed for the current adulthood state, as well as retrospectively, regarding one's experiences in adolescence and childhood. Examining this data revealed that on all four subscales, respondents reported significantly lower levels (most had disrupted and disruptive embodied experiences) during adolescence (Teall, 2006).

Stage VIII: Validation of the Developmental Theory of Embodiment—a prospective qualitative study with girls   This research aimed to study the validity of the core constructs of the developmental theory of embodiment through utilizing a prospective qualitative methodology with girls (Piran et al., 2006, 2007, 2009). Applying a prospective qualitative approach gives the opportunity to document the shifts in social, body, and self experiences over the critical years of transitions from pre-puberty to adolescence among the young group and from early to late adolescence among the older group. The study included three to four interviews, conducted annually for a period of 4 years, with 27 girls. Of those girls, 11 were between 9 and 11 years old (pre-puberty) and 16 were 13 to 14 (post-puberty) at the first year of the study, for a total of 89 interviews. The girls were from diverse backgrounds in terms of ethnic heritage, social class, family arrangements, and rural versus urban geographical sites. Participants were recruited through posted advertisements in diverse urban and rural community settings. Parental consent and child assent forms were reviewed and completed with all of the participants and their parents prior to beginning the interview. Participants were interviewed in their home or, on a couple of occasions when this was not available, in a quiet room at a community centre.

The interview process started by sharing with participants the main focus of the study: exploring girls' self and body experiences in relation to their social environment. The first interview centred on early childhood and led up to their current age with regard to social, body, and self experiences. The following three interviews were conducted annually and involved questions about relational, social, as well as self and body experiences during the past year. At each interview, a summary of the previous interview was constructed by the research team and read back to each girl to check the researchers' understanding of the interview material. Data analysis involved hierarchical theme extraction (Miles & Huberman, 1994). High inter-rater reliability on the major coding categories was established. The hierarchical theme extraction led to the emergence of the same core categories: Physical Freedom (versus Physical Corseting), Mental Freedom (versus Mental Corseting), and Social Power (versus Social Disempowerment), as three key constructs shaping the embodied experiences of girls. Further, the study has provided rich developmental information, this time collected prospectively rather than retrospectively, about the changes that occurred annually with each girl (see the next section for greater detail).

Phase 3: Planned Further Validation Studies of the Developmental Theory of Embodiment
This phase represents a set of planned studies that include a prospective quantitative study examining the quantitative predictive power of the key constructs of the Developmental Theory of Embodiment with girls, a qualitative prospective study with boys, and a larger psychometric study of the Embodiment Scale for Women.

Key Constructs
The Developmental Theory of Embodiment addresses a number of constructs. The first construct relates to the Experience of Embodiment and includes an exploration of the constructs of positive/connected embodiment as well as disrupted embodiment (Piran et al., 2002, 2007, 2009; Piran, Legge, Nagasawa, & Foster, 2010). Utilizing a constant comparison approach to the thematic analysis of research narratives (Glaser, 1994; Miles & Huberman, 1994) in studies with girls (Stage VIII; Piran et al., 2009) and women (Stage VI; Piran et al., 2002) revealed that positive/connected embodiment is a complex construct that includes: feeling "at one" with the body, embodied power and agency, body functionality/competence, a "subjective" experience of living in the body with limited external consciousness, the freedom to act/take space/move especially in private and public spheres, the freedom to challenge external standards, body-anchored joy/passion/comfort/other positive feelings, body care and protection, clarity of needs/rights/desires/internal states, connection to others regarding needs/desires/rights, the freedom to express individuality through the body, connection with the physical environment, and the openness to use the body as a source of knowledge in interacting with the world. A short example of such a narrative is provided by a 10-year-old

girl: "I don't care what I look like I just want to do stuff... I'm the best on my team. I am the only one who can jump up high enough to block a goal like this... and it is fun" (Piran et al., 2009). Similarly, disrupted embodiment is a complex construct that includes the following dimensions: body/ self disconnection, body as a site of disempowerment/vulnerability/constrained space, body as a site of low functionality/competence, external consciousness about the body/harsh evaluative gaze, preoccupation with fitting external standards of appearance/behaviour, predominance of body practices dictated by external standards, self-harming behaviours/self-neglect, the association of the body with negative feelings, difficulty identifying needs/desires/internal states, disconnection from others regarding needs/desires/rights, limiting individuality in order to fit in, disconnection from the physical environment, and not utilizing the body as a source of knowledge in interacting with the world (Piran et al., 2002, 2009). A short example of such a narrative by a 25-year-old woman is "I hate my body and I want my body to die... I... I have to overcome my body" (Piran et al., 2002).

Two qualitative research programs, with a total of 117 interviews with girls and women (Stages VI and VIII in the previous section), therefore provide the first research-based articulation of the construct of embodiment. Further, translating the Experience of Embodiment narrative themes to a quantitative scale (Stage VII in the previous section; Teall, 2006) revealed that the Experience of Embodiment Subscale of the Embodiment Scale for Women was positively related to measures of alexithymia, body and self esteem, and disordered eating.

The second set of constructs relates to the social factors that lead to states of connected and disrupted embodiment in girls and women. Utilizing a constant comparison approach to the thematic analysis of research narratives (Glaser, 1994; Miles & Huberman, 1994) in the qualitative studies with girls (Stage VIII in the previous section) and women (Stage VI in the previous section) led to the creation of a hierarchical categorical structure in which all social experiences that occur during girls' and women's developmental journeys and that are related to embodiment were divided into three core constructs coined in this project as: Physical Freedom (versus Physical Corseting), Mental Freedom (versus Mental Corseting), and Social Power (versus Social Disempowerment) (Piran et al., 2002, 2009). All of these experiences are mediated through varied relational contexts at the familial, peer, school, community, and larger cultural levels and shaped by social location, including gender, social class, ethno-cultural group membership, disability, sexual orientation, and other factors. The positive labels of Physical Freedom, Mental Freedom, and Social Power

reflect the emphasis in the Developmental Theory of Embodiment on protective, as well as on risk, factors, unlike most research, for example, in
eating disorder etiology, which has focused on risk factors (Piran, 2002;
Stice, 2001). These constructs show theoretical convergence with the participatory action study with girls in a dance school (see Figures 1 and 2).

The first factor, Physical Freedom (versus Physical Corseting) relates
to experiences that enhance a girl's and a woman's sense of her body
as a physical site of: (1) safety, care, and respectful ownership; (2) freedom of, and competence in, movement; and (3) comfort with physical
desires, appetites, and age-related changes. Examples of Physical Freedom
include, among others, experiences of safety and equity when exploring
the natural environment in the private and public spheres, immersion
in physical games and activities, wearing unconfining, non-objectifying,
non-sexualizing clothes, or age appropriate and equitable engagement in
family chores. An example of a Physical Freedom narrative from a young
woman about her life as a girl states: "So having that freedom to go off and
do... because I think some of the other girls wanted to play... I mean some
girls wore dresses every day, little pretty shoes, and their hair was all done
up, and they couldn't go home messy... you're not allowed to come home
dirty" (Piran et al., 2009). Physical Corseting, in contrast, relates to situations that make a girl or a woman experience her body as a physical site:
(1) which is unsafe, neglected, and/or a target of violations to body ownership; (2) with limited freedom of movement and low functionality; and
(3) which restricts physical desires, appetites, and disrupts comfort with
age-related changes. Examples of Physical Corseting include the whole
range of violation to body ownership, including sexual harassment and the
marketing of exposing, sexualizing clothing to girls—clothing that also
restricts their ability to move (Piran et al., 2006). An example of Physical
Corseting from one girl's narrative about a comment received from a peer
in the school corridor: "You have the biggest butt in the world. Like, seriously. Like, save some room in the hallway for me... like, seriously, your
boobs have to shrink just a little bit" (Piran et al., 2009). In addition to the
three qualitative studies with girls and women described earlier (Stages I,
VI, & VIII of the embodiment research program), the research program
provides further quantitative validation to the construct of Physical Free-
dom/Corseting. First, the structural equation modelling studies conducted
with university and community samples (Stages II, III, & IV in the previous
section; Piran & Thompson, 2008) have validated the association of a range
of experiences of Violation of Body Ownership, specifically sexual abuse,
sexual harassment, and sexual violation during childhood, adolescence, and
early adulthood, with disordered eating patterns (Piran & Thompson, 2008).

Moreover, the Physical Freedom Subscale of the Embodiment Scale for Women, which provides a quantified measure of Physical Freedom (Stage VII; Piran & Teall, 2006; Teall, 2006) was found to be positively related to one's overall state of embodiment and negatively related to self-surveillance, a subscale of the Objectified Body Consciousness Scale (McKinley & Hyde, 1996; Teall, 2006).

The importance of a sense of Physical Freedom has been well documented in the literature. For example, Young (1990, p. 154) also noted the importance of Physical Freedom and observed that

> girls and women are not given the opportunity to use their full bodily capacities in free and open engagement with the world, nor are they encouraged as much as boys are to develop specific bodily skills. Girls' play is often more sedentary and enclosing than the play of boys. In school and after-school activities girls are not encouraged to engage in sport, in the controlled use of their bodies in achieving well-defined goals.

Young thus highlights that girls and women are often deprived of the same sport, physical activities, and leisure opportunities that help one to achieve a state of connection with their body. Moreover, these opportunities are even sparser during adolescence as participation in sports for females declines further at this time, likely because sports are perceived as not fitting with an acceptable feminine comportment (Ewing & Seefeldt, 1996). Lack of participation in sport and other leisure activities is also problematic because such participation has been known to provide girls and women with a sense of empowerment and the freedom to take space (Theberge, 2003; Young, 1990). For example, Theberge (2003, p. 504) notes in her study of adolescent girl hockey players that "in these girls' accounts, playing hockey involved taking initiative and being powerful and sometimes fearless in the use of their body." Another finding related to Physical Freedom is that women have been noted to spend a significant amount of time devoted to making the body comply with social expectations for a feminine appearance (see, for example, Roberts & Waters, 2004). While this effort alone implies a degree of disembodiment, time devoted to "body work" also allows girls and women less time for leisure, sport, and other physical activities (Wearing, 1998). Another study conducted in this area is by Menzel and Levine (2010).

The second factor, Mental Freedom (versus Mental Corseting), relates to the freedom to explore and determine one's own sense of identity—in particular, the freedom not to belong to socially created and labelled groups (such as "tomboy"/"girlie girl," "butch"/"girlie," "slut"/"prude," "nice"/"bitch"). Oppressive social discourses, and, in particular, dichotomous social labels, disrupt girls' and women's connections with their bodies by forcing their embodied experiences into tight and unfitting moulds, both idealizing and deprecating in nature (Piran et al., 2006). In addition, Mental Freedom involves a critical stance towards these social moulds. An example of Mental Corseting is included in this narrative by a 12-year-old girl who loved sports with a great passion prior to puberty (third interview in the prospective girls study, Stage VIII). However, in line with idealized discourses of a "feminine" body, she claimed that "pretty girls don't sweat" and elaborated that

> It's weird to think about girls' sweating. I try to avoid it...I try not to run too much and not to move too much. Usually in gym if you do not work too hard your grades will go down. So I have to keep my grades up. So it is a balance...I think it's more like boys are having so much fun because they don't care what they look like. When girls want to play something they look so stiff trying not to sweat too much. If I did not care about sweating, I will have so much more fun. If I didn't sweat I will be playing sports like every day. I love sports.

Here, discourses of "femininity" are controlling her ability to fully engage in physical activities once she enters puberty. Another example of Mental Corseting relates to compliance with the "girlie-girl" mould, which involves a particular way of living in the body, as a 13-year-old girl explained: "Like, I wear tight shirts and tight pants. I have friends that are total girlie girls—they don't play sports at all" (Piran et al., 2009). Girls and young women who demonstrated positive embodiment in the three qualitative studies of the Embodiment Research Program (Stages I, VI, and VIII) were able to resist oppressive discourses, as the following narrative by a strong young woman who challenged, as a girl, the tomboy/girlie-girl (or "masculine/feminine") dichotomy indicates: "He [father] had a tough time trying to make me like this little girl with skirts and stuff. I wasn't a tomboy but I just liked being a girl but a powerful girl. That's all. I'd just pick guys' characteristics and be like, 'Yeah, I'll take those. Those are good'" (Stage VI; Piran et al., 2002). In the participatory action research study with students in the dance school (Stage I), the development of critical perspective towards social expectations and moulds was a key component in transforming the school environment (Piran, 2001). In line with the three qualitative studies with girls and women in the Embodiment Research Program (Stages I, VI, & VIII in the previous section), two quantitative studies provide quantitative validation of this construct. A quantitative study with a community sample of young women found a relationship between the internalization of discourses of femininity and disordered eating patterns

(Stage V; Piran & Cormier, 2005). Further, the Mental Freedom Subscale of the Embodiment Scale for Women (Stage VII; Teall, 2006) was found to be positively related to self-acceptance, a subscale on the How I See Myself Scale (Ryff, 1989) and one's overall state of embodiment, and negatively related to body shame, a subscale on the Objectified Body Consciousness Scale (McKinley & Hyde, 1996; Teall, 2006).

Studies to date support the impact of Mental Freedom on embodiment. For example, in a meta-analysis of 22 studies, Murnen and Smolak (1997) found both a small positive relationship between feminine identity and eating problems and a negative relationship between masculinity and eating problems. A further meta-analysis by the same authors also found a positive relationship between feminist identity and positive body attitudes (Murnen & Smolak, 2009). Similarly to Piran and Cormier (2005), Morrison and Sheahan (2009) found that gender-related discourses of self-objectification, self-silencing, and anger suppression related to disordered eating patterns. The concept of Mental Freedom as it relates to a woman's embodiment was also addressed in Guthrie and Castelnuovo's (2001) study of physically active women who also had physical mobility disabilities. They noted that, for those women who viewed both the mind and the body as being equally important, they were also able to develop "their identities for the most part, according to their own criteria, as opposed to those considered acceptable by able bodied society" (p. 14). This demonstrates the Mental Freedom of these women. Similarly, Zitzelsberger (2005, p. 400) in her study of women with physical disabilities, discussed the importance of Mental Freedom:

> Throughout their lives, participants also exposed and evaluated the constructed narrow ranges of bodily being and knowing, and redefined their physical disabilities or differences through constructing, for themselves, more fluid and empowering representations of their bodily differences. In doing so, they experienced a different relationship to their bodies and alternative ways of seeing themselves.

Thus, the development of a strong sense of Mental Freedom was a significant factor in the achievement of a positive connection with the body for these women.

The third factor, Social Power (versus Social Disempowerment), relates to experiences in the life of girls that reflect equity, social power, and connection to desired communities as well as either freedom from being cast in the role of a marginalized "other" or having the opportunity to stand up to inequitable treatment. Embodying privilege is associated with positive embodiment, which includes all of the aspects of social location in terms of gender, social class, ethno-cultural group membership, and other factors. For example, a 14-year-old girl who is blond, blue-eyed, and thin explained the experience of having privilege, in the context of fearing losing it: "I am scared of not being attractive anymore... Probably I would feel that I don't have that right to be who I am anymore. [Interviewer: Who would you be instead?] I don't know, quiet... like not as big, you know [Interviewer: Personality-wise?] Yeah" (Piran et al., 2009). In contrast, embodying inequity related to social location disrupts one's body experience and may involve wishes to alter the body in order to restore social power. For example, a 12-year-old girl of Aboriginal heritage of low socio-economic status who developed a pattern of self-starvation explained it in this narrative: "I had to fit into my favourite pair of jeans" (she could not afford to buy another pair), she added, 'I was fat. Sarah was also fat but she could not be teased because she has a boyfriend... He has red hair and he has blue, crystal blue eyes'" (Piran et al., 2009). Related to her challenged social status, which was associated with her low socio-economic status standing and her ethnic heritage, she felt that losing weight would be her only way to not be "an alien" in her peer group. The structural equation modelling study with the university and community samples (Stages III, IV, & V of the Embodiment Research Program) suggested that both gender and weight harassment loaded significantly onto the Social Power latent construct and were significantly related to disordered eating patterns (Piran & Thompson, 2008). The Social Power Subscale of the Embodiment Scale for Women (Stage VII) was found to be positively related to Autonomy, a subscale on the How I See Myself scale and one's overall state of embodiment (Ryff, 1989; Teall, 2006).

Indeed, research suggests that social power relates to mental and physical health. For example, Zitzelsberger (2005) demonstrated how social disempowerment can cause a greater challenge for maintaining embodiment in her study of women with physical disabilities and differences. She explained that the women's physical differences caused them to receive intrusive and rude reactions from others, such as through gaze and comments, which made them feel shunned and ignored. This reaction led to a state of disembodiment as the women often interiorized these judgments and developed a personal dislike towards their own bodies. In addition, Silverstein and Blumenthal (1997) demonstrated how a lack of gender equity in the home was positively associated with higher levels of somatic depression. Moreover, Piran's (2001) study of young women dancers demonstrated that a lack of social power greatly contributed to difficulties with being able to accept one's body. She noted that

> it seemed that, for the young women who participated in the project, body weight and shape preoccupation worsened when their sense of ownership over their body was disrupted, when their bodies were used as a medium to express pervasive societal prejudices, and when the social construction of women constrained and demeaned ways of being in the body that did not comply with perceived societal expectations. (pp. 227-228)

Finally, Howe (2003) noted that women, who related to less privileged social locations, have less access to experiences in sport that could enhance embodiment. Thus, it is clear that a young woman's degree of social power can significantly affect her ability to live in her body in a connected manner.

The Developmental Theory of Embodiment is based on a number of studies that have delineated in great detail the changes in the Experience of Embodiment over time within the same girl or woman as they relate to shifts in relational and social experiences (Stages VI & VIII; Piran et al., 2002, 2009; Teall, 2006). The construct of the Body Journey reflects this process of change. Examining themes under the core construct of the Experience of Embodiment as delineated retrospectively in the life history study with young women (Stage VI; Piran et al., 2002) and as delineated prospectively for a period of four years for girls, ages 9 to 14, in the first year of the study (Stage VIII; Piran et al., 2007, 2009), reflected shifts from a place of embodied agency, competence, and responsiveness to body needs in childhood to a disrupted Experience of Embodiment during adolescence and beyond. However, these studies also found during the late teens and early adulthood processes of reconnection with the body (Piran et al., 2002). Indeed, the Experience of Embodiment Subscale of the Embodiment Scale for Women (Piran & Teall, 2006; Teall, 2006), which gives women the opportunity to rank the same items not only in reference to their current experience but also retrospectively to their adolescence and childhood, revealed that women's Experience of Embodiment was most positive in childhood, worst during adolescence, and had a mid-level position during adulthood. These shifts in the Experience of Embodiment could be understood in light of the changes occurring in girls' shifting social experiences over time. For example, in the domain of Physical Freedom versus Corseting, girls experienced major reductions in the opportunity to be involved in physical activities, as well as in the experience of safety in their bodies, as they moved from childhood to early adolescence (Stage VIII; Piran et al., 2007, 2009).

In the Mental Freedom versus Corseting domain, girls experienced an intensification of pressures to fit different moulds of femininity and the ostracizing of girls who resisted these moulds post puberty (e.g., post-puberty, "tomboys" became "losers," "butches," or "manly girls") (Stage

VIII; Piran et al. 2007, 2009). In the Social Power domain, girls post-puberty experienced a clearer stratification of social standing related to social location, so that the white (blond, blue-eyed) girls of a higher socio-economic status who had access to varied body-grooming facilities and to shopping at brand name stores (hence, girls who embodied privilege) were the most "popular." Trying to embody this privileged position through alterations in body appearance was experienced as a way of acquiring some form of social power (Stage VIII; Piran et al., 2007, 2009).

Conclusion and Implications

The presentation of the Developmental Theory of Embodiment in the context of a volume on body weight and shape preoccupation and disordered eating relates to viewing these disorders within the spectrum of challenges to the experience of embodiment. The chapter suggests that the construct of embodiment may be more suitable to encompassing the range of body weight and shape preoccupation, disordered eating patterns, and co-existing disruptions in the body domain than the construct of body image. Related to this notion, the chapter suggests the value of developing measures of the construct of embodiment. Further, the chapter suggests that the Developmental Theory of Embodiment helps bridge the gap between social critical theory about the body and society and developmental psychological theory at the level of the individual. This theory suggests the complexity of social experiences related to embodiment and that the reason some individuals develop disordered eating patterns, while others do not, may relate to different embodied journeys in diverse social contexts. The findings of the embodiment research program described in this chapter suggest the possibilities inherent in research studies that concurrently examine risk and protective factors to the development of body weight and shape preoccupation. Further, the findings suggest that research programs should consider the complexity of the social arena in shaping the experience of the body (Piran, 2010).

The Developmental Theory of Embodiment has multiple implications for the treatment and prevention of eating disorders. Starting with treatment, the Developmental Theory of Embodiment suggests that the assessment of individuals presenting with disordered eating should include a broad evaluation of their experience of embodiment, including, for example, a broad range of behaviours related to self-harm and care, the ability to be aware of, and in tune with, their bodies, and the emotional components of body experience. Further, the theory suggests that the chronological social experiences of individuals who present with disordered eating patterns be explored in great detail, especially along the dimensions of Physical

Freedom, Mental Freedom, and Social Power. For example, through work in our research centre and our clinical work, we have found individuals who have been treated for eating disorders whose histories of persistent sexual harassment (namely Violation to Body Ownership in the physical domain), of teasing and shame for not complying with the feminine ideal (such as shame about being labelled "a butch" in the mental domain), or of exposure to racism and socio-economic prejudice (social power domain) were not flagged as significant etiological factors, limiting treatment relevance and effectiveness.

In terms of prevention, the Developmental Theory of Embodiment is useful in that it explores both the risk and protective factors along the three core dimensions of Physical Freedom, Mental Freedom, and Social Power. For example, related to the research-derived Physical Freedom construct, the Developmental Theory of Embodiment suggests that significant adults in the life of children, as well as educational institutions, should provide girls with multiple opportunities to connect positively with their bodies, including active and joyful engagement in non-objectifying physical activities while wearing comfortable, non-sexualizing uniforms or clothes (Piran et al., 2002, 2009). Similarly, connection with the physical environment, through hiking or wilderness trips for girls, is a source of such positive immersion in physical activities. Girls also have to grow in a context that strongly supports their right for safety, respects their body ownership, and guides them in self-care. It is imperative that policies against body-based harassment (gender, weight, and ethnicity) be stated and implemented. Educational experiences of abuse prevention that target adults are important. Girls also need guidance regarding bodily changes during puberty. Similarly, they need adults' encouragement in feeling comfortable with physical desires and appetites. Teaching and modelling respect for body signals and encouraging self-care in relation to these signals are important. Informed discussions of sexual desire in girls, respecting desire in girls, and self-care in the expression of desire are important.

Regarding the research construct of Mental Freedom, girls should have the opportunities in varied relational forums to develop an awareness of, and a critical stance towards, social scripts that disrupt their embodied experiences and their sense of self (Piran et al., 2002, 2007, 2009). Developing critical awareness is most effective when interventions are aimed at creating alternative and liberating peer norms (Becker, Ciao, & Smith, 2008; Piran, 2001). Even further, schools can provide a whole-school educational environment that enhances students' critical perspectives on disruptive cultural norms and prejudices and normalizes the process of challenging social scripts and labels.

In terms of the research construct of Social Power, it is essential to develop critical awareness towards the social processes whereby the body is used as a medium to express social privilege and work to curtail such expressions in educational settings and other communities (Piran, 2001; Piran, 2002; Piran et al., 2007, 2009). In this regard, all aspects of the school environment should be examined, including policies (harassment) and norms (who gets access to the schoolyard; who gets voted to be school representatives; who gets teased). It is most valuable if the school becomes a community that counters dominant social structures regarding gender, social class, ethnicity, health, and other aspects of social locations.

References

Allan, H. T. (2005). Gender and embodiment in nursing: The role of the female chaperone in the infertility clinic. *Nursing Inquiry, 12*, 175-183.

Bagby, R. M., Parker, J. D. A., & Taylor, G. J. (1994). The twenty-item Toronto alexithymia scale: I. Item selection and cross-validation of the factor structure. *Journal of Psychosomatic Research, 38*, 33-40.

Bartky, S. L. (1997). Foucault, femininity, and the modernization of patriarchal power. In K. Conboy, N. Medina, & S. Stanbury (Eds.), *Writing on the body: Female embodiment and feminist theory* (pp. 90-110). New York: Columbia University Press.

Becker, C. B., Ciao, A. C., & Smith, L. M. (2008). Moving from efficacy to effectiveness in eating disorders prevention: The Sorority Body Image Program. *Cognitive and Behavioral Practice, 15*, 18-27.

Biddle, S. J. (1993). Children, exercise, and mental health. *International Journal of Sport Psychology, 24*, 200-216.

Blood, S. K. (2005). *Body work: The social construction of women's body image.* Hove, East Sussex: Routledge.

Bordo, S. (1993). *Unbearable weight: feminism, western culture, and the body.* Berkeley, CA: University of California Press.

Bordo, S. (1997). The body and the reproduction of femininity. In K. Conboy, N. Medina, & S. Stanbury (Eds.), *Writing on the body: Female embodiment and feminist theory* (pp. 90-110). New York: Columbia University Press.

Bradley, C. B., McMurray, R. G., Harrell, J. S., & Deng, S. (2000). Changes in common activities of third through tenth graders: The CHIC study. *Medicine and Science in Sports and Exercise, 32*(12), 2071-2078.

Briere, J., Kaltman, S. M., & Green, B. (2008). Accumulated childhood trauma and symptom complexity. *Journal of Traumatic Stress, 21*, 223-226.

Brown, L. M. (1998). *Raising their voices: The politics of girls' anger.* Cambridge, MA: Harvard University Press.

Bruch, H. (1962). Perceptual and conceptual disturbances in anorexia nervosa. *Psychosomatic Medicine, 24*, 187-194.

Butler, J. (1988). Performative acts and gender constitution: An essay in phenomenology and feminist theory. *Theatre Journal, 40*(4), 519-531.

Crossley, N. (1995). Merleau-Ponty, the elusive body and carnal sociology. *Body and Society, 1,* 43-63.

Csordas, T. J. (1994). *Embodiment and experience, the existential ground of culture and self.* Cambridge: Cambridge University Press.

Dionne, M. (2002). *The variability of body image: The influence of body-composition information and emotional reactivity on young women's body dissatisfaction* (Ph.D. dissertation, psychology department, York University, Toronto).

Ewing, M., & Seefeldt, V. (1996). Patterns of participation and attrition in American agency-sponsored youth sports. In F. Smoll & R. E. Smith (Eds.), *Children and youth in sport: A biopsychosocial perspective* (pp. 31-45). Madison, WI: Brown and Benchmark.

Falgairette, G., Deflandre, A., & Gavarry, O. (2004). Habitual physical activity, influences of gender and environmental factors. *Science and Sports, 19,* 161-173.

Favazza, A. R., DeRosear, L., & Conterio, K. (1989). Self-mutilation and eating disorders. *Suicide and Life Threatening Behaviors, 19(4),* 352-361. Finkelhore, D. (1979). *Sexually victimized children.* New York: Free Press.

Fitzgerald, L. F., Gelfand, M. J., & Drasgow, F. (1995). Meauring sexual harassment: Theoretical and psychometric advances. *Basic and Applied Social Psychology, 17,* 425-445.

Foucault, M. (1979). *Discipline and punish: The birth of the prison.* New York: Vintage.

Fredrickson, B. L., & Roberts, T. (1997). Objectification theory: Toward understanding women's lived experiences and mental health risks. *Psychology of Women Quarterly, 21,* 173-206.

Gadalla, T. M., & Piran, N. (2007). Eating disorders and substance abuse in Canadian men and women: A national study. *Eating Disorders: Journal of Treatment and Prevention, 15,* 189-203.

Garner, D. M., Olmsted, M. P., Bohr, Y., & Garfinkel, P. E. (1982). The eating attitudes test: Psychometric features and clinical correlates. *Psychological Medicine, 12,* 871-878.

Gilligan, C. (1991). Women's psychological development: Implications for psychotherapy. In C. Gilligan, A. G. Rogers, & D. L. Tolman (Eds.), *Women, girls and psychotherapy: Reframing resistance* (pp. 5-31). Binghamton, NY: Harington Park Press.

Glaser, B. G. (1994). *More grounded theory methodology: A reader.* Mill Valley, CA: Sociology Press.

Guthrie, S., & Castelnuovo, S. (2001). Disability management among women with physical disabilities. *Sociology of Sport Journal, 18,* 5-20.

Howe, L. A. (2003). Athletics, embodiment, and the appropriation of the self. *Journal of Speculative Philosophy, 17,* 92-107.

Jack, D., & Dill, D. (1992). The silencing the self scale. *Psychology of Women Quarterly, 16,* 97-106.

Jick, T. D. (1979). Mixing qualitative and quantitative methods: Triangulation in action. *Administrative Science Quarterly, 24*(4), 602-611.

Johnson, C. (1985). Initial consultation for patients with bulimia and anorexia nervosa. In D. M. Garner & P. E. Garfinkel (Eds.), *Handbook of psychotherapy for anorexia nervosa and bulimia* (pp. 19-51). New York: Guilford Press.

Jöreskog, K., & Sörbom, D. (1993). *New features in LISREL 8.* Chicago: Scientific Software International.

Katzman, M. A., & Lee, S. (1997). Beyond body image: The integration of feminist and transcultural theories in the understanding of self starvation. *International Journal of Eating Disorders, 22*, 385-394.

Legge, R. (2008). *If I am thin, I am safe: Speaking through the body following trauma* (Proceedings of the Fourth Critical Multicultural Counselling and Psychotherapy Conference, Ontario Institute for Studies in Education, University of Toronto, Toronto, ON).

McKinley, N. M., & Hyde, J. S. (1996). The objectified body consciousness scale: Development and validation. *Psychology of Women Quarterly, 20*, 181-215.

Mendelson, B. K., Mendelson, M. J., & White, D. R. (2001). Body-esteem scale for adolescents and adults. *Journal of Personality Assessment, 76*, 90-106.

Menzel, J., & Levine, M. P. (2010). Competitive athletics as a context for embodying experiences and the promotion of positive body image. In R. Calogero, S. Tantleff-Dunn, & J. K. Thompson (Eds.), *Self-objectification in women: Causes, consequences, and counteractions* (pp. 163-186). Washington, DC: American Psychological Association.

Merleau-Ponty, M. (1962). *Phenomenology of perception.* New York: Humanities Press.

Miles, M. B., & Huberman, A. M. (1994). *Qualitative data analysis.* Thousand Oaks, CA: Sage.

Morse, J. M., & Mitcham, C. (1998). The experience of agonizing pain and signals of disembodiment. *Journal of Psychosomatic Research, 44*, 667-680.

Morrison, T. G., & Sheahan, E. E. (2009). Gender-related discourses as mediators in the association between internalization of the thin-body ideal and indicants of body dissatisfaction and disordered eating. *Psychology of Women Quarterly, 33*, 374-383.

Murnen, S. K., & Smolak, L. (1997). Femininity, masculinity, and disordered eating: A meta-analytic review. *International Journal of Eating Disorders, 22*, 231-242.

Murnen, S. K., & Smolak, L. (2009). Are feminist women protected from body image problems? A meta-analytic review of relevant research. *Sex Roles, 60*, 186-197.

Piran, N. (1999). Eating disorders: A trial of prevention in a high-risk school setting. *Journal of Primary Prevention, 20*(1), 75-90.

Piran, N. (2001). Re-inhabiting the body from the inside out: Girls transform their school environment. In D. L. Tolman & M. Brydon-Miller (Eds.), *From subjects to subjectivities: A handbook of interpretive and participatory methods* (pp. 218-238). New York, NY: New York University Press.

Piran, N. (2002). Prevention of eating disorders. In C. G. Fairburn & K. D. Brownell (Eds.), *Eating disorders and obesity: A comprehensive handbook* (2nd ed., pp. 367-371). New York: Guildford Press.

Piran, N. (2006). *The end point: Maximizing participants' verification of emergent understanding in a feminist-informed qualitative study* (Paper presented at the Association for Women in Psychology Annual Conference, Ann Arbor, MI)

Piran, N. (2010). Social critical theory, embodiment and counseling. In *Building bridges for wellness through counselling and psychotherapy* (pp. 77-89). Bangalore, India: Center for Diversity in Counselling and Psychotherapy Sampura-Montfort; and Toronto: Center for Diversity in Counselling, Ontario Institute for Studies in Education, University of Toronto.

Piran, N., Antoniou, M., Legge, R., McCance, N., Mizevich, J., Peasley, E., & Ross, E. (2006). On girls' disembodiment: The complex tyranny of the "ideal girl." In D. L. Gustafson and L. Goodyear (Eds.), *Proceedings of the Women, health, and education: CASWE sixth bi-annual international institute* (pp. 224-229). St. John's, NL: Memorial University.

Piran, N., Buttu, D., Damianakis, M., Legge, R., Nagasawa, S., & Mizevich, J. (2007). *Understanding intensified disruptions in girls' self and body experiences during adolescence* (Annual Convention, Canadian Psychological Association, Ottawa, ON, June).

Piran, N., Carter, W., Thompson, S., & Pajouhandeh, P. (2002). Powerful girls: A contradiction in terms? Young women speak about the experience of growing up in a girl's body. In S. Abbey (Ed.), *Ways of knowing in and through the body: Diverse perspectives on embodiment* (pp. 206-210). Welland, ON: Soleil Publishing.

Piran, N., & Cormier, H. (2005). The social construction of women and disordered eating patterns. *Journal of Counseling Psychology, 52*(4), 549-558.

Piran, N., & Gadalla, G. (2006). Eating disorders and substance abuse in Canadian women: A national study. *Addiction, 102,* 105-113.

Piran, N., Legge, R., Nagasawa, S., & Foster, M. (2010). From body agency to shame? Delineating girls' embodied states through adolescence carves paths for alternative outcome (Annual Convention, Canadian Psychological Association, Winnipeg, MB).

Piran, N., & Teall, T. (2006). *The embodiment scale for women* [Unpublished manuscript; on file with the author].

Piran, N., & Thompson, S. (2008). A study of the adverse social experiences model to the development of eating disorders. *International Journal of Health Promotion and Education, 46*(2), 65-71.

Piran, N., Thompson, S., Legge, R., Carter, W., Nagasawa, S., & Teall, T. (2009). *The body journey* [Unpublished manuscript; on file with the author].

Rehorick, D. A. (1986). Shaking the foundations of life world: A phenomenological account of an earthquake experience. *Human Studies, 9,* 379-391.

Richman, E. L., & Shaffer, D. R. (2000). If you let me play sports: How might sport participation influence the self-esteem of adolescent females? *Psychology of Women Quarterly, 24,* 189-199.

Roberts, T., & Waters, P. (2004). Self-objectification and that "not so fresh feeling": Feminist therapeutic interventions for healthy female embodiment. In P. J. Caplan (Ed.), *From menarche to menopause* (pp. 5-21). Binghamton, NY: Haworth Press.

Rohde, P., Lewinson, P. M., & Seeley, J. R. (1991). Comorbidity of unipolar depression: Comorbidity with other mental disorders in adolescents and adults. *Journal of Abnormal Psychology, 100,* 214-222.

Ryff, C. D. (1989). Happiness is everything, or is it? Explorations on the meaning of psychological well-being. *Journal of Personality and Social Psychology, 57,* 1069-1081.

Sansone, R. A., & Levitt, J. L. (2004). The prevalence of self-harm behavior among those with eating disorders. In J. L. Levitt, R. A. Sansone, & L. Cohn (Eds.), *Self-harm behavior and eating disorders: Dynamics, assessment and treatment* (pp. 3-13). New York: Routledge.

Shields, S., Mallory, M., & Simon, A. (1989). The body awareness questionnaire: Reliability and validity. *Journal of Personality Assessment, 53,* 802-815.

Silverstein, B., & Blumenthal, E. (1997). Depression mixed with anxiety, somatization, and disordered eating: Relationship with gender-role-related limitations experienced by females. *Sex Roles, 36,* 709-724.

Spielberger, C. D. (1996). *State-trait anger expression inventory: Professional manual.* Odessa, FL: Psychological Assessment Resources.

Stice, E. (2001). Risk factors for eating pathology: Recent advances and future directions. In H. R. Striegel-Moore & L. Smolak (Eds.), *Eating disorders: Innovative directions in research and practice* (pp. 51-73). Washington, DC: APA Press.

Strauss, M. A. (1979). Measuring intrafamilial conflict and violence: The conflict tactics scales. *Journal of Marriage and the Family, 41,* 75-86.

Taylor, G. J., Bagby, R. M., & Parker, J. D. A. (1991). The Alexithymia construct: A potential paradigm for psychosomatic medicine, *Psychosomatics, 32,* 153-164.

Taylor, M. J., Gilligan, C., & Sullivan, A. M. (1995). *Between voice and silence: Women and girls, race and relationships.* Cambridge, MA: Harvard University Press.

Teall, T. (2006). *The construction of the embodiment scale for women* (Master's thesis, University of Toronto, Toronto, ON) [unpublished].

Theberge, N. (2003). "No fear comes:" Adolescent girls, ice hockey, and the embodiment of gender. *Youth and Society, 34,* 497-516.

Tolman, D. (1994). Doing desire: Adolescent girls' struggles for/with sexuality. *Gender and Society, 8*(3), 324-342.

Wearing, B. (1998). *Leisure and feminist theory.* Thousand Oaks, CA: Sage.

Young, I. M. (1990). Throwing like a girl: A phenomenology of feminine body comportment, mobility, and spatiality. In I. M. Young (Ed.), *Throwing like a girl and other essays in feminist philosophy and social theory* (pp. 141-159). Bloomington, IN: Indiana University Press.

Young, L. (1992). Sexual abuse and the problem of embodiment. *Child Abuse and Neglect, 16,* 89-100.

Zitzelsberger, H. (2005). (In)visibility: Accounts of embodiment of women with physical disabilities and differences. *Disability and Society, 20,* 389-403.

CHAPTER EIGHT

Gender and the Prevention of Eating Disorders

Linda Smolak, *Kenyon College*
Niva Piran, *Ontario Institute for Studies in Education, University of Toronto*

American boys stage fights and rescues with muscular "action figures" (which are never called "dolls"), while American girls change the clothes of thin but large-breasted Barbie dolls to suit their work and leisure activities. This single difference captures many of the issues to be addressed in this chapter. Children grow up with gendered "ideal" body image prototypes, muscular for boys and thin for girls. But, at least as importantly, they grow up with differing understandings of the meaning of bodies. Boys' and men's bodies are active and engaged in a variety of sports and heroic and strength-based activities. Girls' and women's bodies, however, are intended to look good and, in fact, to look "sexy" (Levin & Kilbourne, 2008; Smolak & Murnen, 2011). These messages come from multiple sources. Indeed, they are virtually ubiquitous. It is not surprising, then, that body image is a heavily gendered phenomenon. Furthermore, the consequences of a negative body image, including eating disorders, depression, and obesity, are also strongly gendered. Thus, it is crucial that gender role and gendered experiences be integrated into etiological models as well as therapeutic and preventive interventions. The overarching goal of this chapter is to provide a framework to facilitate the incorporation of gender into programs designed to prevent eating-related problems and disorders. Towards this end, the chapter is divided into three sections. In the first section, we describe the gender differences in body image, including engagement in differing body shape management techniques and differential consequences of negative body image. The second section is a discussion of the gender differences in the etiology of negative body image. Here we aim to undermine the conceptualization of gender as a "fixed" variable. We instead emphasize the "lived experiences" of boys and girls and how differences in such experiences might contribute to the gendering of body image and disordered eating. In particular, we present a model that aims to integrate a range of adverse gender-based social experiences that could contribute to the development of disordered eating patterns. The final section is a consideration of how the gender differences in the definition of body image and in risk and protective factors might help shape efforts to prevent eating disorders.

Gender Differences in Body Image

Body image is a broad term that can encompass satisfaction with, and perceptual experiences of, overall appearance, weight and shape, specific body parts, and post-surgical functioning and appearance (Cash & Pruzinsky, 2002). In this chapter, the focus is on weight and shape. Thus, while boys and girls may not differ on overall body satisfaction, there are sizeable and consistent differences in their concerns about weight and shape (Ricciardelli, McCabe, Mussap, & Holt, 2009; Wertheim, Paxton, & Blaney, 2009). Girls are more concerned about being thin than boys are. This gender difference may start to emerge by 5 years of age among American and Australian children and becomes clearly evident during the elementary-school years (Lowes & Tiggemann, 2003; Musher-Eizenmann, Holub, Edwards-Leeper, Persson, & Goldstein, 2003). By mid-late elementary school, studies frequently find that 40% of girls are concerned that they are, or will become, too fat (Smolak, Levine, & Schermer, 1998; Wertheim et al., 2009). This number rises to 70% or more during adolescence and includes girls who are "normal" weight (Paxton et al., 1991). While some studies indicate small ethnic group differences in weight and shape concerns (Grabe & Hyde, 2006), the gender difference is evident within all American ethnic groups that have been studied (e.g., Croll, Neumark-Sztainer, Story, & Ireland, 2002). Furthermore, elementary-school-aged girls (approximately 6 to 11 years old) are aware of ways to maintain or lose weight, including calorie-restrictive dieting and purging (Hill, Weaver, & Blundell, 1990; Murnen, Smolak, Mills, & Good, 2003). The use of weight management techniques is, in and of itself, problematic. These can result in both short-term negative effects such as headaches, fatigue, and gastrointestinal distress as well as long-term problems including growth stunting. While it is not clear how strongly correlated elementary-school girls' body dissatisfaction is with adolescent or adult body image concerns (Smolak & Levine, 2001; Wertheim et al., 2009), there is evidence to suggest that eating issues, such as "picky" eating, that emerge during this time are related to the later development of disordered eating (Marchi & Cohen, 1990).

Middle school (ages 11 to 13 years) brings additional developments. First, body dissatisfaction increases around the time of puberty. While this is true for both boys and girls, the dissatisfaction among boys abates more rapidly and more thoroughly as puberty moves boys towards the "ideal" body type, while it takes girls away from the feminine "ideal." Importantly, body dissatisfaction appears to become more stable during middle school, bringing with it health risk behaviours such as dieting and smoking (Neumark-Sztainer, Paxton, Hannan, Haines, & Story, 2006). Over a dozen longitudinal studies have found that weight and shape concerns among middle-school girls predict the later development of eating problems, including clinically significant disorders (Wertheim et al., 2009). Furthermore, body dissatisfaction among middle-school girls predicts the later development of depression (e.g., Stice & Bearman, 2001; Stice, Hayward, Cameron, Killen, & Taylor, 2000). The gender difference in body dissatisfaction among middle-school students also predicts the later gender difference in depression (Bearman & Stice, 2008). The use of "naturalistic" calorie restrictive dieting among middle-school girls, which is a response to their desire to be thin, ironically predicts weight gain with dieters more likely to be overweight later on than non-dieters are, even when controlling for initial body mass index (Neumark-Sztainer et al., 2006; Stice, Cameron, Hayward, Taylor, & Killen, 1999). Thus, by about 13 years of age, girls' body dissatisfaction is not only a serious problem in and of itself (see Chapter 7 in this volume), but it is also related to the development of a variety of later psychological and physical health problems.

Problems related to body dissatisfaction clearly do not decrease for women through emerging adulthood. Indeed, it is during adolescence and early adulthood that the eating disorders of bulimia nervosa and anorexia nervosa most commonly onset. By the peak onset ages of about 18 to 20 years, the ratio of female to male sufferers may be as large as nine to one, whereas childhood differences in eating disorders are more in the range of five to one (Bryant-Waugh & Lask, 2007). Although the importance of body dissatisfaction for self-definition may decline somewhat after the college years (McKinley, 1999), women typically continue to struggle with weight and shape issues until age 65 or beyond (Tiggemann, 2004).

None of this should be interpreted as implying that boys and men are without body image issues. Research increasingly demonstrates that boys and men do have body concerns. While they are significantly less likely than girls and women to want to be thin, particularly if they are at or below their recommended weight for height and age, they are considerably more likely to want to be muscular (Ricciardelli & McCabe, 2007). This gender difference is clearly in place by early adolescence, and it does have some serious implications. For example, adolescent boys are much more likely than girls to use steroids or food supplements to try to gain muscle mass (Irving, Wall, Neumark-Sztainer, & Story, 2002; Ricciardelli et al., 2009). Investment in muscularity could lead to muscle dysmorphic disorder, a form of body dysmorphic disorder that is considerably more common in men than in women (Thompson & Cafri, 2007). However, boys' investment in muscularity has not been clearly linked to the onset of other disorders such as depression or anxiety disorders.

Thus, the definition of a "good" body differs for women, who want to be thin, and men, who want to be muscular. What one hopes to achieve from a good body—including athletic prowess, social success, or being deemed attractive—may differ for individuals as well as by gender, ethnicity, and social class. For example, a woman from a lower social class may be trying to meet middle class standards in order to be more accepted at school or work (Piran et al., 2006). The level of investment in achieving the "ideal" body may also vary as might the negative implications of those efforts. Such differences need to be considered in developing prevention programs aimed at reducing body image and eating problems. Furthermore, it is possible that the etiology of body image disturbances is gendered.

Gender and the Etiology of Body Image

Philosophers have long argued that the meaning of the body differs for men and women (e.g., Bordo, 1993). Men's bodies are agentic. Their bodies are supposed to be capable, strong, and powerful—able to accomplish athletic, military, and work-related feats. Arguments against women's participation in these realms are often based on putative physical limitations. This portrayal of the male body is directly related to social constructions of masculinity such as dominance and leadership. Indeed, researchers have demonstrated a link between drive for muscularity and the male gender role, beginning in adolescence (Mahalik et al, 2003; McCreary, Saucier, & Courtenay, 2003; Smolak & Stein, 2006, 2010).

Women's bodies, on the other hand, are meant to be looked at, particularly for the pleasure of men. They are supposed to be "sexy" (McKinley & Hyde, 1996; Murnen et al., 2003). This is increasingly true even of the bodies of young girls (American Psychological Association, 2007; Levin & Kilbourne, 2008; Smolak & Murnen, 2011). With midriff tops and bikinis for preschool and elementary-school-age girls, young girls are in training to be sex objects. The trend towards introducing girls to the demands of a sexy appearance is also evident in the popularity of the pouty, heavily made-up, and scantily clad Bratz dolls.

However, does exposure to "sexy" dolls actually impact girls' body image? Despite Bratz and other newcomers, Barbie continues to be a popular toy for American girls. The average 3-to-11-year-old American girl owns 10 Barbies (Burns, 2008). Barbie is a global presence available in over 150 countries, with sales exceeding $1 billion (Burns, 2008; Collectdolls .about.com, 2012). Barbie's physical proportions are unrealistic; her bust is extraordinarily large relative to her tiny waist (Dittmar, Halliwell, & Ive, 2006). Although Barbie has had over 80 careers in her 50-plus years, currently available dolls include a Dallas Cowboys Cheerleader. Further, about a billion fashions have been produced for Barbie and her friends (Collectdolls.about.com, 2012). Thus, Barbie's image is often sexualized and is fashion oriented.

Dittmar and her colleagues (2006) conducted an experiment in which they exposed 5- and 8-year-old girls to Barbie and Emme dolls or to no dolls. Emme dolls have more realistic body proportions, those of a size 16 adult woman. The 5-year-olds who were exposed to Barbie reported lower body esteem as well as a greater desire to be thin than did the girls in the other conditions. This immediate negative effect was not evident among the 8-year-old girls, but the reaction of the younger girls suggests that a foundation for body dissatisfaction may have already been laid by exposure to Barbie dolls (Dittmar et al., 2006). This effect of short-term exposure is likely intensified by the consistent, continuous play with Barbie that most American girls experience over the course of several years. This early socialization underscores recent conceptualizations of the feminine gender role that include components focusing on attractiveness and thinness as part of what it means to be feminine (Mahalik et al., 2005).

Women are, of course, active participants in sexualization. For example, girls opt to wear suggestive clothing and may even badger reluctant parents in order to get it (American Psychological Association, 2007). This fact, combined with the pervasiveness of sexualization, can make sexualization seem natural or innate. However, there are other reasons that women might adhere to the "sexy" woman stereotype (Glick, Larsen, Johnson, & Branstiter, 2005). Sexuality is potentially a source of power for women. Some third-wave feminists argue that female sexuality is an important source of women's empowerment that should be celebrated (McGhan, 2007). Girls and women who are judged as being more attractive do indeed experience greater social and career success. Thus, there are clear societal rewards for women who participate in their own sexualization. These rewards are yet another indicator that sexualization is part of the societally sanctioned definition of femininity.

On the other hand, the masculine gender role includes power and dominance and is, therefore, consistent with a lean, muscular body shape. Yet muscularity, much less hyper-muscularity, is not an integral part of masculinity. There are other ways to achieve power and dominance as numerous businessmen (e.g., Bill Gates), entertainers (e.g., Vince Vaughn), and even athletes (e.g., C.C. Sabathia) demonstrate. Thinness and interest in attractiveness are part of femininity. Even middle-aged entertainers as powerful as Oprah Winfrey or the women on *Desperate Housewives* are required to attempt to be thin and attractive. Female professional athletes are not immune from this pressure as evidenced by the tennis players and race car driver (Danica Patrick) who routinely appear in the *Sports Illustrated* swimsuit issue. These differences in gender role demands appear to contribute to gender differences in body image.

Objectification Theory

Objectification Theory (Fredrickson & Roberts, 1997; McKinley & Hyde, 1996) builds on the differential cultural meaning of men's and women's bodies. Within these cultural meanings, women's bodies are sexualized objects, meant to be looked at by men for men's sexual pleasure. It is possible to treat a body as an object without sexualizing it, as in the case of slaves' bodies being seen as more appropriate to heavy labour than those of their owners. It is also possible to sexualize without treating someone's body as an appropriate target of sexual desire, as when young girls are dressed in sexy clothes and play make-up despite social rules regarding pedophilia (American Psychological Association, 2007; Goodin, Van Denberg, Murnen, & Smolak, 2011; Smolak & Murnen, 2011). However, the processes of sexualization and objectification are combined in many cultures' current definitions of adolescent girls' and adult women's bodies. Both Fredrickson and Roberts (1997) and McKinley and Hyde (1996) have developed psychological theories that tie the sexualized societal objectification of women to self-objectification. In self-objectification, women have internalized the gaze of the outside observer/evaluator. This means that women will judge and monitor their own bodies to make sure that they are sufficiently attractive and that they meet societal standards. Even elementary-school girls are aware of, and have internalized, these standards. A substantial minority of elementary-school girls—studies commonly report 40% by fourth and fifth grade—are concerned about being, or becoming, too fat (see, e.g., Smolak & Levine, 2001, for a review). Self-objectification is believed to have psychological consequences, including body shame, anxiety, lack of "peak" emotional states, and lack of internal body awareness. These phenomena, in turn, are predicted to put women at risk for eating disorders.

Fredrickson and Roberts' (1997) model has been tested through correlational and experimental research using the Self-Objectification Questionnaire (SOQ) (Fredrickson, Roberts, Noll, Quinn, & Twenge, 1998). In this measure, the participant rates the importance of five physical competence attributes (e.g., health, strength) and five appearance attributes (e.g., weight). The difference between the total scores of competence and appearance attributes is used to indicate self-objectification. McKinley and Hyde (1996) developed the Objectified Body Consciousness (OBC) Scale as a way to measure a similar set of ideas. They argued that objectification increases as girls develop sexually during puberty and that over time some women internalize the objectification, resulting in self-surveillance. Since the beauty standards are so unrealistic, self-surveillance can lead to body shame. Women are told they are responsible for how they look so that they think they should control their bodies, which leads to the third dimension, control beliefs. Thus, the three components measured by the OBC scale are body surveillance, body shame, and appearance control beliefs.

SOQ and OBC scores have been linked to low body esteem and eating problems in cross-sectional, longitudinal, and experimental research (e.g., Calogero, Davis, & Thompson, 2005; Fredrickson et al., 1998; McKinley, 1999; Moradi & Huang, 2008; Muehlenkamp & Saris-Baglama, 2002; Slater & Tiggemann, 2002). Research also indicates that, as predicted by the Objectification Theory, women are more likely than men to engage in self-surveillance. For example, Frederick, Forbes, Grigorian, and Jarcho (2007) reported a moderate d of .48 among 2,206 undergraduate students. While 43 percent of the women in this study reported high levels of self-surveillance, only 25 percent of men did. The association between self-surveillance and body dissatisfaction was particularly strong for heavier and ethnic minority women—that is, for women who do not meet the white, thin ideal (Frederick et al., 2007).

There is also evidence that objectified body consciousness emerges in adolescence and that even at this point there are significant gender differences. In a sample of 10- and 11-year-old children, girls demonstrated significantly higher self-surveillance ($d = .49$) and body shame ($d = .12$) (Lindberg, Grabe, & Hyde, 2007; Lindberg, Hyde, & McKinley, 2006). Two years later, these differences were even more pronounced: $d = .64$ for self-surveillance and $d = .50$ for body shame. Furthermore, among girls, Pubertal Development Scale scores correlated with higher levels of peer sexual harassment, which correlated positively with self-surveillance (Lindberg et al., 2007).

In addition, more advanced puberty itself is associated with higher levels of self-surveillance (Lindberg et al., 2007). Finally, self-surveillance is correlated with body shame (Lindberg et al., 2007). Importantly, pubertal development was not significantly related to either peer sexual harassment or body surveillance among the boys. Thus, although longitudinal data are needed to definitively describe the relationships among puberty, sexual harassment, and self-surveillance in girls, correlational data suggest that an adult female body is associated with adult concerns about meeting societal attractiveness demands. This is not equally true for boys. Further, it may be that at least part of this association for girls is enforced by adolescent boys who indeed believe that thinness influences a girl's attractiveness (Paxton, Norris, Wertheim, Durkin, & Anderson, 2005).

Objectification Theory also offers an explanation of the consistent evidence that media images negatively impact girls' body image (e.g., Groesz, Levine, & Murnen, 2002; Grabe, Ward, & Hyde, 2008). Research suggests that 60% of middle-school girls read "teen" magazines at least 2 to 5 times per month (Field et al, 1999). The majority of print advertisements in these magazines portray women as sexual objects (Stankiewicz & Rosselli, 2008). In fact, only men's magazines are more likely to sexually objectify women in advertisements, perhaps shaping boys' ideas about how girls ought to behave, look, and be treated (Stankiewicz & Rosselli, 2008). Media messages may combine with other common experiences, such as sexual harassment and peer teasing, to produce gender differences in self-objectification.

Culturally valued physical attractiveness is associated with youth. It is noteworthy that self-objectification may decline as women age. This may be because of decreased sexualization of older women (McKinley, 1999). In US culture, younger women are seen as being more sexual and more sexually desirable. Indeed, we expect women to permanently gain weight as they experience pregnancies and menopause as well as in normal aging. Furthermore, middle-aged and older women are more likely to be in very long-term relationships, a situation that may allow them to be less focused on the importance of attractiveness to the success of their core romantic relationship. Indeed, the length of a relationship is negatively correlated with self-surveillance among middle-aged women (McKinley, 1999). This evidence underscores the role of trying to be sexy in order to attract men in increasing self-surveillance in younger women. Similarly, positive attitudes towards menopause and an aging body are negatively related to self-surveillance and positively related to self-esteem in middle-aged women (50 to 68 years old) (McKinley & Lyon, 2008). This suggests that a rejection of the cultural definitions of sexual attractiveness and the meaning of women's bodies may reduce self-objectification, although the direct links need to be investigated in future research.

Everyday Sexism

The everyday, lived experiences of being a boy or a girl are different in important ways. As was discussed earlier, gender role socialization requires differential treatment of boys and girls. Some of these experiential differences are likely related to body image and eating disorders, particularly given the meanings of men and women's bodies. In addition, women face a lower social status in the United States, in terms of political power, corporate positions, economic earnings and opportunities, and even personal safety. Sexual harassment and sex discrimination are means of enforcing this lower status (Glick & Fiske, 1996; Sheffield, 2007). Thus, it is possible that everyday experiences of sexism, including harassment and discrimination contribute to gender differences in body image and eating disorders.

When researchers survey students, there is typically little or no gender difference in reports of peer, but not necessarily cross-gendered, sexual harassment (American Association of University Women, 2001; Hill & Silva, 2006; Murnen & Smolak, 2000). Sometimes boys actually report more sexual harassment than girls do (e.g., Lindberg et al., 2006). For example, in a survey of over 2,000 college students, 62% of the women and 61% of the men reported sexual harassment experiences. Slightly more women (35%) than men (29%) reported experiences with physical harassment (e.g., being grabbed or touched) (Hill & Silva, 2006). In a survey of 2,064 eighth graders through eleventh graders, 83% of the girls and 79% of the boys reported sexual harassment experiences (American Association of University Women, 2001). A survey of 10-12-year-olds found that boys were somewhat more likely than girls to report sexual harassment ($p < .10$) (Lindberg et al., 2006). In an interview study of third-to-fifth-grade children, boys reported a greater variety of sexual harassment episodes than girls did, although the difference was not significant (Murnen & Smolak, 2000). Thus, there is a seemingly anomalous set of findings: a putatively "female" experience actually occurs with comparable frequency in males. But the meaning of sexual harassment appears to vary by gender.

Adolescent girls retrospectively report that they were first sexually harassed in elementary school (Bryant, 1993). In a study using cross-gender sexual harassment vignettes, Murnen and Smolak (2000) found that girls who reported higher frequency of sexual harassment also demonstrated lower global self-esteem and weight-shape self-esteem. These associations were not evident among the boys. Perhaps more importantly, girls were significantly more likely to believe that victims of cross-gender sexual harassment would be "scared." This is potentially important because self-surveillance is related not only to appearance anxiety but also to anxiety about safety (Fredrickson & Roberts, 1997). Thus, early sexual harassment experiences may contribute to the development of self-surveillance as well as to negative body image. Establishing such relationships will require longitudinal data as well as measures of self-surveillance that can be used with elementary-school-age children.

Up to 90% of high-school girls (and boys) report sexual harassment experiences (American Association of University Women, 2001; Leaper & Brown, 2008). The most frequent forms of sexual harassment during high school, reported by 50-67% of the girls as occurring at least once, include unwanted romantic attention, demeaning comments about gender, teasing about appearance, and unwanted physical contact (Leaper & Brown, 2008). Such experiences do affect behaviour and attitudes. Compared to boys, girls report feeling more self-conscious and less confident following sexual harassment (American Association of University Women, 2001). It is easy to imagine that such reactions translate to increases in self-surveillance. Prospective data are needed to test these relationships. Furthermore, girls who perceive themselves as being less typically feminine and less content with the feminine gender role are more likely to perceive themselves as victims of sexism, primarily from male peers (Leaper & Brown, 2008). One possibility is that male peers who notice adolescent girls who stray from the culturally defined path attempt to bring them back in line via sexual harassment and sexist comments about academics and sports (e.g., "girls can't do physics" or "some sports are too rough for girls"). This issue also deserves additional research.

Women have to contend with everyday instances of sexual objectification that threaten their psychological health. Klonoff and Landrine (1995) found that some of the most common experiences involved being exposed to sexually degrading jokes (94% of women reported this experience), being sexually harassed (experienced by 82%), being called sexual names (experienced by 82%), and being the victim of unwanted sexual advances (experienced by 67%). In a daily diary study, women experienced more "everyday sexism" (e.g., comments or jokes that are derogatory to one's gender) than men with an average of between one and two experiences per week and that these experiences were related to feelings of anger, depression, and lowered self-esteem (Swim, Hyers, Cohen, & Ferguson, 2001). Experiencing sexist events has been associated with eating disordered attitudes (Sabik & Tylka, 2006). The recently developed Interpersonal Sexual Objectification Scale (ISOS) measures the experience of sexual objectification (e.g., having one's body evaluated by others experiencing unwanted sexual advances), without having participants label the events as specifically sexist (Kozee, Tylka, Augustus-Horvath, & Denchik, 2007). Total scores on the ISOS were associated with higher self-objectification, which, in turn, related to higher body shame lending support to predictions derived from the Objectification Theory (Kozee et al., 2007). Thus, the everyday experience of being treated like a sexualized body might encourage women to self-objectify, which puts women at risk for body shame and eating disorders.

Abuse and Violence
Girls are more likely than boys to be victims of child sexual abuse. Women are more likely than men to be victims of rape. Among girls and women, such experiences of sexual violence are indeed related to the later development of eating disorders, particularly bulimia nervosa (Smolak & Levine, 2007; Thompson & Wonderlich, 2004). This relationship, which is not as clearly evident for men, may be mediated by neurochemical or psychological factors initiated by the trauma of sexual violence (Smolak & Levine, 2007). It is noteworthy that other forms of trauma may not have the same effects on women's body image and eating problems (e.g., Faravelli, Giugni, Salvatori, & Ricca, 2004).

The Gendered Lived Experience of the Body: The Need for Integrated Theories in Gender-Informed Prevention
Thus far, this chapter has delineated different gender-based social experiences and their relationship to body image and disordered eating patterns. However, in order to understand the meaning of having a gendered body, it is important to explore the shared meaning of different types of gender-based social experiences, their interrelationships, and their intersection with other aspects of social location, such as ethno-cultural heritage or socio-economic standing. The advantage of a multifactorial, integrated model is that it allows the simultaneous consideration of pathways that may link gender-based social experiences to negative body image and disordered eating patterns as well the pathways' interrelationships and aggregated impact. In turn, such a model can help guide prevention work.

Piran (2001, 2008) has suggested an integrated model linking adverse gender-based experiences with body weight and shape preoccupation and disordered eating patterns and refers to it as "Disrupted Embodiment Through Inequity: The Adverse Social Experiences Model to the Development of Disordered Eating" (see Figure 1). This model has been studied so far among girls and women. The model suggests that three broad types of gender-related social experiences contribute to the development

FIGURE 1: DISRUPTED EMBODIMENT THROUGH INEQUITY: THE ADVERSE SOCIAL EXPERIENCES MODEL TO THE DEVELOPMENT OF DISORDERED EATING PATTERNS

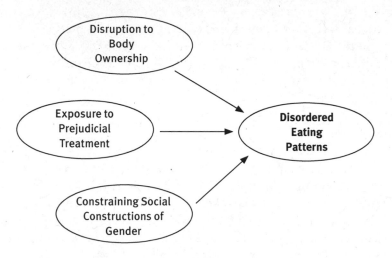

Source: Piran (2001); Piran and Thompson (2008).

of body dissatisfaction and disordered eating among girls and women. Each of these types of social experiences intersects with other social variables. The first class of adverse social experiences, Disruption to Body Ownership, includes a range of experiences that violate the experience of a rightful and safe ownership of one's body, such as the objectification and sexualization of the body, external dictations of appearance or eating standards, breaching of one's privacy, sexual harassment, and a range of sexual and physical violations. The second class of adverse social experiences, Exposure to Prejudicial Treatment, relates to experiences whereby the individual is exposed to prejudices such as sexism, weightism, racism, classism, or heterosexism, which target one's body as a way to demean the individual within the hierarchy of social privilege. At times, prejudicial treatment reflects the intersections of these prejudices. The third class of adverse social experiences, Constraining Social Constructions of Gender, relates to the multiple ways in which the social construction of femininity constrains the way girls and women can inhabit their body. These experiences include, for example, a more limited access to physical experiences of competence and functionality compared with boys, a struggle between self-nurturance and the care of others or the discomfort with their own sexual desire and the negative labeling of women's sexuality (as opposed to the social sanctioning of women being an object of sexual desire).

This model was derived from a large-scale qualitative study with girls (Piran, 2001), as an aspect of a feminist ecological study of a prevention program that led to a significant change in eating disorders among the girls and to their school system (Piran, 1999a). The model (the direct pathways of Violation of Body Ownership and Exposure to Prejudicial Treatment) has been further studied using structural equation modelling in two quantitative studies with a university student sample and a separate community-based sample (Piran & Thompson, 2008), confirming the model and its stability. Both the factor loadings and the factor structure were similar across the samples. The pathway of Constraining Social Constructions of Gender was investigated in a separate study (Piran & Cormier, 2005). Components of this constraining construction—including self-silencing, internalizing anger, and objectified body consciousness—accounted for 32% of the variability in Eating Attitudes Test scores in a sample of university women.

More recently, the model has been supported by a five-year prospective of 27 diverse adolescent girls (Piran, 2008). The model is consistent with the previously discussed findings concerning sexual violence and objectification as well as other research on self-silencing (e.g., Smolak & Munstertieger, 2002) but is more comprehensive and integrative. The model needs further study utilizing a prospective quantitative design with girls and young women. The model may apply to boys and men, and this issue requires further study. Moreover, this model examined adverse social experiences. However, a comprehensive social theory needs to examine protective factors as well (see Piran, Carter, Thompson, & Pajouhandeh, 2002; Chapter 6 in this volume).

The model therefore generates different pathways to eating disorders, such as the early sexualization and objectification of the body or a range of sexual violations (Disrupted Ownership of Body Ownership), exposure to the combined impact of sexism, racism, and weightism (verbal teasing such as "fat brown cow") (Exposure to Prejudicial Treatment), or the penalizing of a girl's natural connection to appetites and desires, both oral and sexual as an aspect of gender socialization (Constraining Social Constructions of Gender). However, the model also suggests that experiences along the different dimensions may aggregate to contribute to the development of disordered eating patterns. For example, a girl who has experienced sexual violation (Disrupted to Body Ownership) that is compounded later by racial teasing (Exposure to Prejudicial Treatment) faces multiple challenges in inhabiting her body. The model highlights the complexity of gender-based social influences and encourages an ecological examination of the embodied experience of youth in multiple social systems (family, school, and the larger social system). This ecological examination, in turn, should guide prevention work.

Implications for Prevention

Research is increasingly clear that girls and women face a variety of typical, frequent experiences that, in combination, may well explain gender differences in body image and eating disturbances. These experiences occur at home, at school, in the workplace, and when reading magazines or watching television. They are pervasive and consistent. If programs aimed at the prevention of body image and eating problems are to be successful on a long-term basis, they must address these experiences.

Program designers should consider adopting a feminist ecological model (Levine & Smolak, 2006; Piran, 1995, 1999b, 2001). A feminist ecological model aims to consider adverse influences in the body domain that are shaped by gender and other social factors and to address their expression at different levels of the social environment (larger social values, local communities such as schools, and families) (Piran, 1999b). Therefore, a feminist ecological model inherently focuses on transformations in the social environment of children. Concurrently, a feminist ecological model aims to foster in youth a critical perspective towards a range of social influences and, through this perspective, both prevent negative internalizations in individuals and use their growing critical awareness as a source of constructive social activism (Piran, 2001). Recognizing that social learning and change occur within a matrix of relationships, a feminist ecological model utilizes relational connections to create constructive changes in the life of youth (Piran, 1999b, 2001). In particular, Piran has emphasized the power inherent in establishing peer norms that are constructive to the sense of self and the body, such as prohibiting forms of peer teasing (Piran, 1999b). Interventions that seek to alter messages and pressures at a variety of levels may be more effective in preventing the development of body image problems, particularly if the messages can be reduced beginning at an early age (see Chapter 6 in this volume).

The integration of feminist perspectives holds promise for prevention. In one of the earliest feminist programs, Piran (1999a, 2001) instituted a longitudinal prevention program in a residential ballet school that embraced all elements of a feminist ecological prevention program. Prior to beginning the program, she secured the school administration's agreement to listen to the girls' concerns and to make appropriate changes in the school to address those issues. Piran emphasized establishing respectful relationships with the students that allowed them to voice their concerns about the elements of their school environment that were damaging to body image. In line with feminist-ecological principles, Piran then worked with the students and staff to actually change the school environment, including peer norms (e.g., no teasing), school policies (e.g., anti-harassment policies), curriculum (e.g., safety training), staff training and hiring (e.g., selecting supportive staff), and the physical setting (e.g., change rooms that allow more privacy), leading to a more constructive environment for students. Overall, students felt an increased sense of safety and rights in relation to their training at the school. Repeated all-school surveys during a ten-year period revealed that the systemic changes documented in the intensive case study analysis were associated with a significant reduction in disordered eating patterns in the school (Piran, 1999b, 2001). Further, over the course of the study, the prevalence of anorexia nervosa dropped tenfold, and there were no new cases of bulimia nervosa. Since this national residential dance school is a unique setting and since the interventions were aimed to address the school community as a whole, no control comparison group was available in Piran's study. However, during the study period, there were no changes in the requirements for thinness in the ballet world. Other prevention programs that have applied specific aspects of the feminist ecological approach also indicate its promise. For example, the Full of Ourselves: Advancing Girl Power, Health, and Leadership program, which was developed by Steiner-Adair and her colleagues (2002) aimed to specifically address a range of adverse influences in the body domain shaped by gender.

To address the disrupted body-self relations, the program emphasizes dialoguing with the body, such as experiential learning through body scanning and writing a journal to the body, and actions that counteract restrictions put on girls (such as "bio-energetic" punching activities, physical exercises, and assertive training). It also addresses weightism as a social issue, identifying and resisting unhealthy media messages. In a controlled evaluation (though without random allocation), the program was found to lead to positive changes to participants' body image, a result not often found in primary prevention programs, which was maintained at the 6-month follow-up. However, changes in eating behaviours were only marginally significant.

Several programs aimed at addressing the peer relational environment, which is one aspect of the larger social environment, have yielded initial positive results. The after-school "Very Important Kids" program responded to students' requests to focus on weight and appearance-related teasing in the school (Haines, Neumark-Sztainer, Perry, Hannan, & Levine, 2006). The program focused on setting no-teasing social norms through a no-teasing campaign and a theatre production. Compared to a control school, the program resulted in reduced weight and appearance-related teasing at the intervention school. At the university level, it is of relevance to highlight the work of Becker and her colleagues who have established prevention programs in sororities, relying on peer facilitators (Becker, Smith, & Ciao, 2005, 2006). As part of the prevention program, the many peer facilitators, all members of the sororities, have agreed to resist the thin ideal and serve as role models and norm setters. For example, similar to Piran's (2001) ballet school students, Becker, Ciao, and Smith (2008) describe that several sororities have established "no commenting on appearance" policies. Becker and her colleagues suggest that this change in the social system of the sororities may have contributed to the findings that the cognitive dissonance prevention program (Stice, Mazotti, Weibel, & Agras, 2000) as implemented in the sororities has led to gains that have been sustained at the 8-month follow-up.

An additional aspect of the feminist ecological prevention approach that has been utilized in prevention is the emphasis on the development of a critical perspective towards cultural pressures. This approach has been used in relation to media literacy, a critical examination of social stereotypes (O'Dea & Abraham, 2000), or the introduction of the cognitive dissonance in universities and sororities (Stice et al., 2000; Becker, Smith, & Ciao, 2006). These successes, limited though they are, underscore the potential value of a feminist approach to prevention. Larkin and Rice (2005) argued that we should "mainstream body equity" into our prevention programs and promote an acceptance of diverse body types. Similarly, Piran (1999b) has argued that we should focus on the many disempowering experiences that women have, including sexual harassment and prejudice. Piran and her colleagues (e.g., 2002; Piran & Cormier, 2005) have further drawn attention to the various ways that women express their disengagement from their bodies ("disembodiment") through behaviours such as smoking for weight control, plastic surgery, self-harm behaviour (such as "cutting"), risky sexual behaviours, and unhealthy weight management practices. In order to fully address such behaviours, we need to add a critique of the culture to our current prevention efforts.

A recent meta-analysis indicates that feminist identity is related to lower levels of thin ideal internalization and body shame (Murnen & Smolak, 2009). Thus, facilitating feminist identity development might protect girls and women against body image and eating problems. This action will include teaching program participants to critique cultural messages and empowering women to be confident and assertive and to actively resist and alter cultural norms and messages (Worell, 2006). Feminist identity alone will not be sufficient, however. The salience of the messages and the power of the rewards for following social norms may often override the feminist identity (Smolak & Murnen, 2011). Indeed, researchers have found such conflicts among college women (Rubin, Nemeroff, & Russo, 2006). Thus, changing the actual social ecology is also crucial.

Conclusion

Gender differences in the extent and nature of body image and eating problems are well documented. The actual role of gender per se in the development of these differences has received less attention. During the past decade, however, accumulating data indicate that gender role, objectification, and everyday sexism all play a role in the gendered nature of body image. Much more research, particularly longitudinal work, is needed to establish the precise nature and timing of these relationships.

These findings underscore the importance of a feminist, ecological approach to prevention (Levine & Smolak, 2006; Piran, 1999b, 2001). In addition to their salutary health effects, such as reducing body dissatisfaction or disordered eating, prevention programs can extend the empirical database. For example, a program that facilitates feminist empowerment can be examined for its effects on thin ideal internalization, self-surveillance, or body shame. Changes may be interpreted as demonstrating a causal link between feminist empowerment and body image. Such work is under way; much more is needed.

Indeed, given the clearly gendered nature of body image and eating problems, it is surprising how few data are available on the role of gender in the development and prevention of these problems. More research is needed on the etiological features of gender, including the frequency and meaning of gendered experiences such as sexual harassment and violence, athletic participation, and self-silencing. The mechanisms that might lead from gendered experiences to body dissatisfaction or disordered eating also need to be delineated and explored. The Adverse Social Experiences Model exemplifies this approach (see Figure 1; Piran, 2001; Piran & Thompson, 2008). Longitudinal data testing this model would be an important addition to the literature. The same might be said of the Objectification Theory.

The consequences of gendered experiences also need to be explored in more detail. Does the age at which the experience occurs matter? Ethnicity and social class are likely to shape the meaning of gendered experiences. How does this happen? Are there personal characteristics or contextual variables that reduce or increase the negative impact of gendered experiences? Recognizing and understanding the contextual importance of gender will significantly advance our ability to prevent body dissatisfaction and disordered eating.

Gender, as a powerful social variable, affects individuals' self and body experiences through shaping social relations at all levels of social organizations. For this reason, the feminist empowerment prevention model aims at transforming the nature of social relations at these multiple levels from policy-level change (such as employing only adult women models who are of healthy weight and diverse in appearance), through increased equity at the community level (such as providing girls and adolescent women with equal opportunity for engagement in physical activities in schools and community centres), to altering peer norms (e.g., prohibiting harassment based on gender, weight, and other social variables in schools). Prevention efforts aimed at system change need to be informed by theoretical perspectives on system frameworks (e.g., Foster-Fishman, Nowell, & Yang, 2007), by a stronger emphasis on contextual factors that shape interventions and their outcome (Trickett, 2009), and by adopting multiple approaches to evaluation, including detailed case analyses (Kraemer Tebes, Kaufman, & Connell, 2003; Trickett, 2009).

References

American Association of University Women. (2001). *Hostile hallways: Bullying, teasing, and sexual harassment in schools.* Washington, DC: Educational Foundation, American Association of University Women.

American Psychological Association. (2007). *Report of the APA Task Force on the sexualization of girls.* Retrieved from http://www.apa.org/pi/women/programs/girls/report-full.pdf

Bearman, S. K., & Stice, E. (2008) Testing a gender additive model: The role of body image in adolescent depression. *Journal of Abnormal Child Psychology, 36,* 1251-1263.

Becker, C. B., Ciao, A. C., & Smith, L. M. (2008). Moving from efficacy to effectiveness in eating disorders prevention: The Sorority Body Image Program. *Cognitive and Behavioral Practice, 15,* 18-27.

Becker, C. B., Smith, L. M., & Ciao, A. C. (2005). Reducing eating disorder risk factors in sorority members: A randomized trial. *Behavior Therapy, 36,* 245-253.

Becker, C. B., Smith, L. M., & Ciao, A. C. (2006). Peer-facilitated eating disorder prevention: A randomized effectiveness trial of cognitive dissonance and media advocacy. *Journal of Counseling Psychology, 53,* 550-555.

Bordo, S. (1993). *Unbearable weight: Feminism, Western culture, and the body.* Berkeley, CA: University of California Press.

Bryant, A. (1993). Hostile hallways: The AAUW Survey on Sexual Harassment in America's schools. *Journal of School Health, 63,* 335-357.

Bryant-Waugh, R., & Lask, B. (2007). Overview. In B. Lask & R. Bryant-Waugh (Eds.), *Anorexia nervosa and related eating disorders in childhood and adolescence* (pp. 35-50). London: Routledge.

Burns, P. (2008). Corporate entrepreneurship: Building the entrepreneural organization. (2nd ed.). Hodgson, UK: Palgrave. Retrived from http://www .palgrave.com/uploaded files/barbie. pdf

Calogero, R. M., Davis, W. N., Thompson, J. K. (2005). The role of self-objectification in the experience of women with eating disorders. *Sex Roles, 52*, 43-50.

Cash, T., & Pruzinsky, T. (2002). *Body image: A handbook of theory, research, and clinical practice.* New York: Guilford.

Collectdolls.about.com (2012). Barbie fun facts. Retrived from http://collectdolls .about.com/library/blbarbie facts.htm

Croll, J., Neumark-Sztainer, D., Story, M., & Ireland, M. (2002). Prevalence and risk and protective factors related to disordered eating behaviors among adolescents: Relationship to gender and ethnicity. *Journal of Adolescent Health, 33*, 166-175.

Dittmar, H., Halliwell, E., & Ive, S. (2006). Does Barbie make girls want to be thin? The effect of experimental exposure to images of dolls on the body image of five-to-eight-year-old girls. *Developmental Psychology, 42*, 283-292.

Faravelli, C., Giugni, A., Salvatori, S., & Ricca, V. (2004). Psychopathology after rape. *American Journal of Psychiatry, 161*, 1483-1485.

Field, A., Camargo, C., Taylor, C., Berkey, C., Frazier, L., Gillman, M., & Colditz, G. (1999). Overweight, weight concerns, and bulimic behaviors among girls and boys. *Journal of the American Academy of Child and Adolescent Psychiatry, 38*, 754-760.

Foster-Fishman, P. G., Nowell, B., & Yang, H. (2007). Putting the system back into system change: A framework for understanding and changing organization and community systems. *American Journal of Community Psychology, 39*, 197-215.

Frederick, D., Forbes, G., Grigorian, K., & Jarcho, J. (2007). The UCLA Body Project I: Gender and ethnic differences in self-objectification and body satisfaction among 2,206 undergraduates. *Sex Roles, 7*, 317-327.

Fredrickson, B. L., & Roberts, T. A. (1997). Objectification theory: Toward understanding women's lived experiences and mental health risks. *Psychology of Women Quarterly, 21*, 173-206.

Fredrickson, B. L., Roberts, T. A., Noll, S. M., Quinn, D. M., & Twenge, J. M. (1998). That swimsuit becomes you: Sex differences in self-objectification, restrained eating, and math performance. *Journal of Personality and Social Psychology, 75*, 269-284.

Glick, P., & Fiske, S. T. (1996). The Ambivalent Sexism Inventory: Differentiating hostile and benevolent sexism. *Journal of Personality and Social Psychology, 70*, 491-512.

Glick, P., Larsen, S., Johnson, C., & Branstiter, H. (2005). Evaluations of sexy women in low- and high-status jobs. *Psychology of Women Quarterly, 29*, 389-395.

Goodin, S., Van Denberg, A., Murnen, S. K., & Smolak, L. (2011). "Putting on" sexiness: A content analysis of the presence of sexualizing characteristics in girls' clothing. *Sex Roles, 65*, 1-12.

Grabe, S., & Hyde, J. S. (2006). Ethnicity and body dissatisfaction among women in the United States: A meta-analysis. *Psychological Bulletin, 132,* 622-640.

Grabe, S., Ward, L. M., & Hyde, J. S. (2008). The role of the media in body image concerns among women: A meta-analysis of experimental and correlational studies. *Psychological Bulletin, 134,* 460-476.

Groesz, L. M., Levine, M. P., & Murnen, S. K. (2002). The effect of experimental presentation of thin media images on body satisfaction: A meta-analytic review. *International Journal of Eating Disorders, 31,* 1-16.

Haines, J., Neumark-Sztainer, D., Perry, C. L., Hannan, P. J., & Levine, M. P. (2006). V.I.K. (Very Important Kids): A school-based program designed to reduce teasing and unhealthy weight-control behaviors. *Health Education Research: Theory and Practice, 21*(6), 884-895.

Hill, C., & Silva, E. (2006). *Drawing the line: Sexual harassment on campus.* Washington, DC: Educational Foundation, American Association of University Women. Retrieved from http://www.aauw.org

Hill, A. J., Weaver, C., & Blundell, J. E. (1990). Dieting concerns of ten-year-old girls and their mothers. *British Journal of Clinical Psychology, 29,* 346-348.

Irving, L., Wall, M., Neumark-Sztainer, D., & Story, M. (2002). Steroid use among adolescents: Findings from Project EAT. *Journal of Adolescent Health, 30,* 243-252.

Klonoff, E. A., & Landrine, H. (1995). The schedule of sexist events: A measure of lifetime and recent sexist discrimination in women's lives. *Psychology of Women Quarterly, 19,* 439-472.

Kozee, H. B., Tylka, T. L., Augustus-Hovath, C., & Denchik, A. (2007). Development and psychometric evaluation of the Interpersonal Sexual Objectification Scale. *Psychology of Women Quarterly, 31,* 176-189.

Kraemer Tebes, J., Kaufman, J. S., & Connell, C. M. (2003). The evaluation of prevention and health promotion programs. In T. P. Gullotta & M. Bloom (Eds.), *Encyclopedia of Primary Prevention and Health Promotion* (pp. 42-61). New York: Kluwer Academic/Plenum Publishers.

Larkin, J., & Rice, C. (2005). Beyond "healthy eating" and "healthy weights": Harassment and the health curriculum in middle schools. *Body Image, 2,* 219-232.

Leaper, C., & Brown, C. (2008). Perceived experiences with sexism among adolescent girls. *Child Development, 79,* 685-704.

Levin, D., & Kilbourne, J. (2008). *So sexy, so soon: The new sexualized childhood and what parents can do to protect their kids.* New York: Ballantine.

Levine, M. P., & Smolak, L. (2006). *The prevention of eating problems and eating disorders: Theory, research, and practice.* Mahwah NJ: Lawrence Erlbaum Associates.

Lindberg, S., Grabe, S., & Hyde, J. S. (2007). Gender, pubertal development, and peer sexual harassment predict objectified body consciousness in early adolescence. *Journal of Research on Adolescence, 17,* 723-742.

Lindberg, S., Hyde, J., & McKinley, N. (2006). A measure of objectified body consciousness for pre-adolescent and adolescent youth. *Psychology of Women Quarterly, 30,* 65-76.

Lowes, J., & Tiggemann, M. (2003). Body dissatisfaction, dieting awareness and the impact of parental influence in young children. *British Journal of Health Psychology, 8,* 135-147.

Mahalik, J. R., Locke, B. D., Ludlow, L. H., Diemer, M. A., Scott, R. P. J., Gottfried, M., & Freitas, G. (2003). Development of the conformity to masculine norms inventory. *Psychology of Men and Masculinity, 4,* 3-25.

Mahalik, J. R., Mooray, E. B. Coonerty-Femiano, A., Ludlow, L. H., Slattery, S. M., & Smiler, A. (2005). Development of the conformity to feminine norms inventory. *Sex Roles, 52,* 417-435.

Marchi, M., & Cohen, P. (1990). Early childhood eating behaviors and adolescent eating disorders. *Journal of the American Academy of Child and Adolescent Psychiatry, 29,* 112-117.

McCreary, D., Saucier, D., & Courtenay, W. (2003). The drive for muscularity and masculinity: Testing the associations among gender-role traits, behaviors, attitudes, and conflict. *Psychology of Men and Masculinity, 6,* 83-94.

McGhan, M. (2007). Dancing toward redemption. In S. Shaw & J. Lee (Eds.), *Women's voices, feminist visions: Classic and contemporary readings* (pp. 284-288). Boston: McGraw-Hill.

McKinley, N. M (1999). Women and objectified body consciousness: Mothers' and daughters' body experience in cultural, developmental, and familial contexts. *Developmental Psychology, 35,* 760-769.

McKinley, N. M., & Hyde, J. S. (1996). The objectified body consciousness scale: Self-objectification, body shame, and disordered eating. *Psychology of Women Quarterly, 22,* 623-636.

McKinley, N. M., & Lyon, L. A. (2008). Menopausal attitudes, objectified body consciousness, aging anxiety, and body esteem: European American women's body experiences in midlife. *Body Image, 5,* 375-380.

Moradi, B., & Huang, Y. (2008). Objectification theory and psychology of women: A decade of advances and future directions. *Psychology of Women Quarterly, 32,* 377-398.

Muehlenkamp, J. J., & Saris-Baglama, R. N. (2002). Self-objectification and its psychological outcomes for college women. *Psychology of Women Quarterly, 26,* 371-379.

Murnen, S. K., & Smolak, L. (2000). The experience of sexual harassment among grade-school students: Early socialization of female subordination? *Sex Roles, 43,* 1-17.

Murnen, S. K., & Smolak, L. (2009). Are feminist women protected from body image problems? A meta-analytic review of relevant research. *Sex Roles, 60,* 186-197.

Murnen, S. K., Smolak, L., Mills, J. A., & Good, L. (2003). Thin, sexy women and strong, muscular men: Grade-school children's responses to objectified images of women and men. *Sex Roles, 49,* 427-437.

Musher-Eizenman, D., Holub, S., Edwards-Leeper, L., Persson, A., & Goldstein, S. (2003). The narrow range of acceptable body types of preschoolers and their mothers. *Applied Developmental Psychology, 24,* 259-272.

Neumark-Sztainer, D., Paxton, S., Hannan, P., Haines, J., & Story M. (2006). Does body satisfaction matter? Five-year longitudinal associations between body satisfaction and health behaviors in adolescent females and males. *Journal of Adolescent Health, 36,* 244-251.

O'Dea, J. A., & Abraham, S. (2000). Improving the body image, eating attitudes, and behaviors of young male and female adolescents: A new educational approach that focuses on self- esteem. *International Journal of Eating Disorders, 28,* 43-57.

Paxton, S. J., Norris, M., Wertheim, E. H., Durkin, S. J., & Anderson, J. (2005). Body dissatisfaction, dating and importance of thinness to attractiveness in adolescent girls. *Sex Roles, 53,* 663-675.

Paxton, S. J., Wertheim, E. H., Gibbons, K., Szmukler, G. I., Hillier, L., & Petrovich, J. L. (1991). Body image satisfaction, dieting beliefs and weight loss behaviors in adolescent girls and boys. *Journal of Youth and Adolescence, 20,* 361-379.

Petersen, A., Crockett, L., Richards, M., & Boxer, A. (1988). A self-report measure of pubertal status: Reliability, validity, and initial norms. *Journal of Youth and Adolescence, 17,* 117-133.

Piran, N. (1995). Prevention: Can early lessons lead to a delineation of an alternative model? A critical look at prevention with school children. *Eating Disorders: Journal of Treatment and Prevention, 3*(1), 28-36.

Piran, N. (1999a). Eating disorders: A trial of prevention in a high-risk school setting. *Journal of Primary Prevention, 20*(1), 75-90.

Piran, N. (1999b). The reduction of preoccupation with body weight and shape in schools: A feminist approach. In N. Piran, M. Levine, & C. Steiner-Adair (Eds.), *Preventing eating disorders: A handbook of interventions and special challenges* (pp. 148-59). Philadelphia, PA: Taylor and Francis.

Piran, N. (2001). Re-inhabiting the body from the inside out: Girls transform their school environment. In D. L. Tolman & M. Brydon-Miller (Eds.), *From subjects to subjectivities: A handbook of interpretive and participatory methods* (pp. 218-238). New York, NY: New York University Press.

Piran, N. (2008). The body journey of girls study report: A five-year prospective study of embodiment in girls [unpublished manuscript; on file with the author].

Piran, N., Antoniou, M., Legge, R., McCance, N., Mizevich, J., Pesley, E., & Ross, E. (2006). *On girls' disembodiment: The complex tyranny of the "ideal girl"* (Presented at the Women, Health, and Education Sixth Bi-Annual International Institute Proceedings, Canadian Association for Social Work Education, St. John's, NL). Available at http://www.med.mun.ca/comhealth/CASWE/pdf_docs/proceeding_july22-06.pdf (http://www.csse.ca/CASWE/Institute/Institute.htm)

Piran, N., Carter, W., Thompson, S., & Pajouhandeh, P. (2002). Powerful girls: A contradiction in terms? Young women speak about the experience of growing up in a girl's body. In S. Abbey (Ed.), *Ways of knowing in and through the body: Diverse perspectives on embodiment* (pp. 206-210). Welland, ON: Soleil Publishing.

Piran, N., & Cormier, H. (2005). The social construction of women and disordered eating patterns. *Journal of Counseling Psychology, 52*, 549-558.

Piran, N., & Thompson, S. (2008). A study of the adverse social experiences model to the development of eating disorders. *International Journal of Health Promotion and Education, 46*, 65-71.

Ricciardelli, L., & McCabe, M. (2007). Pursuit of muscularity among adolescents. In J. K. Thompson & G. Cafri (Eds.), *The muscular ideal* (pp. 199-216). Washington, DC: American Psychological Association.

Ricciardelli, L., McCabe, M., Mussap, A., & Holt, K. E. (2009). Body image in preadolescent boys. In L. Smolak & J. K. Thompson (Eds.), *Body image, eating disorders, and obesity in youth: Assessment, prevention, and treatment* (2nd ed., pp. 77 96). Washington, DC: American Psychological Association.

Rubin, L. R., Nemeroff, C. J., & Russo, N. F. (2004). Exploring feminist women's body consciousness. *Psychology of Women Quarterly, 28*, 27-37.

Sabik, N. J., & Tylka, T. L. (2006). Do feminist identity styles moderate the relation between perceived sexist events and disordered eating? *Psychology of Women Quarterly, 30*, 77-84.

Sheffield, C. J. (2007). Sexual terrorism. In L. L. O'Toole, J. R. Shiffman, & M. L. K. Edwards (Eds.) *Gender violence: Interdisciplinary perspectives* (2nd ed., pp. 111-130). New York: New York University Press.

Slater, A., & Tiggemann, M. (2002). A test of the objectification theory in adolescent girls. *Sex Roles, 46*, 343-349.

Smolak, L., & Levine, M. P. (2001). Body image in children. In J. K. Thompson & L. Smolak (Eds.), *Body image, eating disorders, and obesity in children: Theory, assessment, treatment, and prevention* (pp. 41-66). Washington, DC: American Psychological Association.

Smolak, L., & Levine, M. P. (2007). Trauma, eating problems, and eating disorders. In S. Wonderlich, J. Mitchell, H. Steiger, & M. deZwaan (Eds.) *Annual Review of Eating Disorders: Part I—2007* (pp. 113-124). New York: Radcliffe/Oxford.

Smolak, L., Levine, M. P., & Schermer, F. (1998). Lessons from lessons: An evaluation of an elementary school program. In G. Noordenbos & W. Vandereycken (Eds.) *The prevention of eating disorders* (pp. 137-172). London: Athlone Press.

Smolak, L., & Munstertieger, B. (2002). The relationship of gender and voice to depression and eating disorders. *Psychology of Women Quarterly, 26*, 234-241.

Smolak, L., & Murnen, S. K. (2011). The sexualization of girls and women as antecedents of objectification. In R. Calogero, S. Tantleff-Dunn, & J. K. Thompson (Eds.), *Self- objectification in women: Causes, consequences, and counteractions.* Washington, DC: American Psychological Association.

Smolak, L., & Stein, J. A. (2010). A longitudinal investigation of gender role and muscle building in adolescent boys. *Sex Roles, 63*, 738-746.

Smolak, L., & Stein, J. (2006). The relationship of drive for muscularity to sociocultural factors, self-esteem, physical attributes gender role, and social comparison in middle school boys. *Body Image, 3*, 121-129.

Stankiewicz, J. M., & Rosselli, F. (2008). Women as sex objects and victims in print advertisements. *Sex Roles, 58*, 579-589.

Steiner-Adair, C., Sjostrom, L., Franko, D. L., Pai, S., Tucker, R., Becker, A., & Herzog, D. (2002). Primary prevention of risk factors for eating disorders in adolescent girls: Learning from practice. *International Journal of Eating Disorders, 32*, 401-411.

Stice, E., & Bearman, S. K. (2001). Body image and eating disturbances prospectively predict increases in depressive symptoms in adolescent girls: A growth curve analysis. *Developmental Psychology, 37*, 597-607.

Stice, E., Cameron, R., Hayward, C., Taylor, C. B., & Killen, J. (1999). Naturalistic weight-reduction efforts prospectively predict growth in relative weight and onset among female adolescents. *Journal of Consulting and Clinical Psychology, 67*, 967-974.

Stice, E., Hayward, C., Cameron, R., Killen, J. D., & Taylor, C. B. (2000). Body image and eating related factors predict onset of depression in female adolescents: A longitudinal study. *Journal of Abnormal Psychology, 109*, 438-444.

Stice, E., Mazotti, L., Weibel, D., & Agras, W.S. (2000). Dissonance prevention program decreases thin-ideal internalization, body dissatisfaction, dieting, negative affect, and bulimic symptoms: A preliminary experiment. *International Journal of Eating Disorders, 27*, 206-217.

Swim, J. K., Hyers, L. L., Cohen, L. L., & Ferguson, M. J. (2001). Everyday sexism: Evidence for its incidence, nature, and psychological impact from three daily diary studies. *Journal of Social Issues, 57*, 31-53.

Thompson, J. K., & Cafri, G. (2007). The muscular ideal: An introduction. In J. K. Thompson & G. Cafri (Eds.), *The muscular ideal* (pp. 3-12). Washington, DC: American Psychological Association.

Thompson, K. M., & Wonderlich, S. (2004). Child sexual abuse and eating disorders. In J. K. Thompson (Ed.), *Handbook of eating disorders and obesity* (pp. 679-694). Hoboken, NJ: Wiley.

Tiggemann, M. (2004). Body image across the adult life span: Stability and change. *Body Image, 1*, 29-41.

Tiggemann, M., & Kuring, J. K. (2004). The role of body objectification in disordered eating and depressed mood. *British Journal of Clinical Psychology, 43*, 299-311.

Trickett, E. J. (2009). Community psychology: Individuals and interventions in community context. *Annual Review of Psychology, 60*, 395-419.

Wertheim, E., Paxton, S., & Blaney, S. (2009). Body image in girls. In L. Smolak & J. K. Thompson (Eds.), *Body image, eating disorders, and obesity in youth: Assessment, prevention, and treatment* (2nd ed., pp. 47-76). Washington, DC: American Psychological Association.

Worell, J. (2006). Pathways to healthy development: Sources of strength and empowerment. In J. Worell & C. D. Goodheart (Eds.), *Handbook of girls' and women's psychological health* (pp. 25-35). New York: Oxford.

CHAPTER NINE

Eating Disorders and Obesity: Epidemiology and the Perception of Risk

Leora Pinhas, *Hospital for Sick Children*
Benjamin Taylor, *University of Toronto*

Risk is difficult to interpret and manage. Even for scientists and clinicians, understanding how risk impacts your life is nearly impossible given the widely varying, and often disparate, messages we receive. Additionally, realizing subtle differences in absolute risk (one's overall chance of developing diabetes, for example) and relative risk (your change in diabetes risk due to a factor such as diet) are nearly impossible, particularly given the type and amount of information we receive. This chapter will provide a context with which to think about risk—from the sources of data to how it is presented and even how the subject matter impacts interpretation and meaning. Specifically, this chapter will focus on the literature and knowledge around obesity and eating disorders and finish with a discussion on how decisions about risk impact prevention and intervention in a clinical setting.

Risk

Risk is defined as a chance or possibility of danger, loss, injury, or other adverse consequence (Allen, 1990). However, in the technical language of epidemiology, risk is simply defined as the probability, or likelihood, that an event, whether positive or negative, will occur within a stated period of time or by a certain age (Last, 2001). Therefore, a risk factor is an attribute or exposure that is associated with an increased probability of a specified outcome. Therefore, we could speak about the risk of leg cramps following swimming, the risk of a hand injury when using a power drill, or the risk of sneezing after pepper exposure. Importantly though, we are not necessarily talking about a causal relationship, where one factor precedes the outcome and is required for that outcome to occur (Last, 2001). Often, when most people speak about risk, they might simply be referring to an association. This can be misinterpreted as causation. For example, women are at greater risk of getting breast cancer than men, but this does not mean that being a woman causes breast cancer. A cause is something that is necessary to produce an effect, while an association is present simply if the probability of an occurrence of an event depends on the occurrence of another event or characteristic, which may or may not be a causal relationship (Last, 2001). So, while being female does not cause breast cancer, there is an association between the two since being female does predict a higher risk of developing breast cancer than being male. Just by examining these definitions, it becomes clear that scientists and the lay public use the word risk to describe quite differing concepts.

Absolute versus Relative Risk

There are two main types of risk—absolute risk and relative risk—and although they are related they can often be wildly different for the same disease. Absolute risk is simply the incidence of a disease in a population. Relative risk is the probability of an event or outcome occurring in an exposed group (to some factor of interest) as compared to the probability of the event in non-exposed people (Gordis, 2004). We will look at an example of adolescent obesity prevalence to illustrate these two concepts.

One of the concerns about obesity is the associated morbidity of certain illnesses such as diabetes. How data are presented can lead to confusion because of the misunderstandings that arise in relation to relative and absolute risk. Canadian incidence studies report that 95% of the new cases of type II diabetes in children and adolescents occur in obese youth (Canadian Paediatric Society, 2008). From these data, we can then say that the risk of type II diabetes is 19 times greater in obese children and adolescents as compared to non-obese youth. In fact, the authors of this study have recommended screening all obese youth for type II diabetes, despite the fact that there are only about 200 new cases per year in all of Canada (Canadian Paediatric Society, 2007). While most of these cases do occur in obese youth, the absolute incidence in obese youth is about 1 per 2,000 individuals (0.0005%) (Shields, 2004). This finding means that physicians would have to screen 1999 obese young people before they found one new case with type II diabetes. It is unlikely that any ten physicians will have that many adolescent patients, let alone obese adolescents. It is rather more likely that the screen will be negative. The absolute risk remains extremely small, but the relative risk is very high. These types of large relative increases, where the absolute risk is still very small, can serve to exaggerate the problem. Type II diabetes remains a rare condition in youth but is often described as an epidemic (Vivian, 2006)—one that is so serious it needs its own prevention programs (Canadian Paediatric Society, 2008). Inadequate explanations of the type of risk being discussed can be a recipe for skewed judgment, and both of these examples of obesity in youth show us that how risk is perceived depends a great deal on how data are presented.

While not technically defining risk, prevalence data can also help us contextualize the numbers being discussed in relation to risk and, thus, help us to better conceptualize the size of the youth obesity problem. For example, the overall prevalence of type II diabetes in adolescents ranges from 0.4 per 1,000 to 4 per 1,000 (Goran et al., 2008; Mayer-Davis, 2008). The prevalence of type II diabetes in the largest children in the United States (adolescents who have a body mass index (BMI) in the ninety-ninth percentile or higher) is 13 per 1,000 (1.3%) (Goran et al., 2008). This finding means that the prevalence of type II diabetes in the largest adolescents is approximately three to 30 times greater than the prevalence in the general population of adolescents. However, in terms of absolute prevalence, it is still quite rare. Consider that 98.7% of the largest adolescents will *not* have type II diabetes as compared to 99.6-99.9% of the general population of adolescents—the numbers do not seem so wildly different now. This prevalence of 1.3% is much lower than many other teen "conditions," including getting pregnant or contracting a sexually transmitted disease such as chlamydia or herpes (Division of Sexually Transmitted Disease Prevention, 1999). The risk of developing type II diabetes can thus be described in very different ways. On the one hand, it can be said that "about 98 percent of obese children do not have type II diabetes." On the other hand, it can be described in relative terms, which, while mathematically correct, may create a picture where the problem appears greater than it is.

Risk: Perception Equals Presentation

The general public tends to think quite differently than scientists about risks—general "feelings" about perceived risk tend to overpower real numbers and statistics about the event actually occurring. For example, are you scared of sharks, bears, snakes? You have every reason to be frightened of these creatures provided the context of your risk is also apparent—that is, do you live near any of these animals? Are they a part of the natural fauna in your town?

Risk perception is the subjective judgment or belief that an individual or group has about the nature of a risk, its severity, its likelihood of occurring, and the timing of its occurrence. These beliefs can be rational or irrational

(Fischhoff, 1995). Risk experts tend to judge risk on the likelihood of an event happening. For example, generally the chance of injury in a hurricane is high, but the actual risk to a farmer in land-locked Saskatchewan is very low due to the fact that hurricanes are non-existent in this province. Vincent Covello, a professor of risk management at Columbia University, writes: "Strong beliefs about risk, once formed, change very slowly and are extraordinarily persistent in the face of contrary evidence" (cited in Walsh, 1998). So let us revisit our fear of sharks and compare it with something you probably have very positive feelings towards—fireworks. Worldwide, the average risk of dying from a fireworks-related accident is one in about 340,000 or 0.000003%. Your risk of dying from a shark attack, on the other hand, is about one in 3.75 million, or more than 10 times less than your fireworks risk, but the *perceived* risk of shark attack in the general population is much greater. The Discovery Channel dedicates an entire week to sharks and their attacks, in fact. Why? Not because the risk is actually anything to worry about but, rather, because it makes for a good story, which is where presentation becomes important. Presentation is really what is driving risk communication in popular media—if the story is sensational, or at least entertaining, it will be written about. If the story is not something your news station or television network thinks is worth hearing about, chances are you will not hear about it as it will not become news.

Risk perception is affected by many things, including the immediacy of risk (Fischhoff, Slovic, Lichtenstein, Read, & Combs, 1978; Fischhoff, Watson, & Hope, 1984), the nature of the risk and how "dreaded" the outcome is (Kasperson et al., 1988), how familiar the risk is (Wilson & Crouch, 2001), and the degree to which there is a voluntariness in undertaking the risk (Starr, 1969). Layered onto this is how someone *feels* about the consequence or benefit of the risk. For example, if consequences carry sharp and strong affective meaning, as is the case with a lottery jackpot (positive affective meaning) or a cancer (negative affective meaning), subjects become insensitive to variation in probability. That is, whether the chance of either occurring goes up or down by 100 times, the feeling about it is the same—people still want to win the lottery and avoid cancer. What is more, when chances of either are extremely low or become even lower than before, such as when the lottery pot increases due to no one winning it for two weeks, the affective meaning may become even stronger, which is counterintuitive—the meaning of the outcome becomes stronger the less likely it is to occur (Slovic, Peters, Finucane, & Macgregor, 2005).

Risk perception is also affected by how the risk is presented (Wilson & Crouch, 2001). If you were to ask a random group of 50 adults, most would agree that one or two glasses of red wine is good for your heart. Therefore, a perceived "healthy choice" for drinking-age people might be to drink wine in this quantity. However, what is seldom regarded is that alcohol is also a proven risk factor for 60 other causes of death and disability, including stroke and a number of well-known cancers, even at the recommended two glasses of wine per day (Bagnardi, Blangiardo, La Vecchia, & Corrao, 2001; Rehm et al., 2003). Additionally, the main benefits of drinking wine are found only in those over 40 years of age and only those in Western cultures, since alcohol is actually associated with an increase in mortality for those under 40 and associated with only negative consequences in non-Western countries, both from a health and social standpoint (Fuchs et al., 1995; World Health Organization, 2004). What is more, it may be most beneficial to those at an already increased risk of coronary heart disease, meaning that for those with a low absolute risk of coronary heart disease already, a couple of glasses of a nice Cabernet Sauvignon is not going to help their heart a great deal (nor hurt it, for that matter), despite the hype (Jackson & Beaglehole, 1995).

The point here is that risk perception (or misperception) and presentation is extremely difficult, even for experts. We drive cars, walk around on busy streets, and play recreational sports, all of which carry inherent risks of death and injury to us, but the risks are so familiar that we gladly accept and/or ignore them. Since they are not discussed as risk factors for death or injury in the same way that the "dreaded consequences" of obesity, alcohol, and smoking are, for example, their risk is seemingly low due to non-coverage and routine. In truth, driving a car is just as modifiable a risk factor as any of the "big three" (obesity, alcohol, and smoking).

Why Is Knowing about True Risk Important?
It is clear that risk communication is complex and multi-dimensional and hard to judge, but it is vitally important to consider because of its influence on health behaviour. We make choices about our health and act accordingly, but there is a real need to have all of the pertinent information. While studies on the relationship between risk perception and health behaviour vary in outcome, meta-analyses support the idea that risk perceptions predict health behaviours—the greater the risk perception, the more likely the health-seeking relationship (Brewer et al., 2007). However, there is great variation in the strength of this relationship. Interpretation of risk is probably more important for behaviours that are thought to reduce a specific health consequence rather than for behaviours that have a wide range of positive health and non-health consequences, such as exercise and diet—that is, most people are more willing to take a cholesterol-lowering drug than work out for an hour per day. Risk perceptions are

also more important when people make voluntary decisions than when strong external influences are present, as with physician recommendations. Finally, when behaviours are easy to carry out, more people do them (Brewer et al., 2007).

For the purpose of this chapter, it should be understood that one's health behaviour is dependent on how risk is perceived, combined with beliefs about the benefits and consequences of the health behaviour—that is, this combination affects decisions about the action to be taken to minimize health risks. Keep in mind, though, that these beliefs do not exist in a vacuum—cultural norms and general consensus about the health behaviour and its inherent benefits and consequences will also affect your health behaviour.

There are so many factors at work when it comes to determining risk for certain conditions, many of which are out of the control of the average consumer, that it becomes very confusing. However, a firmer understanding of what risk is should become apparent in the following pages. We will be first illustrating and highlighting, in terms of measurement and scientific studies, the culture of risk perception and risk presentation in the highly contentious world of child and adolescent obesity. What is more, we will see how risk presentation and perception has an impact on clinical experts and decision-makers in the clinical world of eating disorders.

Body Weight and BMI as a Measure

Let us discuss first how weight is measured in adults and children. Weight is typically categorized by a BMI (weight in kilograms divided by height in metres squared) into six categories for adults: underweight (BMI under 18.5); normal weight (BMI between 18.5 to 24.9); overweight (BMI between 25.0 to 29.9); obese, class I (BMI between 30.0 to 34.9); obese, class II (BMI between 35.0 to 39.9); and obese, class III (BMI of 40 or greater) (Statistics Canada, 2010). What is more, these categories were developed for use in adults. BMIs for children and adolescents change markedly throughout the maturation process in as little as a couple of years, so BMI percentiles are used instead for children and adolescents. For example, a BMI of greater than 30 in children corresponds to a BMI that is at the ninety-fifth percentile or higher for age and sex (Statistics Canada, 2005).

In Canada, 8.2% of children up to the age of 18 years would meet the definition of obesity, 18.3% would meet criteria for overweight, and the rest, 73.4%, are classified as "neither overweight or obese" (Statistics Canada, 2005). Interestingly, data for the underweight category are not provided, and these children are included in the "neither overweight or obese" category, indicating the priorities of Statistics Canada (the Canadian

National Government Agency that collects this data) (Statistics Canada, 2005). Regardless, there has been much debate about whether or not these categories are meaningful when assessing an individual's particular risk for certain conditions or even when assessing an individual person clinically. The issue is that, even as early as 1972, a BMI was identified as the most useful index of relative body weight that would allow for comparisons of body weight across populations, not across individual people. This means that a BMI was useful for population-based studies, not for individual "judgment" (Keys, Fidanza, Karvonen, Kimura, & Taylor, 1972). Mean BMIs represent an average in a population, and this does not mean that everyone in that population has, or should have, exactly the same BMI. Most characteristics that are measured in humans fall on a bell curve, so what is normal for one person may not be for the next. "Healthy" can come in many shapes and sizes, so using a population-based measure to determine an individual's health is fraught with potential errors.

Limitations in a BMI as a Measure of Individual Risk

Early on, a BMI was shown to account for only two-thirds of the variance in obesity. This means that a significant minority of subjects are misclassified as fat using the BMI scale, even among adults (Keys, Fidanza, Karvonen, Kimura, & Taylor, 1972). This misclassification is easily demonstrated through recognizable celebrities such as Brad Pitt and Arnold Schwarzenegger. Both of these actors are considered to be "fit" and are clearly examples of, if not icons of, manliness. However, these two examples of male "perfection" have BMIs in the overweight and obese categories respectively (Center for Consumer Freedom, 2010). These measurements are a result of the fact that a BMI does not distinguish between differing body compositions. It does not matter if you have a high muscle mass or high fat mass because only absolute weight impacts weight in kilograms and, thus, a BMI. This finding has been supported by more recent studies in children and adolescents. A study by Kurt Widhalm and his colleagues concluded that the relationship between body fat percentage and BMI varies widely and that while BMI is a useful parameter in epidemiologic studies, it is limited in use for the individual pediatric patient in identifying the individual's degree of adiposity (Freedman, Ogden, Berenson, & Horlick, 2005; Wickramasinghe et al., 2005; Widhalm, Schonegger, Huemer, & Auterith, 2001; Pietrobelli et al., 1998). Since a BMI does not explain "fatness" very well (Pietrobelli et al., 1998), many studies caution against using a BMI to categorize an individual child's adiposity (Freedman et al., 2005; Wickramasinghe et al., 2005; Widhalm et al., 2001; Pietrobelli et al., 1998).

TABLE 1

	Boy 1 (aged 8 years)	Boy 2 (aged 10 years)
Height	138.5 cm	138.5 cm
Weight	34.5 kg	34.5 kg
BMI	17.9	17.9
BMI percentile	85%	72%

An example of how BMI scales may adversely categorize children into normal and overweight groups is illustrated in Table 1 using the example of two boys only a couple of years apart in age (8 years old and 10 years old). Keep in mind that both of these boys look identical. Moreover, although both boys have a BMI of 17.9, the 10-year-old boy is considered to be within a healthy weight range, whereas the younger of the two would be considered overweight, in the eighty-fifth percentile of BMI.

What are the health and behavioural outcomes of classifying children at early stages of development? Should we put an eight-year-old on a diet (see Table 1)? Should we place him on an exercise regime? Is he just a very active, strong child, such that his muscles are placing him in a higher BMI percentile? Chances are the younger boy is not fat. BMI does not predict body fat composition in children very well, with widely varying adiposity and body composition for a given BMI (Pietrobelli et al., 1998). In fact, one of the obesity/overweight prevention measures—exercise—has the ability to change body fat into lean muscle and reduce mortality risk for many adiposity-related diseases without changing measured BMI at all (Ebbeling & Ludwig, 2008; Sigal, Kenny, Wasserman, Castaneda-Sceppa, & White, 2006). So, not all high BMI kids reflect the actual predictors of disease such as adiposity, and body composition (ratio of fat to lean muscle) may not be reflected well at all. In fact, Ebbeling and Ludwig (2008, p. 2443) suggest that "BMI is no more than a screening tool, the relevance of which to any patient must be considered in light of the medical history, physical examination, and presence of comorbidities." Here, finally, we see some suggestion of context. Before rushing our eight-year-old off to a nutritionist and personal trainer, we should consider his individual situation and not paint him with the same brush as another child since the BMI cut-points are not indicative of the individual and may be arbitrary.

The BMI cut-points developed by the Centre for Disease Control (CDC) were based on expert committees and can be regarded as a "best guess" (Kuczmarski et al., 2000). Decisions by experts are still decisions that are at the mercy of competing interests, money, and finding some consensus within a reasonable amount of time. They are conversations ending in concessions and compromises that form the basis of health policy. Recently, an expert group at the CDC even recommended that those in the eighty-fifth percentile, previously described as "at risk for overweight," have their status changed to "overweight" (Barlow & Expert, 2007). When this definition is changed, then, immediate increases in the perception of risk will rise (being at risk of something is not as bad as actually having the condition), with no actual change in this population—it would be an artifact of changing definitions, not changing BMIs. The context of the reporting obviously becomes very important in this case. It will remain a question whether or not this context will be reported. When definitions changed previously in 1998, no such background was given (Kuczmarski & Flegal, 2000). In the United States, roughly a doubling of the rates of obesity for men and women was seen, with most major news outlets demonstrating little regard for the explanation that it was due to definitions of obesity, not changes in the population. These large, sweeping increases are indeed an indicator of an epidemic on the surface, but they may cloud true judgment of what is really going on.

Risk Presentation and Perception in Action: The Obesity Epidemic

The childhood obesity epidemic is a strong signal on the public health radar, but there is some concern about the use of this term. Epidemics are a very particular kind of spread of disease—alarm bells should be going off about nasty, high death toll diseases that are sweeping across countries. Everyone is at risk, and no one is safe. Does childhood obesity fit within that framework?

The "epidemic" of childhood and adolescent obesity is a well-worn and oft-used phrase that has evoked a strong reaction in the popular press, but it is actually a misnomer. An epidemic is the occurrence, in a community or specified population, of deaths or cases of a condition in numbers greater than usual expectation for a given period of time (Last, 2001). Nevertheless, even Steven Galson (2008), the acting surgeon general of the United States, in his address on 3 April 2008 entitled "Adolescent Obesity: Everyone's Business," spoke about "the youth obesity epidemic," citing that "an estimated 17 percent of adolescents between the ages of 12 and 19 are overweight." This type of language misuses the term "epidemic," which is really defined by a *recent* and *transient* increase in *incidence*, not a solitary, non-contextualized prevalence estimate. What is more, most recent estimates of adolescent obesity from the CDC show no significant changes in the prevalence of obesity from 1999 to 2006 for either boys or girls, meaning that the term "epidemic" simply does not apply (Ogden, Carroll, & Flegal, 2008). The statistics even get confusing—the report stated that 16% of the population was at or above the ninety-fifth percentile. Mathematically, this number is difficult to comprehend. It is unclear, even to an epidemiologist, what this means and why this number should be anything other than 5% (Jensen & Steele, 2009).

Changes in standards and definitions have a role in the reporting of incidence and prevalence figures. The only way that more than 5% of a distribution could exceed the ninety-fifth percentile of a distribution is if the distributions are not the same. This means, however, that the BMI cut-offs on which the surgeon general's claims were based may be invalid. The BMI percentiles were based on data from the 1960s and 1970s, meaning that the current height and weight charts do not correspond to current distributions of children being assessed and evaluated (Jensen & Steele, 2009). Adolescents in the 1960s and 1970s were certainly smaller than they are now, but the increases seen are roughly a 10% mean difference in BMI from 1960 to 2002 in the 40 years of study (Ogden, Fryar, Carroll, & Flegal, 2004). Additionally, most of the major increases are seen in the heaviest children, which means that the increases that occurred in the adolescents who were already obese, and who got bigger, had a larger relative impact on the mean BMI in this analysis than the normal weight individuals did. The mean BMI in the population did not increase to obese, or even to overweight categories in this age group, so the average BMI of all US adolescents has been maintained at a so-called healthy BMI. Many other health outcomes have increased to similar or higher rates of increases than obesity over the same time period. Life expectancy, for example, has also risen since the 1960s from about 69 years to about 77, a rise of roughly 11.5%. Can this be termed an "epidemic of health"? What is more, is it correct to report that increases in BMI in adolescents are associated with a corresponding increase in average life expectancy in the United States? Is this finding just as valid a message?

This chapter cannot stress enough that numbers alone cannot speak for themselves. They require context and explanation, often in the form of time periods and clearly articulated comparisons in order to function as decision-making tools, specifically for prevention policy. Numbers cannot come at the expense of a well-defined overall investigation, and comparisons cannot be made without a sense of the magnitude of the numbers being compared, as problems can arise very quickly, often lending themselves to incorrect interpretations.

Large Problems in Small Numbers

One of the concerns about childhood obesity is the associated morbidity of certain illnesses such as diabetes, hypertension, and ischemic heart disease. As adults, they must live with these chronic conditions and must shoulder the high social, health, and financial burden of these illnesses for the rest of their lives. What often goes unmentioned, however, is that although these diseases occur more frequently in obese adolescents, they are still relatively rare, leading to more confusion between relative and absolute risk. Remember the example of type 2 diabetes.

This is indicative of another problem in risk perception and presentation—the comparison of very small numbers to indicate changes in risk. The very small numbers used to describe incidence or prevalence (0.4 per 1,000, which is equivalent to four people in every 10,000, for example) are actually very difficult for the general public to understand (Walsh, 1998). The term used to describe this inability to understand magnitude in numbers has been coined "number numbness" and goes hand in hand with another term described by Walsh (1998). "Technical intensity" refers to a situation in which measurement in very precise and very accurate ways actually obscures risk assessment (Walsh, 1998). Thus, in a given situation (say, obesity), heights and weights can be measured very precisely to ten significance figures (or to up to ten billionths of a unit) anthropometrically using very sophisticated devices to reduce error. If the incidence of two diseases can be measured accurately in a similar population, then the result will be a very precise measure of correlation between the two. However, this "exactness" is actually completely misleading—wrong in fact—when we are talking about risk. A cross-sectional correlation is merely the co-occurrence of two things in the same time space—it says nothing about what factor caused the other, whether the two are biologically related, and whether the removal of one of these would lead to the other decreasing or disappearing. True risk can really only be quantified when the temporality of two events occurring is known *and* when there is a biological relationship in addition to other criteria (Rothman, Greenland, & Lash, 2008).

All too often, the public, reporters, and even the scientific community are "numb to the numbers" and get lost in precision and technical intensity of measures. What is ultimately important is causality, not correlation, when talking about disease risk. This important separation is necessary when planning, implementing, and evaluating prevention strategy—after all, the temporality, or developmental sequence, of a disease must be known in order to find ways to stop it from occurring. However, the numbers exist and come from somewhere—reputable scientific journals in most cases—and are then transmitted to the general public, clinicians, and interest groups.

The Relationship between Research and the Media

Research is a business like anything else, but the altruism of science as a whole sometimes may suffer since the focus of research and, therefore, the allocation of clinical and public health resources can be affected by how risk is presented. The science may not be wrong, but it just may not be generating readers, citizen concern, and political attention. Researchers and clinicians may be rewarded based on how they present risk, so framing obesity as a public health threat promotes an investment of public funds into research and treatment and can be an argument for relaxing concerns about specific medical interventions designed to treat perceived negative health conditions (Saguy & Almeling, 2008). For example, the risks of high-revenue weight-loss treatments, drugs, or surgery may be clouded by the perception that the health consequences of obesity are so great that it is worth any risk in order to reduce one's weight (Oliver, 2006; Saguy, & Riley, 2005).

Consider an example in the research-funding world. The National Institute of Health (NIH) working group on the setting of funding priorities places public health needs in first place on its list of five major criteria for the allocation of research funds (National Institutes of Health, 1997), and an Institute of Medicine panel has endorsed the NIH criteria as an appropriate framework for funding (Committee on the NIH Research Priority-Setting Process, 1998). However, this panel also recommended that the NIH use health data, such as burdens and costs of diseases, in applying these criteria to health research funding priorities (National Institutes of Health, 1997). Therefore any area of research can increase its likelihood of receiving funding if it can demonstrate a significant burden of illness or significant mortality rates (Gross, Anderson, & Powe, 1999). Obesity research appears to be such an area and has successfully increased its funding. The obesity experts who were raising the alarm about the health consequences of obesity were also the ones directly benefiting from the resultant increase in funding for research and clinical services (Oliver, 2006). In 2003-04, the surgeon general declared war on obesity, and public health officials began quoting research articles and warning that obesity was killing 400,000 Americans per year (Campos, 2004; Mokdad, Marks, Stroup, & Gerberding, 2000; Oliver, 2006). At the same time, with the assistance of obesity experts, the NIH developed a strategic plan for NIH obesity research (National Institutes of Health, 2004).

Is it any surprise that that by 2005 the US federal government had allocated US$440 million annually for obesity research funding (Obesity in America, 2008)? This is nearly a 13-fold increase from US$34 million in 1997 (Shape up America, 1996). Is there a conflict of interest when researchers who stand to benefit from the money allocated to obesity research are the ones who inform the funding strategy? Does this affect how researchers present risk? The idea that obesity is responsible for hundreds of thousands of deaths a year has been refuted, but obesity research funding is unaffected (Flegal, Grabaud, Williamson, & Gail, 2007).

The responsibility for understanding and operating effectively and ethically within this state of affairs does lie solely with the research community though because popular sources of media are prone to extrapolating population-level studies to the individual and often relate obesity to how individuals eat and other personal choices people make (Saguy & Almeling, 2008). This perception actually frames the "obesity epidemic" in a unique way—in this age of personal health responsibility, everyone is at risk because everyone has to eat. Therefore, everyone has the potential for eating too much and becoming overweight or obese. As well, obesity, like more traditional epidemics, is characterized as contagious (Christakis & Fowler, 2007). As such, everyone is expected to be highly vigilant about what they eat and expected to never take a day off from obsessing about eating and exercising (behaviour that some might consider eating disordered). Thin waifs and lean men are held up to be the ideal warriors fighting their own personal battle against the "risks of obesity" (Boero, 2007). If everyone is at risk of obesity, as recently suggested by a scholarly article that projected all Americans would be overweight or obese by 2048 (Wang, Beydoun, Liang, Caballero, & Kumanyika, 2008), curing or preventing obesity is often characterized as being within individual control—you just have to diet and exercise more (in spite of evidence to the contrary) (Boero, 2007; Campos, Saguy, Ernsberger, Oliver, & Gaesser, 2006).

Children are characterized as not being in control of their environment, so parents are often blamed by both the media and experts for their child's shortcomings (Saguy & Almeling, 2008; Shape Up America, 1996). Calls for policies to prevent obesity in children raise the alarm that something must be done. This heightened sense of risk adds to the experience that bodies are out of control and chaos rules. The natural feelings of blame are so pervasive now—weight-based guilt is associated with both parents and children and is indicative of the view of the larger society as a whole. Fat is out, way out, and the thin ideal persists.

Biases against obesity are widespread and on the increase (Andreyeva, Puhl, & Brownell, 2008). The prevalence of weight/height discrimination has increased from 7% in 1995-96 to 12% in 2004-06. While the prevalence is relatively close to reported rates of race and age discrimination, there are virtually no legal or social sanctions against weight discrimination (Andreyeva et al., 2008). Obesity is also viewed negatively by children and adolescents (Latner & Stunkard, 2003; Strauss & Pollack, 2003). Overweight adolescents are socially marginalized, and in the last forty years the stigmatization of obesity by children has only increased (Latner & Stunkard, 2003; Strauss & Pollack, 2003). Fat children and adolescents are viewed as the least desirable playmates (Strauss & Pollack, 2003; Latner & Stunkard, 2003). The stigma of obesity also affects how parents view their children and how children feel about themselves. As early as 5 years of age, girls with a higher weight status have a lower self-concept. In addition, parents' concern about their child's weight and resultant restriction of access to food are associated with negative self-evaluations among girls (Davison & Birch, 2001). Teachers and healthcare providers also hold negative stereotypes of obese children (Foster et al., 2003). Teachers view overweight students as untidy, less likely to succeed, and more emotional. They also have lower expectations of overweight students (Puhl & Heuer, 2009). Unfortunately, the effects of weight-based fears are overlooked. Weight stigma can have a significant effect on psychological health of young people and can lead to missed days at school, unhealthy eating patterns, and avoidance of physical activity (Puhl & Heuer, 2009).

Similar biases exist in health care. Many physicians view obese patients as awkward, unattractive, ugly, and non-compliant (Foster et al., 2003). Patients are aware of these biases, and larger-sized women report that barriers related to their weight, including disrespectful treatment, embarrassment at being weighed, negative attitudes of providers, unsolicited advice to lose weight, and medical equipment that is too small to be functional, contribute to their delay in accessing health care (Amy, Aalborg, Lyons, & Keranen, 2006). Obese patients consequently delay seeking treatment (Amy et al., 2006). Is it possible that this delay in treatment holds the potential for negatively affecting the health of this marginalized group of patients? Among women, an increased BMI is also associated with decreased preventive health care services, which may exacerbate or even account for some of the increased health risks of obesity (Fontaine, Faith, Allison, & Cheskin, 1998). These biases are not only limited to clinicians but also affect researchers. Obesity researchers show very strong weight bias, indicating pervasive and powerful stigma (Schwartz, Chambliss, Brownell, Blair, & Billington, 2003). The question of how much these biases impact health care clinical outcomes or the interpretation of results remains not only unanswered but also unexamined (Puhl & Brownell, 2001).

Eating Disorders Are Also on the Rise

Recently, it has been suggested that negative body esteem can be helpful in the war against obesity. After all, if one feels bad about oneself and certain aspects of one's body, he or she may work harder to lose weight. This disconcerting trend considers the stigma of obesity in a positive light. This attitude is seen by some experts as a positive outcome because these experts fear that, after all, a young girl without negative self-esteem may not realize the need to control her weight and may not be protected against obesity (Saguy & Almeling, 2008). After all, as discussed earlier, these experts believe that the best way to avoid obesity is to be ever vigilant in regard to what one eats. Focusing on weight and body shape, counting calories, reading labels, and never going a day without exercise—essentially being fearful of getting fat—are considered to be important behaviours to stave off increasing weight gain. However, these are also the symptoms of an eating disorder (American Psychiatric Association, 2004). Yet, the risk of an eating disorder, which is considered a rare disorder, seems tolerable given the "greater risks" of obesity.

However, the science does not support this claim. The long-term consequences of obesity in adolescence do not compare to the severe immediate physical and psychological consequences of an eating disorder (let alone their long-term effects) in this same age group (Papadopoulos, Ekbom, Brandt, & Ekselius, 2009; Steinhausen, 2009). However, with heightened concern about the "obesity epidemic," it becomes almost impossible for individuals to make a balanced judgment about competing risks, whether they are experts, journalists, or the lay public. Even if eating disorders are serious illnesses, are they so rare as to be irrelevant to obesity prevention and treatment? In the balance of pros and cons, it may be reasonable to risk a rare illness in order to correct what is presented as a much more common health scourge.

Are eating disorders truly so rare? When the prevalence of eating disorders in children and adolescents is presented, reports often refer to only anorexia nervosa or bulimia nervosa, and the range presented is 0.5-2%. Epidemiological data for the category of Eating Disorders Not Otherwise Specified (EDNOS) are rarely reported, and the statistics available are provided by very expensive studies that do diagnostic assessments. These studies are laborious to implement and not cost effective since the diagnostic categories describe such a small part of the eating-disordered population that they are not practical. Instead, large community-based studies looking at prevalence tend to rely on self-reports. Those who report eating-disordered behaviours such as food restriction, binging, and purging are then described as having "disordered eating" rather than "having an eating disorder" as they have not undergone an official diagnostic clinical assessment. The behaviour reported can be quite severe, require clinical care, and would likely meet criteria for EDNOS, if not for anorexia nervosa or bulimia nervosa. However, these individuals are rarely labelled as having a "disorder." Large community-based self-report surveys suggest that in adolescents the rates of disordered eating that are severe enough to warrant clinical evaluation are approximately 15-20% in girls and 2-4% in boys (Austin et al., 2008; Jones, Bennett, Olmsted, Lawson, & Rodin, 2001; Pinhas, Heinmaa, Bryden, Bradley, & Toner, 2008). This rate is supported by the few studies where the prevalence of EDNOS is actually reported (Isomaa, Isomaa, Marttunen, Kaltiala-Heino, & Bjorkqvist, 2009; Keski-Rahkonen et al., 2007; Kjelsas, Bjornstrom, & Gotestam, 2004). These percentages are certainly as high as the rates of obesity in Canada in this age group.

Although these adolescents with EDNOS are using extreme, potentially dangerous methods to manage their weight and are at risk for impaired health, the majority would not be represented in data that report only the prevalence or incidence of anorexia nervosa or bulimia nervosa. A second confounder is the lack of identification of these disorders by health care providers. Less than one in ten adolescent girls with significantly disordered eating is assessed for an eating disorder (Jones, Bennett, Olmsted, Lawson, & Rodin, 2001). These difficulties with diagnosis effectively obscure and minimize the severity and range of the problem. While up to one in five adolescent girls may be potentially affected by the medical and psychological consequences of disordered eating, the rates of eating disorders are often focused only on those that meet the full criteria for anorexia nervosa or bulimia nervosa and are reported as 1-2%. One in 100 is much less worrisome and much less urgent than one in five or even one in ten. Remember, less than one in ten adolescent girls meet the definition of obesity.

Why Should We Care?

The reasons that professionals interested in preventing eating disorders should be concerned are numerous. First and foremost, if we believe that the obesity epidemic exists and is costing lives and health care dollars, then we—clinicians, public health officials, parents, and politicians—should feel compelled to act and in so acting may do more harm than good (Neumark-Sztainer et al., 2006; University of Arkansas for Medical Sciences, 2006).

Prevention programs for eating disorders show some promise (see Chapters 1, 2, and 3 in this volume). Recent meta-analyses suggest that they can have a meaningful effect in reducing eating-disordered behaviours and cognitions (Cororve Fingeret, Warren, Cepeda-Benito, & Gleaves, 2006; Piran, 2005; Stice, Shaw, & Marti, 2007). This finding is not true for prevention programs to prevent obesity, which is discouraging given the enormous amount of resources that are being allocated to its prevention (Foster et al., 2008; Kropski, Keckley, & Jensen, 2008; Plachta-Danielzik et al., 2007; Summerbell et al., 2002). What is more concerning is the possibility that these programs may actually cause harm—remember the risk that developing disordered eating may be seen as acceptable. A recent review concluded that the existing evidence did not support the view that childhood obesity prevention programs are associated with unintended psychological harm. However, no definitive evidence exists, in part due to the fact that these variables were so poorly assessed (Carter & Bulik, 2008). Consequently, conclusions about the possible negative (i.e., iatrogenic) effects of these programs were considered premature (Carter & Bulik, 2008). One of the difficulties may lie in the length of time to follow-up, as many obesity prevention programs and their follow-up assessments last only a year or less (Jansen et al., 2008; Summerbell et al., 2002), and adverse effects of dieting and weight focus can take up to five years to evolve (Neumark-Sztainer et al., 2006).

The possibility that obesity prevention programs may cause harm rests on results from large prospective studies of high-school populations that suggest that adolescents who are focused on their weight and are attempting to lose weight in adolescence are more likely to develop disturbed or disordered eating and are heavier than those who are not attempting to lose weight (Neumark-Sztainer et al., 2006). These findings would suggest that interventions that are focused on anthropomorphic measurements and nutritional restriction with the goal of weight loss, as many obesity prevention programs are, may actually cause harm (Jansen et al., 2008). Based on the current evidence in the literature, there is little reason to allocate resources towards obesity prevention programs in children and adolescents, as there is little or no evidence of their success. It might even be considered a waste of resources, given how poor the outcomes are.

Regardless of these results, in some situations, the presentation of the data makes it appear otherwise. For example, a statewide legislated obesity prevention program was introduced in Arkansas in 2002 (University of Arkansas for Medical Sciences, 2006). It included multi-faceted nutritional and physical education programming, including raising awareness about, and limiting access to, unhealthy food choices in schools (University of Arkansas for Medical Sciences, 2006). It also included a "BMI report card" that involved weighing all students annually and reporting to families whether their child was underweight, normal weight, overweight, or obese. After 3 years, the program was declared a success as the rates of obesity and overweight had levelled off (University of Arkansas for Medical Sciences,

2006). Proponents of the program argued that, prior to the implementation of the program, rates of overweight and obesity had for some time been on the rise and now this trend had been halted. Interestingly, what the researchers failed to address is that, at the same time the rates of obesity had reached a plateau in children and adolescents in Arkansas, they had also levelled off across the United States and across all age groups, even in states without any obesity prevention programs (Ogden, Carroll, & Flegal 2008; Ogden, Carroll, McDowell, & Flegal, 2007). It is hard to argue that the obesity prevention program had a significant effect if those not exposed to the intervention had a similar outcome.

The Arkansas program cost just over US$1 million the first year alone, including state funds and grants from private sources. The program cost about a third of that in the following year (Chmelynski, 2005). There are no similar state programs to combat eating disorders in Arkansas. This is unfortunate, given the fact that after 5 years of running this program, young people in Arkansas are just as likely to be fat as anywhere else in the United States—and adolescents in Arkansas eat fewer vegetables, drink less milk, and drink more soda. Moreover, adolescent girls in Arkansas are more likely to engage in risky weight loss behaviours, including fasting, using diet pills, and using laxatives and vomiting as methods of weight loss (National Center for Chronic Disease Prevention & Health Promotion, 2007, 2010). More than one-third of parents reported that their children were more concerned about their weight than they should be, and more children reported being the victims of weight-based bullying than before the BMI report cards were instituted (University of Arkansas for Medical Sciences, 2006). In the prevention and treatment of eating disorders, one must consider the effects of the "obesity epidemic." In fact, countering the unsubstantiated and potentially dangerous claims of the obesity epidemic experts might be an important tool in preventing eating disorders.

Closer to home, schools have created policies about what foods are acceptable to bring to school from home. In some communities, should children bring an unapproved snack they will be asked to put it away uneaten (Region of Peel, 2010). This is problematic in many ways. First, it sends the message that it is better to be hungry than to eat a granola bar with chocolate chips. This notion is cause for concern because being hungry can impede learning (Kleinman et al., 2002; Taras, 2005). Second, it can be shaming to the child to be singled out. Third, it undermines parental authority and sends the message that parents cannot be trusted to feed their kids. What if this is the only snack the family can afford? What if the child is a picky eater or needs to gain weight? How does the school board decide what is a good food and what is a bad one? What if a parent disagrees?

Recently, even the president and the first lady of the United States have turned their attention to the childhood obesity epidemic and have reported to the press that they have been worried their daughters were getting too fat (Reporter, 2010; Stolberg, 2010). They also reported how they began to limit their daughters' eating as a result. The obesity epidemic has become so commonplace that it is now deemed appropriate to judge these young developing bodies and comment on their weight in a public arena. What would it be like for young girls on the cusp of puberty to have the whole world know their parents felt compelled to control their not yet fully grown bodies? Could we blame either of these girls if they developed disordered eating or a negative body esteem? Would we care or would we just be happy they were not fat? In a world where experts, journalists, teachers, and physicians are all in the trenches fighting in the war against obesity and where the message is clear that eating behaviours that approximate or lead to eating disorders are acceptable if they help avoid overweight and obesity, eating disorder prevention programs cannot ignore the messages stemming from the obesity programs. The Western world's bias against fat(ness) and fat people, and how it has affected our perspectives on health and well-being, must be factored into any program that seeks to protect youth from disordered eating and weight and shape distress.

Conclusion

Risk is a complicated concept. We have shown how numbers, whether large or small in value, may not accurately reflect the risk of certain illnesses or diseases. Alone, numbers contain no intrinsic value and are meaningless—they need accompanying *context, explanation*, and *correct interpretation* from qualified individuals. Additionally, it is up to those individuals to transmit these interpretations in a format that can be easily understood and that is free from the politics of healthcare, government, and special interest groups. However, it is also up to clinicians and decision-makers to understand the forces and inherent biases acting on the presentation and interpretation of risk and to make informed decisions accordingly for their patients or population. Risk presentation has a huge impact in risk perception, clouding and affecting judgment and behaviour accordingly, so it is vital that these choices and conclusions are correct.

The obesity and eating disorder worlds are intimately connected in both the clinical and public health realm. Media scare tactics, publication bias in research, and clinical and public perception of overweight have drastically altered behavioural and cultural norms towards a thinner ideal, without a large and thorough evidence base to support it. The desire to be thin and the fear, if not terror, of fat permeate our media, and pressures to adhere to prevailing ideas about body shape are aggressive and targeting younger age groups with potentially severe, though unintended, consequences. Adolescents and children are at a severe disadvantage in terms of their ability to fit into an adult "ideal weight category" due to the onset and duration of puberty, and they are not able to exert a large amount of control in their lives. Thus, in order to fit into the messages they receive about weight and shape, these vulnerable populations may be at a higher risk for disordered eating and/or eating disorders.

Time will tell whether this shift will persist or whether a healthier, more holistic approach to, and message on, health will be taken. As clinicians, we must be vigilant about the messages we send, and as decision-makers and defenders of public health we must be mindful of the policies we make. Individually, and especially collectively, our voices are relatively loud and the public tends to listen when we speak. We affect individual health behaviours and practices, so accurate transmission of risk information plays a huge role in maintaining the well-being of the populations we serve. Always keep context, explanation, and correct interpretation at the forefront of your messages and be mindful of separating junk science, anecdotes, and media clips from reliable evidence. Risk and how it affects our daily lives is complicated, but it is up to us to get it right because it is so important.

References

Allen, R. E. (Ed.) (1990). *The concise oxford dictionary of current English* (8th ed.). Oxford: Clarendon Press.

American Psychiatric Association. (2004). Diagnostic and statistical manual of mental disorders: DSM-IV-TR (4th ed.). Washington, DC: American Psychiatric Association

Amy, N. K., Aalborg, A., Lyons, P., & Keranen, L. (2006). Barriers to routine gynecological cancer screening for White and African-American obese women. *International Journal of Obesity, 30*(1), 147-155.

Andreyeva, T., Puhl, R. M., & Brownell, K. D. (2008). Changes in perceived weight discrimination among Americans, 1995-1996 through 2004-2006. *Obesity, 16*(5), 1129-1134.

Austin, S. B., Ziyadeh, N. J., Forman, S., Prokop, L. A., Keliher, A., & Jacobs, D. (2008). Screening high school students for eating disorders: Results of a national initiative. *Preventing Chronic Disease, 5*(4), A114.

Bagnardi, V., Blangiardo, M., La Vecchia, C., & Corrao, G. (2001). Alcohol consumption and the risk of cancer: A meta-analysis. *Alcohol Research and Health, 25*(4), 263-270.

Barlow, S. E., & Expert, C. (2007). Expert committee recommendations regarding the prevention, assessment, and treatment of child and adolescent overweight and obesity: Summary report. *Pediatrics, 120*(4), S164-S192.

Boero, N. (2007). All the news that's fat to print: The American obesity epidemic and the media. *Qualitative Sociology, 30,* 41-60.

Brewer, N. T., Chapman, G. B., Gibbons, F. X., Gerrard, M., McCaul, K. D., & Weinstein, N. D. (2007). Meta-analysis of the relationship between risk perception and health behavior: The example of vaccination. *Health Psychology, 26*(2), 136-145.

Campos, P. F. (2004). *The obesity myth: Why America's obsession with weight is hazardous to your health.* New York: Gotham Book.

Campos, P., Saguy, A., Ernsberger, P., Oliver, E., & Gaesser G. (2006). The epidemiology of overweight and obesity: Public health crisis or moral panic? *International Journal of Epidemiology, 35*(1), 55-60.

Canadian Paediatric Society. (2007). *Canadian Paediatric Surveillance Program 2010.* Retrieved from http://www.web.cps.ca/English/surveillance/CPSP/Studies/2007Results.pdf

Canadian Paediatric Society. (2008). *Canadian Paediatric Surveillance Program 2008.* Retrieved from http://www.web.cps.ca/English/surveillance/CPSP/Studies/2008Results.pdf

Carter, F. A., & Bulik, C. M. (2008). Childhood obesity prevention programs: How do they affect eating pathology and other psychological measures? *Psychosomatic Medicine, 70*(3), 363-371.

Center for Consumer Freedom. (2005). *Pitt stained by bogus BMI.* Retrieved from http://www.consumerfreedom.com/news_detail.cfm/h/2820-pitt-stained-by-bogus-bmi

Chmelynski, C. (2005). *States weigh idea of BMI reports as they tackle obesity epidemic.* National School Boards Association. Retrieved from http://www.nsba.org/Board-Leadership/SchoolHealth/SelectedNSBAPublications/Healthy Eating/obesityepidemic.txt

Christakis, N. A, & Fowler J. H. (2007). The spread of obesity in a large social network over thirty-two years. *New England Journal of Medicine, 357*(4), 370-379.

Committee on the NIH Research Priority-Setting Process. (1998). *Scientific opportunities and public needs: Improving priority setting and public input at the National Institutes of Health,* Health Sciences Policy Program, Health Sciences Section. Washington, DC: National Academy Press.

Cororve Fingeret, M., Warren, C. S., Cepeda-Benito, A., & Gleaves, D. H. (2006). Eating disorder prevention research: A meta-analysis. *Eating Disorders, 14*(3), 191-213.

Davison, K. K., & Birch, L. L. (2001). Weight status, parent reaction, and self-concept in five-year-old girls. *Pediatrics, 107*(1), 46-53.

Division of Sexually Transmitted Disease Prevention. (1999). *Sexually transmitted disease surveillance, 1998.* Atlanta, GA: Center for Disease Control and Prevention.

Ebbeling, C. B., & Ludwig, D. S. (2008). Tracking pediatric obesity: An index of uncertainty? *Journal of the American Medical Association, 299*(20), 2442-2443.

Fischhoff, B. (1995). Risk perception and communication unplugged: Twenty years of process. *Risk Analysis, 15*(2), 137-145.

Fischhoff, B., Slovic, P., Lichtenstein, S., Read, S., & Combs, B. (1978). How safe is safe enough? A psychometric study of attitudes towards technological risks and benefits. *Policy Sciences, 9*(2), 127-152.

Fischhoff, B., Watson, S. R., & Hope C. (1984). Defining risk. *Policy Sciences, 17*(2), 123-139.

Fontaine, K. R., Faith, M. S., Allison, D. B., & Cheskin, L. J. (1998). Body weight and health care among women in the general population. *Archives Family Medicine, 7*(4), 381-384.

Flegal, K. M., Graubard, B. I., Williamson, D. F., & Gail, M. H. (2007). Cause-specific excess deaths associated with underweight, overweight and obesity. *Journal of the American Medical Association, 298*(17), 2028-2037.

Foster, G. D., Sherman, S., Borradaile, K. E., Grundy, K. M., Vander Veur, S. S., Nachmani, J., Karpyn, A., Kumanyika, S., & Shults, J. (2008). A policy-based school intervention to prevent overweight and obesity. *Pediatrics, 121*(4), e794-e802.

Foster, G. D., Wadden, T. A., Makris, A. P., Davidson, D., Sanderson, R. S., Allison, D. B, & Kessler, A. (2003). Primary care physicians' attitudes about obesity and its treatment. *Obesity Research, 11*(10), 1168-1177.

Freedman, D. S., Ogden, C. L., Berenson, G. S., & Horlick, M. (2005). Body mass index and body fatness in childhood. *Current Opinion in Clinical Nutrition and Metabolic Care, 8*(6), 618-623.

Fuchs, C. S., Stampfer, M. J., Colditz, G. A., Giovannucci, E. L., Manson, J. E., Kawachi, I., Hunter, D. J., Hankinson, S. E., Hennekens, C. H., & Rosner, B. (1995). Alcohol consumption and mortality among women. *New England Journal of Medicine, 332*(19), 1245-1250.

Galson, S. (2008). Adolescent obesity: Everyone's business. In D. Paxman (Chair), *Remarks to the College of Physicians of Philadelphia* (Conducted at the Meeting of the College of Physicians of Philadelphia, Philadelphia, PA). Retrieved from http://www.surgeongeneral.gov/news/speeches/sp20080403a.html

Goran, M. I., Davis, J., Kelly, L., Shaibi, G., Spruijt-Metz, D., & Soni, S. M., Weigensberg, M. (2008). Low prevalence of pediatric type 2 diabetes: Where's the epidemic? *Journal of Pediatrics, 152*(6), 753-755.

Gordis, L. (2004). *Epidemiology* (3rd ed.). Philadelphia, PA: Saunders.

Gross, C. P., Anderson, G. F., & Powe, N. R. (1999). The relation between funding by the National Institutes of Health and the burden of disease. *New England Journal of Medicine, 340*(24), 1881-1887.

Isomaa, R., Isomaa, A. L., Marttunen, M., Kaltiala-Heino, R., & Bjorkqvist, K. (2009). The prevalence, incidence and development of eating disorders in Finnish adolescents: A two-step three-year follow-up study. *European Eating Disorders Review, 17*(3), 199-207.

Jackson, R., & Beaglehole, R. (1995). Alcohol consumption guidelines: Relative safety versus absolute risks and benefits. *Lancet, 346*(8977), 716.

Jansen, W., Raat, H., Zwanenburg, E. J., Reuvers, I., van Walsem, R., & Brug, J. (2008). A school-based intervention to reduce overweight and inactivity in children aged six to twelve years: Study design of a randomized controlled trial. *BMC Public Health, 8,* 257.

Jensen, C. D., & Steele, R. G. (2009). Body dissatisfaction, weight criticism, and self-reported physical activity in preadolescent children. *Journal of Pediatric Psychology, 34*(8), 822-826.

Jones, J. M., Bennett, S., Olmsted, M. P., Lawson, M. L., & Rodin, G. (2001). Disordered eating attitudes and behaviours in teenaged girls: A school-based study. *Canadian Medical Association Journal, 165*(5), 547-552.

Kasperson, R., Renn, O., Slovic, P., Brown, H., Emel, J., Goble, R., Kasperson, J. X., & Ratick, S. (1988). The social amplification of risk: A conceptual framework. *Risk Analysis, 8*(2), 177-187.

Keski-Rahkonen, A., Hoek, H. W., Susser, E. S., Linna, M. S., Sihvola, E., Raevuori, A., Bulik, C., Kaprio, J., & Rissanen, A. (2007). Epidemiology and course of anorexia nervosa in the community. *American Journal of Psychiatry, 164*(8), 1259-1265.

Keys, A., Fidanza, F., Karvonen, M. J., Kimura, N., & Taylor, H. L. (1972). Indices of relative weight and obesity. *Journal of Chronic Diseases, 25*(6), 329-343.

Kjelsas, E., Bjornstrom, C., & Gotestam, K. G. (2004). Prevalence of eating disorders in female and male adolescents (fourteen to fifteen years). *Eating Behaviors, 5*(1), 13-25.

Kleinman, R. E., Hall, S., Green, H., Korzec-Ramirez, D., Patton, K., Pagano, M. E., & Murphy, J. (2002). Diet, breakfast, and academic performance in children. *Annals of Nutrition and Metabolism, 46*(1), 24-30.

Kropski, J. A., Keckley, P. H., & Jensen, G. L. (2008). School-based obesity prevention programs: An evidence-based review. *Obesity, 16*(5), 1009-1018.

Kuczmarski, R. J., & Flegal, K. M. (2000). Criteria for definition of overweight in transition: background and recommendations for the United States. *American Journal of Clinical Nutrition, 72*(5), 1074-1081.

Kuczmarski, R. J., Ogden, C. L., Grummer-Strawn, L. M., Flegal, K. M., Guo, S. S., Wei, R., Mei, Z., Curtin, L. R., Roche, A. F., & Johnson, C. L. (2000). CDC growth charts: United States. *Advance Data, 8*(314), 1-27.

Last, J. M. (2001). *A dictionary of epidemiology* (4th ed.). New York: Oxford University Press.

Latner, J. D., & Stunkard, A. J. (2003). Getting worse: The stigmatization of obese children. *Obesity Research, 11*(3), 452-456.

Mayer-Davis, E. J. (2008). Type 2 diabetes in youth: Epidemiology and current research toward prevention and treatment. *Journal of the American Dietetic Association, 108*(4), 45-51.

Mokdad, A. H., Marks, J. S., Stroup, D. F., & Gerberding, J. L. (2004). Actual causes of death in the United States, 2000. *Journal of the American Medical Association, 291*(10), 1238-1245.

National Center for Chronic Disease Prevention and Health Promotion. (2007). *Results for Arkansas 2007 compared with United States 2007.* Youth Risk Behavior Surveillance System. Retrieved from http://www.cdc.gov/Healthy Youth/yrbs/index.htm

National Center for Chronic Disease Prevention and Health Promotion. (2010). *Data and statistics.* Youth Risk Behavior Surveillance System. Retrieved from http://www.cdc.gov/HealthyYouth/yrbs/index.htm

National Institutes of Health. (1997). *Setting research priorities at the National Institutes of Health* (Report no. 97-4265). Bethesda, MD: National Institutes of Health.

National Institutes of Health. (2004). *NIH Obesity Research Task Force.* Retrieved from http://dpcpsi.nih.gov/council/pdf/CoC-112008-Nabel-Rodgers-ORTF .pdf

Neumark-Sztainer, D., Wall, M., Guo, J., Story, M., Haines, J., & Eisenberg, M. (2006). Obesity, disordered eating, and eating disorders in a longitudinal study of adolescents: How do dieters fare five years later? *Journal of the American Dietetic Association, 106*(4), 559-568.

Obesity in America. (2008). *Government Gives Money for Obesity.* Retrieved May 11, 2010, from http://www.obesityinamerica.org/funding.html

Ogden, C. L., Carroll, M. D., & Flegal, K. M. (2008). High body mass index for age among US children and adolescents, 2003-2006. *Journal of the American Medical Association, 299*(20), 2401-2405.

Ogden, C. L., Carroll, M. D., McDowell, M. A., & Flegal, K. M. (2007). Obesity among adults in the United States—no statistically significant chance since 2003-2004. *National Center for Health Statistics Data Brief,* (1), 1-8.

Ogden, C. L., Fryar, C. D., Carroll, M. D., & Flegal, K. M. (2004). Mean body weight, height, and body mass index, United States 1960-2002. *Advance Data, 27*(347), 1-17.

Oliver, J. E. (2006). *Fat politics: The real story behind America's obesity epidemic.* New York: Oxford University Press.

Papadopoulos, F. C., Ekbom, A., Brandt, L., & Ekselius, L. (2009). Excess mortality, causes of death and prognostic factors in anorexia nervosa. *British Journal of Psychiatry, 194*(1), 10-17.

Pietrobelli, A., Faith, M. S., Allison, D. B., Gallagher, D., Chiumello, G., & Heymsfield, S. B. (1998). Body mass index as a measure of adiposity among children and adolescents: A validation study. *Journal of Pediatrics, 132*(2), 204-210.

Pinhas, L., Heinmaa, M., Bryden, P., Bradley, S., & Toner, B. (2008). Disordered eating in Jewish adolescent girls. *Canadian Journal of Psychiatry, 53*(9), 601-608.

Piran, N. (2005). Prevention of eating disorders: A review of outcome evaluation research. *Israel Journal of Psychiatry and Related Sciences, 42*(3), 172-177.

Plachta-Danielzik, S., Pust, S., Asbeck, I., Czerwinski-Mast, M., Langnase, K., Fischer, C., Bosy-Westphal, A., Kriwy, P., & Muller, M. (2007). Four-year follow-up of school-based intervention on overweight children: The KOPS study. *Obesity, 15*(12), 3159-3169.

Puhl, R., & Brownell, K. D. (2001). Bias, discrimination, and obesity. *Obesity Research, 9*(12), 788-805.

Puhl, R. M., & Heuer, C. A. (2009). The stigma of obesity: A review and update. *Obesity, 17*(5), 941-964.

Region of Peel. (2010). Public health: Food and beverages — making healthy food accessible. Retrieved from http://www.peelregion.ca/health/baew/lunches -snacks/healthyfood/healthy-snacks/snacksinclassroom.html

Rehm, J., Room, R., Graham, K., Monteiro, M., Gmel, G., & Sempos, C. T. (2003). The relationship of average volume of alcohol consumption and patterns of drinking to burden of disease: An overview. *Addiction, 98*(9), 1209-1228.

Reporter, D. M. (2010). Reform begins at home: Michelle Obama puts daughters on a diet as she launches anti-obesity campaign. *Daily Mail.* Retrieved from http://www.dailymail.co.uk/news/article-1247254/Michelle-Obama-puts -daughters-diet-launching-obesity-campaign-U-S.html

Rothman, K. J., Greenland, S., & Lash, T. L. (2008). *Modern epidemiology* (3rd ed.) Philadelphia, PA: Wolters Kluwer Health/Lippincott Williams and Wilkins.

Saguy, A. C., & Almeling, R. (2008). Fat in the fire? Science, the news media, and the "obesity epidemic." *Sociological Forum, 23*(1), 53-83.

Saguy, A. C., & Riley, K. W. (2005). Weighing both sides: Morality, mortality, and framing contests over obesity. *Journal of Health Politics Policy and Law, 30*(5), 869-923.

Schwartz, M. B., Chambliss, H. O., Brownell, K. D., Blair, S. N., & Billington, C. (2003). Weight bias among health professionals specializing in obesity. *Obesity Research, 11*(9), 1033-1039.

Shape Up America. (1996). *Dr. Koop supports goals to increase obesity research.* Retrieved from http://www.shapeup.org/about/arch_pr/021196.php

Shields, M. (2004). *Measured Obesity: Overweight Canadian children and adolescents.* Ottawa: Statistics Canada. Retrieved from http://www.statcan.gc.ca/ pub/82-620-m/2005001/pdf/4193660-eng.pdf

Sigal, R. J., Kenny, G. P., Wasserman, D. H., Castaneda-Sceppa, C., & White, R. D. (2006). Physical activity/exercise and type 2 diabetes. *Diabetes Care, 29*(6), 1433-1438.

Slovic, P., Peters, E., Finucane, M. L., & Macgregor, D. G. (2005). Affect, risk, and decision making. *Health Psychology 24*(4), 35-40.

Starr C. (1969). Social benefit versus technological risk. *Science, 165*(899), 1232-1238.

Statistics Canada. (2005). *Canadian community health survey: Obesity among children and adults.* Retrieved from http://www.statcan.gc.ca/daily-quotidien/ 050706/dq050706a-eng.htm

Statistics Canada. (2010). *Health indicators: Adult body mass index.* Retrieved from http://www.statcan.gc.ca/pub/82-221-x/2011002/def/def1-eng.htm#hc1abm

Steinhausen, H. C. (2009). Outcome of eating disorders. *Child and Adolescent Psychiatric Clinics of North America, 18*(1), 225-242.

Stice, E., Shaw, H., & Marti, C. N. (2007). A meta-analytic review of eating disorder prevention programs: Encouraging findings. *Annual Review of Clinical Psychology, 3,* 207-231.

Stolberg, S. G. (2010). Childhood obesity battle is taken up by first lady. *New York Times,* February 9, 2010.

Strauss, R. S., & Pollack, H. A. (2003). Social marginalization of overweight children. *Archives of Pediatrics and Adolescent Medicine, 157*(8), 746-752.

Summerbell, C. D., Waters, E., Edmunds, L. D., Kelly, S., Brown, T., & Campbell, K. J. (2002). Interventions for preventing obesity in children. *Cochrane Database of Systematic Reviews 2,* CD001871 (update 2005(3): CD001871).

Taras H. (2005). Nutrition and student performance at school. *Journal of School Health, 75*(6), 199-213.

University of Arkansas for Medical Sciences. (2006). *Year three evaluation: Arkansas Act 1220 of 2003 to combat childhood obesity.* Fay W. Boozman College of Public Health. Retrieved from http://www.uams.edu/coph/reports/2006 Act1220_Year3.pdf

Vivian, E. M. (2006). Type 2 diabetes in children and adolescents: The next epidemic? *Current Medical Research and Opinion, 22*(2), 297-306.

Walsh, J. (1998). *True odds: How risk affects your everyday life.* Los Angeles, CA: Silver Lake Publishing.

Wang, Y., Beydoun, M. A., Liang, L., Caballero, B., & Kumanyika, S. K. (2008). Will all Americans become overweight or obese? Estimating the progression and cost of the US obesity epidemic. *Obesity, 16*(10), 2323-2330.

Wickramasinghe, V. P., Cleghorn, G. J., Edmiston, K. A., Murphy, A. J., Abbott, R. A., & Davies, P. S. (2005). Validity of BMI as a measure of obesity in Australian white Caucasian and Australian Sri Lankan children. *Annals of Human Biology, 32*(1), 60-71.

Widhalm, K., Schonegger, K., Huemer, C., & Auterith, A. (2001). Does the BMI reflect body fat in obese children and adolescents? A study using the TOBEC method. *International Journal of Obesity, 25*(2), 279-285.

Wilson, R., & Crouch, E. A. C. (2001). *Risk-benefit analysis* (2nd ed.). Cambridge, MA: Harvard Center for Risk Analysis.

World Health Organization. (2004). Global status report on alcohol 2004. Department of Mental Health and Substance Abuse. Retrieved from http://www.who.int/substance_ abuse/publications/global_status_report_2004_overview.pdf

CHAPTER TEN

Socio-Economic Position, Social Inequality, and Weight-Related Issues

Lindsay McLaren, *University of Calgary*
Janet deGroot, *University of Calgary*
Carol E. Adair, *University of Calgary*
Shelly Russell-Mayhew, *University of Calgary*

From a public health perspective, social inequalities in health are a pressing concern (CSDH 2008). Social inequalities in health refer to variation in health outcomes (i.e., morbidity, mortality) that occurs within and between countries, which reflects variation in economic and social circumstances that are unjust, or avoidable (Commission on the Social Determinants of Health, 2008).[1] A foundation of the research literature on social inequalities in health is a phenomenon known as the social gradient in health, which refers to the linear or stepwise relationship between socio-economic position (SEP), which refers to one's position in society as influenced by social and economic factors, and health status, favouring those of higher SEP (Mackenbach et al., 2008; Marmot, 2006; Shaw et al., 2008). The social gradient in health is a robust phenomenon in the developed world. It has been observed for both men and women, it is apparent across a variety of health outcomes, it persists over historical time, and it is not reducible to health behaviours and clinical risk factors such as cholesterol, smoking, blood pressure, and physical activity (Dunn 2010; McIntosh, Finès, Wilkins, & Wolfson, 2009; Rose & Marmot, 1981; Stringhini, 2010).

Knowledge of the social gradient in health underscores the importance of taking social inequalities into consideration when developing prevention efforts, and the prevention of weight-related health issues is no exception. To inform the socio-economically sensitive prevention of weight-related health issues, the objective of this chapter is to review and discuss what is known about the relationship between SEP and, first, obesity and body mass index (BMI) and, second, eating disorders and disordered eating attitudes and behaviours, including patterns of association and plausible underlying mechanisms. We focus on inequalities by SEP, although we acknowledge that inequalities can occur along various axes (e.g., race/ethnicity, gender, immigration, demographic, and so on), which furthermore interact with one another (e.g., Adler et al., 2008; Galabuzi, 2009). We conclude by identifying suggestions for research and prevention.

Socio-Economic Position and Obesity

The prevalence of obesity (typically defined as a BMI greater than or equal to 30 kilograms per square metre) has risen dramatically during the past two to three decades in parts of North America, the United Kingdom, Eastern Europe, the Middle East, the Pacific Islands, Australasia, and China (World Health Organization, 2003). The increase has been particularly rapid in developing countries, where obesity often, in an apparent paradox, coincides with under-nutrition (Popkin, 2002; World Health Organization, 2003).

Within developed and developing countries, the association between SEP and obesity is complex, gendered, and changing. In a review of the literature, McLaren (2007) observed a graded inverse pattern among countries. For both women and men, as one moves from countries of high- to medium- to low-development status (based on the UN Development Programme's human development index), the proportion of inverse associations (higher SEP, lower obesity likelihood) decreases and the proportion of positive associations (higher SEP, higher obesity likelihood) increases. This pattern was also observed by Monteiro and his colleagues (2004, 2007) who reported that the burden of obesity in a developing country tends to shift towards the lower SEP groups as a country's gross national product increases. McLaren (2007) observed that patterns of association further varied by the indicator of SEP. For example, the predominantly positive association for women in developing countries was most striking for materially based indicators of SEP, such as income and material possessions. The inverse association for women in countries of high development status was particularly prominent when education and occupational status were used as indicators of SEP. Similar, though attenuated, patterns were observed for men, reflecting the greater proportion of non-significant or non-linear effects observed in male samples. The differential relationship of obesity with indicators of SEP in different contexts likely speaks to the differential relevance of material, socio-cultural, and symbolic processes underlying variation in body weight, a point we return to below (McLaren 2007; McLaren & Godley 2009).

In general, associations between SEP and BMI/obesity among adults in developed countries are more often inverse than positive, and this is particularly true for women (McLaren, 2007; Senese Almeida, Fath, Smith, & Loucks, 2009). However, even within wealthier countries, the SEP indicator chosen appears to matter. For example, population-based data from several developed countries indicates an inverse association between education and BMI in both men and women (higher education, lower BMI/obesity), but this association is stronger and/or more consistent for women (Garcia-Alvarez et al., 2007; Groth, Fagt, Stockmarr, Matthiessen, & Biltoft-Jensen, 2009; McLaren, 2007; McLaren, Auld, Godley, Still, & Gauvin, 2009; Tjepkema, 2006). Published associations with income are less straightforward. In the McLaren 2007 review, of associations observed between income and obesity in developed countries, 49% were inverse for women, with most of the remaining associations (45%) being non-significant or curvilinear. Canadian data, for example, show the highest BMI/obesity among women in the middle-income category (Kuhle & Veugelers, 2008; Tjepkema, 2006). Among men, 14% of the associations between income and obesity in developed countries reported by McLaren (2007) were inverse, 24% were positive, and the remainder (majority) were non-significant or curvilinear. Recent Canadian data demonstrate an association of a positive nature between income and BMI in men, with the highest income men being the heaviest (Kuhle & Veugelers, 2008; McLaren & Godley, 2009; Shields & Tjepkema, 2006; Tjepkema, 2006). Other studies have highlighted moderation by race/ethnicity—for example, an inverse income-obesity association among US white women and a positive income-obesity association among US black men (Chang & Lauderdale, 2005).

Returning to the social gradient in health, generally speaking—that is, not specific to weight-related issues—research on the mechanisms underlying the gradient is accumulating, which suggests that health inequalities reflect inequalities in opportunities, resources, and constraints for both men and women (Commission on the Social Determinants of Health, 2008; Frohlich, Ross, & Richmond, 2006; Marmot & Wilkinson, 2005; Raphael, 2009). In other words, it is argued that persons of lower SEP face systematic barriers to achieving optimal health, such as fewer opportunities (e.g., fewer opportunities to attain higher education, due to lower expectations and/or financial constraints), fewer resources (e.g., limited income with which to acquire health-promoting assets such as adequate housing or nutrition), and more constraints (e.g., less flexible and/or insecure occupational circumstances). Certain processes are unique to women, such as gendered norms and expectations around domains such as educational attainment, family, and labour force participation (Bartley, Sacker, & Schoon, 2002). Against this backdrop, we next consider plausible mechanisms underlying the relationship between SEP and obesity.

In the developing world, we see perhaps the clearest example of absolute material deprivation, with insufficient food causing under-nutrition and malnutrition. The observation of a positive association between SEP and obesity in the poorest countries touches on both material and psychosocial processes: wealth amid extreme poverty marks one's possession of essentials such as food as well as (sedentary) leisure (McLaren, 2007). As such, a large body and the abundance it symbolizes acquire social value in many cultures—it is considered beautiful and a marker of social distinction, particularly in women (Sobal, 1991; Sobal & Stunkard, 1989).

Although this pattern is robust, it is arguably becoming increasingly complex with globalization. Referring basically to a "process of worldwide integration," which encompasses changes in, among other things, communication technology and trade relations, globalization and associated processes have had significant implications for the socio-economic patterning of obesity within and between countries worldwide (Sobal, 2001, p. 1137). For example, as Corinna Hawkes (2006) points out, inequalities in diet between the rich and poor have worsened, largely due to global changes in the production and trade of agricultural goods, foreign direct investment in food processing and retailing, and global food advertising and promotion. This shift has resulted in a situation in which inexpensive and lower quality (e.g., highly processed) foods are increasingly available in poorer countries and to the poor within richer countries. Whereas high income groups (especially in poorer countries) tend to benefit from a more dynamic marketplace brought on by these global changes, lower income groups are more likely to experience the disproportionate negative impact of economic and cultural convergence towards low quality diets (e.g., inexpensive vegetable oils and trans fats) with heavily promoted products whose desirability reflects earlier popularity among wealthier groups (Hawkes, 2006).

These dynamics are powerfully illustrated through case studies of cultures in social and economic transition. For example, the nearly 90% prevalence of overweight in Kosrae, Micronesia, has been attributed to a constellation of factors related to foreign dependence and influence, global food trade (that is, foods imported from the United States became extremely inexpensive and, in fact, cheaper in some cases than food produced locally) and associated social change (e.g., generations of residents began to prefer processed food imports, both for its taste and for its prestige through association with the wealthy US benefactor).[2] The interaction of these myriad influences is epitomized by the popularity and prestige associated with imported processed foods such as Spam and potato chips on an island where breadfruit and coconut are plentiful and whose shores are one of the world's richest sources of tuna (Cassels, 2006; Ruppel & Shell, 2002).

Within wealthy countries, evidence of a primarily inverse obesity gradient (that is, lower SEP, higher likelihood of obesity) has prompted several lines of inquiry into underlying reasons or mechanisms (McLaren, 2007). One line of inquiry focuses on food insecurity, which refers to "the inability to acquire or consume an adequate diet quality or sufficient quantity of food in socially acceptable ways, or the uncertainty that one will be able to do so" (McIntyre, 2004, p. 174). It is the term used to describe hunger in developed countries, reflecting the fact that low income in rich countries does not necessarily mean insufficient intake but, rather, a reliance on poor-quality, highly-processed foods that are often calorie-dense and inexpensive (McIntyre, 2004). Reflecting these processes, several studies have observed a seemingly paradoxical positive association between food insecurity and obesity (i.e., elevated risk of obesity among those who are food insecure), particularly for women (versus men) in wealthy countries such as the United States (Dinour, Bergen, & Yeh, 2007) and Finland (Sarlio-Lahteenkorva & Lahelma, 2001). Findings in Canada are more equivocal, which may reflect genuine contextual differences or methodological limitations of survey data used (Che & Chen, 2001; Vozoris & Tarasuk, 2003). One explanation put forth to explain the phenomenon is the "food stamp cycle" hypothesis, whereby an injection of new funds (e.g., from social assistance) and/or food stamps (in the United States) and therefore food at the beginning of the month to a food-depleted household could lead to overconsumption and weight gain (e.g., Dinour et al., 2007; Townsend, Peerson, Love, Achterberg, & Murphy, 2001). The fact that the association is more consistent in women than in men may reflect a predominant focus on women in research on this topic. However, it may also have to do with the fact that despite structural changes in gender roles, women often remain responsible for food purchase and preparation (Jansson, 1995; Kemmer, 2000) and are thus more often engaged with food, which, in turn, magnifies the opportunity for a food insecurity-obesity relationship. Studies have also shown that in food insecure households, mothers may sacrifice their own intake so that their children will be less affected (Dinour et al., 2007; McIntyre, Glanville, Raine, Anderson, & Battaglia, 2003). Although a food insecurity-obesity relationship is apparent and intriguing, it is important to note that the association between food insecurity and weight might be curvilinear, such that extreme levels of food insecurity (i.e., hunger) are associated with lower weight, as would be intuitively expected (McIntyre, 2004; Olson, 1999).

Another line of inquiry to understand socio-economic patterning of weight-related issues mainly within wealthy countries focuses on the physical and social aspects of one's residential environment (i.e., the neighbourhood or community). For example, based on the observation of significant disparities in obesity by economic and racial/ethnic minority status in the United States, Paula Ford & David Dzewaltowski (2008) reviewed research on the retail food environment (i.e., the availability, accessibility, and pricing of foods associated with healthy eating behaviours) and its implications for these disparities. Overall, their review supported the position that socio-economically disadvantaged areas in the United States tend to have poor-quality retail food environments (e.g., fewer chain groceries, higher costs of foods, more limited availability of fresh fruits and vegetables) and that these environments may thereby contribute to increased risk of obesity among those of limited personal finances. Ford and Dzewaltowki's (2008) review builds on existing research showing that food pricing patterns, whereby the lowest-cost sources of calories, including refined grains and added sugars/fats, discourage healthy eating among low SES individuals (Drewnowski, 2004; Drewnowski & Darmon, 2005).

The stress response (i.e., the activation of the hypothalamic-pituitary-adrenal axis and the sympathetic nervous system) has been associated with the development of several risk factors for chronic disease, including abdominal obesity (Bjorntorp, 2001). Neuroendocrine markers of chronic stress have also been observed in persons living in circumstances characterized by social/economic marginalization and limited power and control, and thus low SEP constitutes a social stressor with plausible biological and bio-behavioural (e.g., coping behaviours, emotional eating) links to body weight (Sapolsky, 2004). Rosmond and Bjorntorp (2000) observed perturbed cortisol secretion in men of lower SEP and demonstrated that such neuroendocrine dysregulation constituted a viable mechanism linking socio-economic status and visceral obesity. Daniel and his colleagues (2006) extended this line of inquiry to women and showed that an inverse association between cortisol rhythm and BMI among a sample of blue collar women was moderated by level of educational achievement, such that the magnitude of the association was smaller in women with more education. Interestingly, elevated cortisol levels (as a marker of physiological stress) have also been associated with dysfunctional cognitions around appearance and body image, such as strong beliefs about the importance of appearance, negative emotions and cognitions about one's own body

(Putterman & Linden, 2006) and dietary restraint (McLean, Barr, & Prior, 2001) among convenience samples of young women, providing a potential biologically plausible link between subclinical eating disorder variables and weight gain/obesity.

In sum, the social gradient in health model applies to obesity to some extent, based on evidence from several studies of an inverse association between SEP and obesity (McLaren, 2007). However, this summary statement must be qualified with the acknowledgement that there is important variation by country (the inverse association is more prominent in the developed than in the developing world), by gender (the inverse association is more consistent for women than men), and by indicator of SEP (the association is more consistent for certain indicators of SEP, such as education, than for others, such as income). Given the consistency of the education-obesity relationship, some consideration of how education as an indicator of SEP may translate into a lower risk of obesity is thus in order. Independent of its relationship with income, education may confer a set of values and beliefs that are generally more health promoting. For example, those with higher (versus lower) education may be more attentive to, and more likely to act on, health promotion messages because they place a higher value on health and related outcomes (Wardle et al., 2002). To the extent that a thinner body is viewed as desirable, from a health point of view or otherwise, such values and associated behaviours could translate into the lower BMI/obesity risk observed among those with a higher education. We view these processes as highly important to understanding the socio-economic patterning of both obesity and disordered eating, and, as such, we return to them in the next section.

SEP and Disordered Eating: Weight as a Social Symbol

Eating disorders and related constructs (e.g., body dissatisfaction, disordered eating) have traditionally been viewed as "Western" illnesses (Hoek, 2002). However, they are increasingly emerging in other societies including Asia, India, South America, and Africa (Lee & Katzman, 2002; Nasser, Katzman, & Gordon, 2001). The relatively few studies that exist on eating disorders in the developing world have highlighted that manifestations may differ—for example, a concern about fat is not always prominent (Hsu & Lee, 1993; Lee & Katzman, 2002). Research in Curaçao in the Caribbean revealed that cases of anorexia nervosa occurred among young women with a higher socio-economic background and with the opportunity to travel overseas, speaking to an apparent epidemiological transition whereby eating disorders, as they emerge in developing countries, appear first among those higher on the socio-economic spectrum

(Hoek et al., 2005; Katzman, Hermans, Van Hoeken, & Hoek, 2004). An increasing global dispersion of disordered eating attitudes and behaviours draws attention to processes associated with globalization as important determinants. For example, Becker (2004; Becker, Burwell, Gilman, Herzog, & Hamburg, 2002) documented the exportation of disordered eating through her anthropological research with schoolgirls in Fiji. At the beginning of the research, the media-naive Fijian culture valued larger body sizes in girls and women as a symbol of abundance. Three years following the introduction of Western television, girls were observed to have learned about and, in some cases, adopted disordered eating behaviour in a desire to become thin like the television characters. Although the internalization of Western ideals of physical beauty is certainly pertinent, Lee and Katzman (2002) caution against accepting a simplified view of eating disorders as simply appearance disorders, which neglects the legitimate concerns experienced by women in settings of rapid social transformation and the power of food refusal as a vehicle for exerting self-control.

Within developed countries, the socio-economic patterning of eating disorders is somewhat unclear, largely because of difficulties in teasing apart these issues in patient samples (e.g., inequalities in illness versus treatment access). Based on a review of studies published between the early 1970s and the early 1990s, Gard and Freeman (1996) concluded that there does not appear to be a social class bias in anorexia nervosa, claiming that previously reported associations reflected clinical stereotype and methodological and referral biases. Emerging work at the time actually pointed to the possibility that bulimia nervosa was more common in lower social class groups (Gard & Freeman, 1996).

Since Gard and Freeman's (1996) review, studies have continued to probe this issue (although studies are far fewer in number than those focused on SEP and obesity). Based on a retrospective survey (1960-93) of patient records from a national centre for assessment and treatment of anorexia nervosa in the United Kingdom, McClelland and Crisp (2001) concluded that the social class distribution of patients was consistently weighted towards the higher social class. The duration of illness at presentation did not differ across the social classes, suggesting that social class was unlikely to have influenced access to service (McClelland & Crisp, 2001). Two other studies examined social class in eating disorder patients using a case-control design. In Sweden, Nevonen and Norring (2004) observed higher parental occupational status and higher SEP of area of residence in the eating disorder group than in the age-matched and sex-matched control group. In Spain, Rodriguez Martin and her colleagues (2004) reported no significant differences in social class distribution in cases versus controls. However, they pointed out that while 12% of cases (anorexia nervosa, bulimia nervosa, and mixed) fell into the highest social class group, only 5% of controls fell into this category. They also concluded that "anorexia nervosa and mixed forms appear to be predominant in the higher SES categories, whereas bulimia is distributed more uniformly across all SES categories" (p. 850). On the other hand, three studies that investigated clinically significant levels of disordered eating among population-based community samples of adolescents did not find any association between these behaviours and SEP (Neumark-Sztainer & Hannan, 2000; Rogers, Resnick, Mitchell, & Blum, 1997; Toselli et al., 2005). A positive SEP-eating disorder association in patient, but not community, samples suggests that there may be some residual SEP bias in terms of service access, treatment referral, or inclination towards care.

Several studies have focused on subclinical levels of disordered eating attitudes and behaviours among population-based or volunteer/convenience samples. Of those that focused on adolescents, several point to a positive association: higher SEP (based on parent or school-level variables) associated with higher levels of restrained eating, weight loss attempts, body dissatisfaction, dieting frequency, and ideals of slimness (Adams et al., 2000; O'Dea & Caputi, 2001; Ogden & Thomas, 1999; Robinson, Chang, Farish, & Killen, 2001; Rogers et al., 1997; Wardle et al., 2004). A smaller number of findings indicate an absence of association between SEP and weight concern, body dissatisfaction, perceived and ideal body size (Adams et al., 2000; Jones, Bennett, Olmsted, Lawson, & Rodin, 2001; Striegel-Moore et al., 2000; Wardle et al., 2004). One study reported a finding in the opposite direction, namely higher SEP (parental education) was associated with a lower score on several eating disorder index subscales including drive for thinness and bulimia nervosa, after adjusting for BMI (Striegel-Moore et al., 2000). Of the studies focused on adults, the most prominent finding is a positive association: higher SEP associated with higher levels of weight concern, restrictive dieting, body dissatisfaction, perceived overweight, weight esteem, and perceived-ideal discrepancy (Jeffery & French, 1996; Lynch et al., 2007; McLaren & Gauvin, 2002; McLaren & Kuh, 2004a; McLaren & Kuh, 2004b; Paeratakul, White, Williamson, Ryan, & Bray, 2002; Wardle & Griffith, 2001; Wardle, Griffith, Johnson, & Rapoport, 2000).

Thus, the relationship between socio-economic position and eating disorders/disordered eating departs from the social gradient in health. While the relationship between SEP and eating disorders is unclear, existing research focusing on subclinical disordered eating variables in the general population suggests that, if anything, higher SEP confers heightened risk for these outcomes. To understand this pattern and to identify plausible underlying mechanisms, we need to consider a framework that embraces the psychosocial aspects of class and weight. Body weight is a prominent and highly value-laden aspect of one's physical appearance (Bell, 1985; Schwartz, 1986; Stearns, 1997), and we need a framework that helps us to understand how attitudes about, and efforts taken to manipulate, weight are socially patterned.

The work of theorist Pierre Bourdieu (1984) is well suited to our task (Power 1999, 2005; Shilling 2005). Of particular relevance is Bourdieu's concept of *habitus*, which refers to the embodiment of social structures. Through sustained exposure to axes of social stratification such as class (but also others, such as gender, race/ethnicity, and so on), one's body (broadly conceptualized, to include appearance, style, size, and mannerisms) becomes a metaphor for one's status. One's class or status, according to Bourdieu, is not just about income but also consists of one's level of various forms of capital—cultural (i.e., capital ensuing from one's educational qualifications and associated dispositions) and social (that is, capital ensuing from one's social networks) as well as economic (income, wealth). One can also accrue symbolic capital if he or she possesses an attribute that is highly valued or sought after in a given society (e.g., a strong work ethic, a particular accent, a certain physical appearance).

This framework can help us to understand some of the plausible mechanisms underlying the positive relationship between SEP and disordered eating outcomes as well as the inverse relationship between certain indicators of SEP (education) and obesity, which is particularly strong for women, as discussed in the first section of this chapter. For example, someone with relatively high levels of cultural capital is able to effectively navigate and adhere to societal norms and expectations, including those having to do with body weight, appearance, and gender. High educational attainment as an indicator of cultural capital may convey an affinity towards the body and health. Such an affinity could manifest in the aforementioned observations that higher SEP women are more likely to diet, to be dissatisfied with their bodies, and also to be thinner. In support of this reasoning, education as an indicator of SEP has shown a more consistent association with body dissatisfaction than other indicators of SEP (McLaren & Kuh, 2004a). Greater body dissatisfaction and lower BMI among women of higher SEP could also reflect social capital, to the extent that network norms (e.g., friends, colleagues, peers) and expectations emphasizing health and thinness, which are known to influence individuals' attitudes and behaviours (e.g., Shomaker & Furman, 2009) are more prominent in higher class groups. The role of social networks could also accommodate a geographical dimension. For example, McLaren and Gauvin (2002) examined body dissatisfaction among a random sample of Canadian women in relation to neighbourhood attributes. We observed that, for a given BMI, women living in more affluent (higher income) neighbourhoods were more likely to be dissatisfied with their own bodies than women living in lower income neighbourhoods. In a follow-up study, this effect was partially explained by the thinner average body size of women in higher income neighbourhoods, speaking to a likely role of social norms within one's area of residence (McLaren & Gauvin, 2003). Similar processes could occur in workplaces, community groups, and other settings.

Bourdieu's (1984) notion of symbolic capital (capital incurred through the possession of attributes that are highly valued in a society) is highly relevant to weight-related issues because not all body types are regarded equally. A thin body in women has enormous symbolic value in Western society, whereas a large body does not and, thus, having a thin body incurs social benefits ("capital") that are not reducible to the economic dimension of class. Thinness as a marker of social distinction in women has deep roots in feminist literature (Malson & Burns, 2009), and the desirability of a thin appearance is reinforced through societal institutions including Western media (Groesz, Levine, & Murnen, 2002; Katzmarzyk & Davis, 2001; Rubinstein & Caballero 2000). Coupled with this is the strong societal disparagement of fat, which has been demonstrated to manifest in socio-economic penalties for larger women (Campos, 2005; Stearns, 1997). For example, using prospective population-based US data, Cawley (2004) demonstrated that excess weight was associated with subsequent lower earnings in white women (adjusting for several other socio-economic attributes as well as general intelligence), to an extent that was approximately equivalent to one and a half years of education. Overall, from the perspective of Bourdieu's theory, the greater value placed on thinness and resources directed towards attaining this goal among women of higher SEP constitutes part of one's social class. As such, these attributes plausibly help to explain the associations observed in the literature between SEP and obesity (inverse, particularly with education as an indicator of SEP) and between SEP and disordered eating (positive, for subclinical variables in the general population of women).

The story is somewhat different for men, but Bourdieu's theory may help us to understand gender differences as well. As noted earlier, the association between education and BMI is stronger for women than men (McLaren, 2007; McLaren et al., 2009), and the association between income and BMI for men is more often positive than negative (McLaren, 2007). To explain these patterns, one must acknowledge that the societal ideal physique differs for men and women. As demonstrated by research on body image among children, thinness is idealized for women, while a larger, more muscular physique is desirable for men (e.g., McVey, Tweed, & Blackmore, 2005). Thus, although men are undoubtedly exposed to some stigma associated with excess weight, there is also a conflicting social pressure—valuation of a larger body size as conveying attributes such as strength, power, and dominance. With men being the traditional earners in families, it is plausible that, in conjunction with other contributory processes, the symbolic value of body size for men accords with this position of household dominance, such that men of higher SEP value and pursue largeness for reasons analogous to why women of SEP value and pursue thinness—because of the status and prestige it conveys. In support of this argument, McLaren and Godley (2009) examined BMI in relation to occupational prestige among a population-based sample of Canadian men and women and observed that men in certain high-prestige occupations (those that involve supervisory or management responsibilities) tended to be heavy. In such positions, it makes sense that larger body size (whether overweight, muscular, or some combination) could be valuable towards asserting one's dominance or authority.

In sum, disordered eating outcomes depart from the social gradient in health, such that, if anything, higher SEP confers heightened risk. To understand this phenomenon, one must adopt a framework that embraces weight as a social symbol and reflects how class relates to its pursuit. We identified Bourdieu's theory of *habitus* as a suitable framework. This framework is also informative for understanding the inverse association between SEP and obesity in women, which is particularly consistent with certain indicators of SEP (e.g., educational attainment) and thus provides a way to bridge the study of socio-economic patterning of the two health outcomes.

Conclusions

We conclude by offering the following suggestions for research and prevention, which we believe emanate from this chapter's discussion of SEP and weight-related issues.

- Knowledge of the association between SEP and weight-related issues draws attention to factors that would need to be incorporated into prevention efforts that yield significant and sustained impact. Examples include income-related barriers to a nutritious diet, and norms and expectations around thinness that appear to be more prominent in higher social class groups. Targeting such determinants requires taking an upstream perspective to prevention, for which a population health approach is suitable (see Chapter 2 in this volume).

- At a basic level, the discussion indicates that it would be important to be aware of the socio-economic circumstances of the individuals/groups being targeted in a prevention initiative and adapting the prevention efforts accordingly. For example, a prevention initiative that centres around social inoculation against harmful messages conveyed through mass media in a higher SEP population of young women is not likely to be effective if their social norms otherwise relentlessly promote those same messages. Likewise, offering instruction in healthy cooking and food preparation in a low-income population misses the mark, as it does not address larger issues such as one's capacity to purchase nutritious foods in the first place. Relatedly, knowledge of a target group's socio-economic circumstances can help to avoid unintended consequences of prevention initiatives. For example, one may need to be particularly attuned to the possibility that obesity prevention messages may inadvertently promote body dissatisfaction and disordered eating behaviours, if the target group includes women of higher SEP (e.g., students in a private school).
- The socio-economic patterning of weight-related issues (particularly disordered eating) departs from the familiar social gradient in health and, as such, continued population-based monitoring of these health outcomes and their socio-economic patterning is important. While population-based data on BMI/obesity is routine in many countries, such data for disordered eating appears less available. In addition to enabling monitoring of population-based trends within and between countries, such data would be useful for evaluating the impact of larger-scale prevention activities (intended or otherwise) such as changes to food policy or private sector initiatives to promote a healthier ideal body size.

Notes

1   The terms inequality and inequity are sometimes used in the public health literature to denote group differences, and group differences that are avoidable or unjust, respectively (Whitehead, 1992).
2   Originally an independent kingdom, Kosrae was subsequently governed by the United States administration after the Second World War and later entered into a relationship of free association in which the United States remained the island's chief benefactor in exchange for granting the United States free military access.

References

Adams, K., Sargent, R. G., Thompson, S. H., Richter, D., Corwin, S. J., & Rogan, T. J. (2000). A study of body weight concerns and weight control practices of fourth and seventh grade adolescents. *Ethnicity and Health*, 5, 79-94.

Adler, N., Singh-Manoux, A., Schwartz, J., Stewart, J., Matthews, K., & Marmot, M. G. (2008). Social status and health: A comparison of British civil servants in Whitehall-II with European- and African-Americans in CARDIA. *Social Science and Medicine, 66*, 1034-1045.

Bartley, M., Sacker, A., & Schoon, I. (2002). Social and economic trajectories and women's health. In D. Kuh & R. Hardy (Eds.), *A life course approach to women's health* (pp. 233-254). Oxford: Oxford University Press.

Becker, A. (2004). Television, disordered eating, and young women in Fiji: Negotiating body image and identity during rapid social change. *Culture, Medicine, and Psychiatry, 28*, 533-559.

Becker, A., Burwell, R. A., Gilman, S. E., Herzog, D. B., & Hamburg, P. (2002). Eating behaviours and attitudes following prolonged exposure to television among ethnic Fijian adolescent girls. *British Journal of Psychiatry, 180*, 509-514.

Bell, R. M. (1985). *Holy Anorexia*. Chicago: University of Chicago Press.

Bjorntorp, P. (2001). Do stress reactions cause abdominal obesity and comorbidities? *Obesity Reviews, 2*, 73-86.

Bourdieu, P. (1984). *Distinction: A social critique of the judgement of taste*. London: Routledge.

Campos, P. (2005). *The diet myth* [previously published as *The Obesity Myth*]. New York: Gotham Books.

Cassels, S. (2006). Overweight in the Pacific: Links between foreign dependence, global food trade, and obesity in the Federated States of Micronesia. *Global Health, 2*, 10.

Cawley, J. (2004). The impact of obesity on wages. *Journal of Human Resources, 39*, 451-474.

Chang, V. W., & Lauderdale, D. S. (2005). Income disparities in body mass index in obesity in the United States, 1971-2002. *Archives of Internal Medicine, 165*, 2122-2128.

Che, J., & Chen, J. (2001). Food insecurity in Canadian households. *Health Reports, 12*, 11-22.

Commission on the Social Determinants of Health. (2008). *Closing the gap in a generation: Health equity through action on the social determinants of health.* Final Report of the Commission on the Social Determinants of Health. Geneva: World Health Organization.

Daniel, M. D., Moore, D. S., Decker, S., Belton, L., DeVellis, B., Doolen A., & Campbell, M. K. (2006). Associations among education, cortisol rhythm, and BMI in blue-collar women. *Obesity, 14*, 327-335.

Dinour, L. M., Bergen, D., & Yeh, M. C. (2007). The food insecurity—obesity paradox: a review of the literature and the role food stamps may play. *Journal of the American Dietetic Association, 107*, 1952-1961.

Drewnowski, A. (2004). Obesity and the food environment: Dietary energy density and diet costs. *American Journal of Preventive Medicine, 27*, 154-162.

Drewnowski, A., & Darmon, N. (2005). The economics of obesity: Dietary energy density and energy cost. *American Journal of Clinical Nutrition, 82*(Suppl): S265-S273.

Dunn, J. R. (2010). Health behavior versus the stress of low socioeconomic status and health outcomes. *Journal of the American Medical Association, 303,* 1199-1200.

Ford, P. B., & Dzewaltowski, D. A. (2008). Disparities in obesity prevalence due to variation in the retail food environment: Three testable hypotheses. *Nutrition Reviews, 66,* 216-228.

Frohlich, K. L., Ross, N., & Richmond, C. (2006). Health disparities in Canada today: Some evidence and a theoretical framework. *Health Policy, 79,* 132-143.

Galabuzi, G. E. (2009). Social exclusion. In D. Raphael (Ed.), *Social determinants of health: Canadian Perspectives* (2nd edition; pp. 252-268). Toronto: Canadian Scholars' Press.

Garcia-Alvarez, A., Serra-Majem, L., Ribas-Barba, L., Castell, C., Foz, M., Uauy, R., Plasencia, A., & Salleras L. (2007). Obesity and overweight trends in Catalonia, Spain (1992-2003): Gender and socio-economic determinants. *Public Health Nutrition, 10,* 1368-1378.

Gard, M. C. E., & Freeman, C. P. (1996). The dismantling of a myth: A review of eating disorders and socioeconomic status. *International Journal of Eating Disorders, 20,* 1-12.

Groesz, L. M., Levine, M. P., & Murnen, S. K. (2002). The effect of experimental presentation of thin media images on body satisfaction: A meta-analytic review. *International Journal of Eating Disorders, 31,* 1-16.

Groth, M. V., Fagt, S., Stockmarr, A., Matthiessen, J., and Biltoft-Jensen, A. (2009). Dimensions of socioeconomic position related to body mass index and obesity among Danish women and men, *Scandinavian Journal of Public Health, 37,* 418-426.

Hawkes, C. (2006). Uneven dietary development: Linking the policies and processes of globalization with the nutrition transition, obesity and diet-related chronic diseases. *Global Health, 2,* 4.

Hoek, H. W. (2002). Distribution of eating disorders. In C. G. Fairburn & K. D. Brownell (Eds.), *Eating disorders and obesity: A Comprehensive Handbook* (2nd ed.; pp. 233-237). New York: Guilford Press.

Hoek, H. W., van Harten, P. N., Hermans, K. M., Katzman, M. A., Matroos, G. E., & Susser, E. S. (2005). The incidence of anorexia nervosa on Curaçao. *American Journal of Psychiatry, 162,* 748-752.

Hsu, L. K., & Lee, S. (1993). Is weight phobia always necessary for a diagnosis of anorexia nervosa? *American Journal of Psychiatry, 150,* 1466-1471.

Jansson, S. (1995). Food practices and division of domestic labour: A comparison between British and Swedish households. *Sociological Review, 43,* 462-477.

Jeffrey, R. W., & French, S. A. (1996.) Socioeconomic status and weight control practices among twenty-to-forty-five-year old women. *American Journal of Public Health, 86,* 1005-1010.

Jones, J. M., Bennett, S., Olmsted, M. P., Lawson, M. L., & Rodin, G. (2001). Disordered eating attitudes and behaviours in teenaged girls: A school-based study. *Canadian Medical Association Journal, 165,* 547-552.

Katzman, M. A., Hermans, K. M., Van Hoeken, D., & Hoek, H. W. (2004). Not your "typical island woman": Anorexia nervosa is reported only in subcultures in Curaçao. *Culture, Medicine, and Psychiatry, 28,* 463-492.

Katzmarzyk, P. T., & Davis, C. (2001). Thinness and body shape of Playboy centerfolds from 1978 to 1998. *International Journal of Obesity, 25,* 590-592.

Kemmer, D. (2000). Tradition and change in domestic roles and food preparation. *Sociology, 34,* 323-333.

Kuhle, S., & Veugelers, P. J. (2008). Why does the social gradient in health not apply to overweight? *Health Reports, 19,* 7-15.

Lee, S., & Katzman, M. A. (2002). Cross-cultural perspectives on eating disorders. In C. G. Fairburn & K. D. Brownell (Eds.), *Eating disorders and obesity: A comprehensive handbook* (2nd ed., pp. 260-264). New York: Guilford Press.

Lynch, E., Liu, K., Spring, B., Hankinson, A., Wei, G. S., & Greenland, P. (2007). Association of ethnicity and socioeconomic status with judgments of body size: The Coronary Artery Risk Development in Young Adults study. *American Journal of Epidemiology, 165,* 1055-1062.

Mackenbach, J. P., Stirbu, I., Roskam, A. J. R., Schaap, M. M., Menvielle, G., Leinsalu, M., & Kunst, A. E. (2008). Socioeconomic inequalities in health in twenty-two European countries. *New England Journal of Medicine, 358,* 2468-2481.

Malson, H., & Burns, M. (Eds.). (2009). *Critical feminist approaches to eating disorders.* London: Routledge.

Marmot, M. (2006). Health in an unequal world. *Lancet, 368,* 2081-2094.

Marmot, M., & Wilkinson, R. (Eds.). (2005). *Social determinants of health* (2nd ed.). Oxford: Oxford University Press.

McClelland, L., & Crisp, A. (2001). Anorexia nervosa and social class. *International Journal of Eating Disorders, 29,* 150-156.

McIntosh, C. N., Finès, P., Wilkins, R., & Wolfson, M. C. (2009). Income disparities in health-adjusted life expectancy for Canadian adults, 1991 to 2001. *Health Reports, 20,* 55-64.

McIntyre, L. (2004). Food insecurity. In D. Raphael (Ed.), *Social determinants of health: Canadian perspectives* (pp. 173-185). Toronto: Canadian Scholars' Press.

McIntyre, L., Glanville, T., Raine, K. D., Anderson, B., & Battaglia, N. (2003). Do low-income lone mothers compromise their nutrition to feed their children? *Canadian Medical Association Journal, 168,* 686-691.

McLaren, L. (2007). Socioeconomic status and obesity. *Epidemiological Reviews, 29,* 29-48.

McLaren, L., Auld, C. M., Godley, J., Still, D., & Gauvin, L. (2009). Examining the association between socioeconomic position and body mass index in 1978 and 2005 among Canadian working-age women and men. *International Journal of Public Health, 55,* 193-200.

McLaren, L., & Gauvin, L. (2002). Neighbourhood- versus individual-level correlates of women's body dissatisfaction: Toward a multilevel understanding of the role of affluence. *Journal of Epidemiology and Community Health, 56,* 193-199.

McLaren, L., & Gauvin, L. (2003). Does the "average size" of women in the neighbourhood influence a woman's likelihood of body dissatisfaction? *Health & Place, 9,* 327-335.

McLaren, L., & Godley, J. (2009). Social class and body mass index among Canadian adults: A focus on occupational prestige. *Obesity, 17,* 290-299.

McLaren, L., & Kuh, D. (2004a). Women's body dissatisfaction, social class, and social mobility. *Social Science and Medicine, 58,* 1575-1584.

McLaren, L., & Kuh, D. (2004b). Body dissatisfaction in midlife women. *Journal of Women and Aging, 16,* 35-54.

McLean, J. A., Barr, S. I., & Prior, J. C. (2001). Cognitive dietary restraint is associated with higher urinary corisol excretion in healthy premenopausal women. *American Journal of Clinical Nutrition, 73,* 7-12.

McVey, G., Tweed, S., & Blackmore, E. (2005). Correlates of weight loss and muscle-gaining behavior in ten-to-fourteen-year-old males and females. *Preventive Medicine, 40,* 1-9.

Monteiro, C. A., Conde, W. L., Lu, B., & Popkin, B. M. (2004). Obesity and inequities in health in the developing world. *International Journal of Obesity and Related Metabolic Disorders, 28,* 1181-1186.

Monteiro, C. A., Conde, W. L., & Popkin, B. M. (2007). Income-specific trends in obesity in Brazil: 1975 2003. *American Journal of Public Health, 97,* 1808-1812.

Nasser, M., Katzman, M. A., & Gordon, R. A. (Eds). (2001). *Eating disorders and cultures in transition.* New York: Brunner-Routledge.

Neumark-Sztainer, D., & Hannan, P. J. (2000). Weight-related behaviors among adolescent girls and boys: Results from a national survey. *Archives of Pediatrics and Adolescent Medicine, 154,* 569-577.

Nevonen, L., & Norring, C. (2004). Socio-economic variables and eating disorders: A comparison between patients and normal controls. *Eating and Weight Disorders, 9,* 279-284.

O'Dea, J. A., & Caputi, P. (2001). Association between socioeconomic status, weight, age and gender, and the body image and weight control practices of six-to-nineteen-year-old children and adolescents. *Health Education Research, 16,* 521-532.

Ogden, J., & Thomas, D. (1999). The role of familial values in understanding the impact of social class on weight concern. *International Journal of Eating Disorders, 25,* 273-279.

Olson, C. M. (1999). Nutrition and health outcomes associated with food insecurity and hunger. *Journal of Nutrition, 129,* 521S-524S.

Paeratakul, S., White, M. A., Williamson, D. A., Ryan, D. H., & Bray, G. A. (2002). Sex, race/ethnicity, socioeconomic status, and BMI in relation to self-perception of overweight. *Obesity Research, 10,* 345-350.

Popkin, B. M. (2002). The shift in stages of the nutrition transition in the developing world differs from past experiences. *Public Health Nutrition, 5,* 205-214.

Power, E. M. (1999). An introduction to Pierre Bourdieu's key theoretical concepts. *Journal for the Study of Food and Society, 3,* 48-52.

Power, E. M. (2005). Determinants of healthy eating among low-income Canadians (Suppl), *Canadian Journal of Public Health, 96*(3), S37-S38.

Putterman, E., & Linden, W. (2006). Cognitive dietary restraint and cortisol: Importance of pervasive concerns with appearance. *Appetite, 47,* 64-76.

Raphael, D. (Ed). (2009). *Social determinants of health: Canadian perspectives* (2nd ed.). Toronto: Canadian Scholars' Press.

Robinson, T. N., Chang, J. Y., Farish, H. K., & Killen, J. D. (2001). Overweight concerns and body dissatisfaction among third-grade children: The impacts of ethnicity and socioeconomic status. *Journal of Pediatrics, 138,* 181-187.

Rodriguez Martin, A., Novalbos Ruiz, J. P., Martinez Nieto, J. M., Escobar Jimenez, L., & Castro de Haro, A. L. (2004). Epidemiological study of the influence of family and socioeconomic status in disorders of eating behaviour. *European Journal of Clinical Nutrition, 58,* 846-852.

Rogers, L., Resnick, M. D., Mitchell, J. E., & Blum, R. W. (1997). The relationship between socioeconomic status and eating-disordered behaviors in a community sample of adolescent girls. *International Journal of Eating Disorders, 22,* 15-23.

Rose, G., & Marmot, M. G. (1981). Social class and coronary heart disease. *British Heart Journal, 45,* 13-19.

Rosmond, R., & Bjorntorp, P. (2000). Occupational status, cortisol secretory pattern, and visceral obesity in middle-aged men. *Obesity Research, 8,* 445-450.

Rubinstein, S., & Caballero, B. (2000). Is Miss America an undernourished role model? *Journal of the American Medical Association, 283*(12), 1569.

Ruppel Shell, E. (2002). *The hungry gene: The science of fat and the future of thin.* New York: Atlantic Monthly Press.

Sapolsky, R. M. (2004). *Why zebras don't get ulcers: The acclaimed guide to stress, stress-related diseases, and coping* (3rd ed.). New York: Owl Books.

Sarlio-Lahteenkorva, S., & Lahelma. E. (2001). Food insecurity is associated with past and present economic disadvantage and body mass index. *Journal of Nutrition, 131,* 2880- 2884.

Schwartz, H. (1986). *Never satisfied: A cultural history of diets, fantasies, and fat.* New York: Free Press.

Senese, L. C., Almeida, N. D., Fath, A. K., Smith, B. T., & Loucks, E. B. (2009). Associations between childhood socioeconomic position and adult obesity. *Epidemiologic Reviews, 31,* 21-51.

Shaw, M., Galobardes, B., Lawlor, D.A., Lynch, J., Wheeler, B., & Davey Smith, G. (2008). *The handbook of inequality and socioeconomic position: Concepts and measures.* Bristol, United Kingdom: Policy Press.

Shields, M., & Tjepkema, M. (2006). Trends in adult obesity. *Health Reports, 17,* 53-59.

Shilling, C. (2005). *The body and social theory* (2nd ed.). London: Sage Publications.

Shomaker, L. B., & Furman, W. (2009). Interpersonal influences on late adolescent girls' and boys' disordered eating. *Eating Behaviors, 10,* 96-106.

Sobal, J. (1991). Obesity and socioeconomic status: A framework for examining relationships between physical and social variables. *Medical Anthropology, 13,* 231-247.

Sobal, J. (2001). Commentary: Globalization and the epidemiology of obesity. *International Journal of Epidemiology, 30,* 1136-1137.

Sobal, J., & Stunkard, A. J. (1989). Socioeconomic status and obesity: A review of the literature. *Psychological Bulletin, 105,* 260-275.

Stearns, P. N. (1997). *Fat history: Bodies and beauty in the modern West.* New York: New York University Press.

Striegel-Moore, R. H., Schreiber, G. B., Lo, A., Crawford, P., Obarzanek, E., & Rodin, J. (2000). Eating disorder symptoms in a cohort of eleven-to-sixteen-year-old black and white girls: The NHLBI Growth and Health Study. *International Journal of Eating Disorders, 27,* 49-66.

Stringhini, S., Sabia, S., Shipley M, Brunner, E., Nabi, H., Kivimaki, M., & Singh-Manoux, M. (2010). Association of socioeconomic position with health behaviors and mortality. *Journal of the American Medical Association, 303,* 1159-1166.

Tjepkema, M. (2006). Adult obesity. *Health Reports, 17,* 9 25.

Toselli, A. L., Villani, S., Ferro, A. M., Verri, A., Cucurullo, I., & Marinoni, A. (2005). Eating disorders and their correlates in high school adolescents of northern Italy. *Epidemiologia e Psichiatria Sociale, 14,* 91-99.

Townsend, M. S., Peerson, J., Love, B., Achterberg, C., & Murphy, S. P. (2001). Food insecurity is positively related to overweight in women. *Journal of Nutrition, 131,* 1763-1745.

Vozoris, N., & Tarasuk, V. (2003). Household food insufficiency is associated with poorer health. *Journal of Nutrition, 133,* 120-126.

Wardle, J., & Griffith, J. (2001). Socioeconomic status and weight control practices in British adults. *Journal of Epidemiology and Community Health, 55,* 185-190.

Wardle, J., Griffith, J., Johnson, F., & Rapoport, L. (2000). Intentional weight control and food choice habits in a national representative sample of adults in the UK. *International Journal of Obesity, 24,* 534-540.

Wardle, J., Robb, K. A., Johnson, F., Griffith, J., Brunner, E., Power, C., & Tovee, M. (2004). Socioeconomic variation in attitudes to eating and weight in female adolescents. *Health Psychology, 23,* 275-282.

Wardle, J., Waller, J., & Jarvis, M. J. (2002). Sex differences in the association of socioeconomic status with obesity. *American Journal of Public Health, 92,* 1299-1304.

Whitehead, M. (1992). The concepts and principles of equity and health. *International Journal of Health Services, 22,* 429-445.

World Health Organization. (2003). Global strategy on diet, physical activity, and health. *Obesity and Overweight fact sheet.* Retrieved from http://www.who.int/hpr/NPH/docs/gs_obesity.pdf

Conclusion

Gail L. McVey, *The Hospital for Sick Children, University of Toronto*
Michael P. Levine, *Kenyon College*
Niva Piran, *Ontario Institute for Studies in Education, University of Toronto*
H. Bruce Ferguson, *The Hospital for Sick Children, University of Toronto*

The chapters in this book emphasize the multiple domains that influence body image and body experiences in children, youth, and adults. Body experiences and body image shape the ways in which individuals live in their bodies, and, in particular, they influence eating patterns, self-care behaviours, and engagement in pleasurable physical activities. Since these connections have a powerful impact on children's well-being and sense of self-worth, we need to both understand and address multiple sources of influence.

One of the principal themes of this book is that this work and the resulting prevention programs must be guided by critical theory that places individuals in the context of social relationships and social structures. Critical theory is critically important because prevention programs should be informed by theoretical perspectives that consider the complexity of inducing change in a multi-layered social environment, while also taking into consideration individuals' developmental levels and the unique social contexts that emerge from multiple domains of influence. We therefore highlight three domains of work that we believe will advance the shared goal of prevention of eating and weight-related disorders.

Contextual Development Research

In line with Bronfenbrenner's theory (1979, 2005) there is a need to examine the impact of the multiple levels of the social environment on children's development and on adult's experiences and behaviours (see Levine

& Smolak, 2006, Chapter 15). Bronfenbrenner's theory looks at a child's development within the context of the system of relationships that form his or her environments. Each layer of environment has an effect on a child's development. For example, the interaction between factors in the child's maturing biology, his or her immediate family/community environment, and the societal landscape fuels and steers his/her development. Changes or conflict in any one layer will ripple throughout other layers.

To date, most developmental research has focused on individuals or "microsystems" such as the relationships and interactions that a child has with his or her immediate surroundings, including family, school, neighbourhood, or childcare environments. For the most part, factors such as socio-economic status, gender, or ethnicity have not been extensively or sufficiently incorporated into these theoretical perspectives. Similarly, and with some notable exceptions within the eating disorder field (see, e.g., Smolak & Murnen, 2004), important social factors that shape the differential prevalence distribution of eating disorders, such as gender, have not received anywhere near sufficient attention in developmental research (Piran, 2010a).

The chapters in the present volume that address the impact of socio-economic factors on body weight and experiences, together with those that consider the intersection of gender with other social factors, suggest that developmental and contextual information can and should serve to guide prevention work. Specifically, evidence suggests that to minimize unintended consequences, there is a need to adapt prevention initiatives according to the socio-economic circumstances of the targeted individuals or groups (e.g., income-related barriers to a nutritious diet; norms and expectations around thinness that appear to be more prominent in higher social class groups). In terms of gender, there is a need to transform the nature of social relations at the multiple levels of our existing social organizations/structures, from policy level change, through increased equity at the community level, to altering peer norms. As the Developmental Theory of Embodiment (Piran, 2010b; Piran & Teall, Chapter 7 of this volume) stipulates, children and youth need to be exposed to opportunities to connect positively with their bodies (e.g., active and joyful engagement in non-objectifying physical activities, wearing comfortable clothing) and with the physical environment. Prevention efforts are required to provide children (girls especially) with a context that supports their right to safety, respects their body ownership, and guides them in self-care. Despite the acknowledgement of gender disparities in negative body image and full-blown eating disorders such as anorexia nervosa and bulimia nervosa, there remains a dearth of programs that address, directly, topics such as

(1) the development of gender roles; (2) the sexualization and objectification of children's bodies and, in particular, girls' bodies; and (3) everyday sexism, including its position in the web of racism, class-based prejudice, and so on. Continued work in these domains is emphatically encouraged.

Ecological Prevention Interventions

This book leaves no doubt that progress in the field of prevention of eating and weight-related disorders will advance in line with a greater emphasis on ecological approaches to prevention. The chapters in the book indicate that important work is currently being done in multiple aspects of the social environment (schools, athletics, media). However, there is a great need to develop this work further. In particular, we are facing challenges in intervening at the higher level of the social environment in ways that take action on underlying causes, create circumstances that facilitate and maintain the desired outcomes, and sustain a focus on funding public health interventions. To accomplish these goals, we will need to become much more proficient in understanding and intervening with cyber-media and in involving all stakeholders in a child's environment, parents in particular.

Engagement and collaboration constitute two important and interrelated themes in this book. In order to ensure that public health messages are consistent with eating disorder and with anti-obesity goals, it is essential that we achieve greater co-operation among the various constituencies that generate public health interventions designed to encourage healthy eating and body image. In order to ensure that time and dollars are well spent on the delivery of health care and education that are truly child-centred, we must pool our resources and be careful neither to confuse the public with conflicting health messaging nor leave professionals feeling confused and ineffective. The 50-year-old war on obesity in North America has clearly not reduced the incidence or prevalence of obesity, and it very likely has contributed to the rise of eating disorders in North America since the 1960s (Gordon, 2000). There is a need for the public to embrace a public health perspective that helps us shift to a healthier, more holistic approach to health. The chapters in this book indicate that incorporating ecological and contextual developmental perspectives will be a complex, but extremely important, part of such public health initiatives and programs (see also Levine & Piran, 2004; Levine & Smolak, 2006, Chapter 15; Piran, 2010a, 2010b; Steiner-Adair, 1994).

In the process of developing such programs, we will need to revisit and grapple with the meanings and implications of the powerful word "feminism" (see, e.g., Bordo, 1993; Brown & Jasper, 1993; Orbach, 1978; Piran, 1999; Smolak & Murnen, 2004; Striegel-Moore & Steiner-Adair, 1998).

One important element of the Feminist Ecological Developmental perspective being advocated here is the need to ground prevention programs and prevention outcome research in ongoing collaborative partnerships with local stakeholders and, in particular, with those who constitute the "ecologies" we seek to understand and alter, notably parents, school personnel, and media professionals. Prevention roll-out in an ideal world would be consistent and integrated in the multiple environments within which children live. As noted previously, the lives of children and adolescents are constructed and influenced by many adults, so optimal outcomes would be achieved if common health-promoting messages are delivered in their home, school, religious, and recreational settings. Although this idea seems true, if not obvious, at a theoretical level, such co-ordination presents significant practical challenges and requires effective bridging across the sectors of education, health, and sport.

Piran's (1999, 2001a, 2001b) decade-long work within a co-educational, competitive residential ballet school—which many people would envision as "an impossible setting" for effective prevention—broke new ground in the field by creating an ecological approach to prevention imbued with a feminist lens. With girls ages 10 to 18, Piran facilitated over 300 groups centred on giving a voice to the girls' descriptions of events that affected how they felt about, and otherwise experienced, their bodies. Next, within these groups, Piran guided the girls to a stage in which the girls derived core critical concepts related to the various events that they shared. Under Piran's guidance as a teacher, mentor, and role model, this interpretive, critical stage was followed by an action-oriented stage in which the girls decided upon, and implemented, plans of action to generate constructive changes within the school.

The rich accounts voiced by the girls to Piran and to each other led to Piran's (2001a) critical theory of body weight and shape preoccupation. Piran's detailed thematic analyses of events shared in these groups yielded three main themes that spoke to inequities in social power within this particular school: violation of body ownership, prejudicial treatment, and constraining social constructions of gender. Action plans developed and enacted by the girls aimed to reduce these inequities throughout the school environment—for example, by changing peer-norms, staff-student norms, the school's committee structure, staff hiring, and even physical aspects of the school environment (Piran, 2001b). Piran's work in this ballet school showed how giving voice to girls' lived experiences of and in the body, then reclaiming power through activism, could allow them to join together to create environments that resist societal oppression of the female body in order to reclaim healthier relationships with food, the body, dance, and each other. Piran's attention to social discourses, at multiple levels in a system (individual, peer, school, family), illustrates not only how social discourses and structures can adversely impact a person's senses of self and body experiences, but also how new discourses and structures can heal.

Respectful dialogue remains a key aspect of Piran's (1991, 2001a, 2001b) feminist approach. At another level, we also need to develop and deepen dialogues between professionals, including "basic" researchers in various fields, notably obesity prevention, education, social media, and public policy. In Canada, collaborative research and national dialogue have been initiated among prevention specialists and researchers on ways to begin the process of integrating obesity and eating disorder prevention work (McVey et al., 2008). Support for this integration stems from longitudinal research that shows that there are common/shared risk factors among these weight-related disorders that can be folded into the same intervention strategy (Neumark-Sztainer et al., 2006; see also Haines & Neumark-Sztainer, 2006). Research is required to identify the most effective ways to initiate the connections and dialogues that will help prepare professionals to carry out integrated, cross-sector prevention work.

In countries such as Australia, Israel, Spain, Argentina, and the United Kingdom, advancements have been made at the government level in terms of establishing regulations to discourage disordered eating among children and youth and to either limit or buffer the widespread exposure of the public to media-based images of severely underweight fashion models. Yet, despite these important strides, we still do not have laws that reinforce these regulations. Thus, there remains considerable work to be done—for example, in making public the harmful effects of weight cycling and in imposing mandatory guidelines on the advertising industry to add disclaimers to images that are retouched in magazines and other media.

There is a need to look back, slow down, and address the dearth of knowledge about key, now-overused constructs, such as "media literacy," "age-appropriate prevention programs," and "being 'at risk.'" Simultaneously, there is a need to look forward, get up to speed, and address the need to know more about what is happening on the World Wide Web and how knowledge, beliefs, and actions are being transformed by experiences in and based on cyberspace. As this book indicates, the digital era offers activists and researchers working in the eating-related disorders field a new and potentially very effective set of tools to learn more about "media effects" as well as to promote awareness, mobilize social groups, and co-ordinate actions to promote social change. The added value to using Web-based technologies as research, advocacy, and activism tools include, but are not limited to, accessibility, time and cost effectiveness, more effective information gathering, and dissemination.

Evaluation Research

Finally, the ecological prevention approach needs to be enhanced by evaluative procedures that acknowledge the complexities of assessing ecological influences. How does the ecological context affect the lives of children, youth, and their families? How do we measure the processes involved in the implementation of multi-level, systemic interventions and their interaction with mediating variables such as critical thinking by key players that lead to the modification and evolution of a program? As this book describes, researchers need to make use of sophisticated study designs that capture outcome indicators other than those associated with individual attitudinal or behaviour changes. These include policy and/or organizational change, changes in weight-related group norms, and feelings of connectedness to, and engagement with, positive, health-promoting features of the social and physical environment.

Drawing from the field of community psychology, we know that "developing such complex models and their appropriate analytic techniques represents a significant conceptual and methodological challenge" (Trickett, 2009, p. 400). Looking at the literature on social determinants of health, we know that it is possible, and indeed likely, that, operating outside of the eating or weight-related interventions we build, there are multiple competing factors that cause individuals to resist change (Commission on Social Determinants of Health, 2008). Alternatively, participants might experience the intervention in ways that were not intended. Capturing these moderating, mediating, and unintended consequences is important to help advance the field of prevention.

Finally, how do we design interventions that are relevant to the circumstances faced by individuals in multiple ecological levels of their community context (e.g., homes, schools, neighbourhoods)? An ecological perspective focuses less on specific programs and more on how interventions are coupled with community contexts (Trickett, 2009; see, e.g., Arthur et al., 2010). For example, attention is focused on the social and cultural context that can affect the implementation of a community intervention. This process necessitates assessing the relevance of existing evidence-based interventions for a particular community or organizational setting and searching for effective ways to mobilize collaborations to agree on a common desired outcome (e.g., improving health and reducing health disparities). How to assess the multiple contexts (social, cultural, gender) and their effects on individuals remains an important area for future study. Trickett (2009) outlines various directions for future research that have relevance to extending knowledge in the field of prevention of weight-related disorders. First, there is a need to delineate effective measures to assess social and/or community settings (e.g., homes, schools, and neighbourhoods). Second, there is a need to assess within-setting processes that describe particular environments (e.g., schools as multi-level settings not captured in classroom-level assessments) and how these processes affect individual behaviour in that setting. Third, research is required to link the varied aspects of the social or community contexts to individual outcomes.

Weight-related disorders carry a heavy burden, socially, psychologically, physically, and economically (Adair et al., 2007). The stress of being stigmatized triggers a maladaptive cycle of poor mental and physical health, which further compromises the uptake of health-promoting behaviours necessary to prevent chronic diseases in the first place (Muennig, 2008). Surprisingly, with some exceptions (Levine & Smolak, 2006, Chapter 9; Maclean et al., 2009), best practice recommendations to incorporate weight discrimination awareness into weight-related prevention efforts have been largely ignored (Puhl & Heuer, 2010). Research is required to identify how best to prepare health professionals to implement evidence-informed decision-making (and practices) that respond to the complex and diverse needs of the community, all the while sensitizing them to multiple factors that can hinder or support the uptake of health-promoting behaviours such as weight bias (Leischow et al., 2008).

A Final Thought on Tension, Challenge, Courage, and Hope

There is no escaping the powerful tensions or frictions that will arise from our conclusions. Under the present systems operating in academia, for instance, how can we define professional achievement in terms of the patient development of effective programs and excellent quantitative and qualitative research? Can the Boulder Model of scientist-practitioner in clinical psychology, along with its parallels in public health, medicine, and dietetics, be transformed to a "bolder model" of the scientist-practitioner-advocate-vocal citizen (Irving, 1999; Levine & Maine, 2010; Maine, 2000)? Can those who are worried by the rising tide of obesity and related health problems find common ground with those who are concerned about the iatrogenic effects of a cultural emphasis on "fear of fat," "drive for thinness," and "undue influence of weight and shape" on self-esteem and social status? Community health problems such as the spectrum of weight-related disorders are often complex in nature and require a comprehensive set of strategies for intervention (Maclean et al., 2009; Perry, 1999). Prevention is a key part of the social, behavioural, and medical sciences—and a strong scientific perspective will need to capture both content and process as they unfold in intersectional and interdisplinary collaborations. With accurate and meaningful data, framed by critical social theories, we will be better equipped to compare spending on intervention versus prevention programming over the long term for the various risky outcomes and health problems we are all concerned about.

References

Adair C. E., McVey, G., deGroot, J., McLaren, L., Gray-Donald, K., Plotnikoff, R., Marcoux, G., & Linder, J. (2007). *Obesity and eating disorders, seeking common ground to promote health: A national meeting of researchers, practitioners, and policymaker.* Discussion document. Retrieved from http://www.ocoped.ca/DNN/PDF/Obesity_eating_disorders_discussion_document_2008.pdf

Arthur, M. W., Hawkins, D., Brown, E. C., Briney, J. S. Oesterle, S., & Abbot, R. D. (2010). Implementation of the Communities That Care prevention system by coalitions in the Community Youth Development Study. *Journal of Community Psychology, 38,* 245-258.

Bordo, S. (1993). *Unbearable weight: Feminism, Western culture, and the body.* Berkeley, CA: University of California Press.

Brown, C., & Jasper, K. (Eds.). (1993). *Consuming passions: Feminist approaches to weight preoccupation and eating disorders.* Toronto: Second Story Press.

Bronfenbrenner, U. (1979). *The ecology of human development: Experiments by nature and design.* Boston: Harvard College.

Bronfenbrenner, U. (2005). *Making human beings human: Bioecological perspectives on human development.* Thousand Oaks, CA: Sage Publications.

Commission on Social Determinants of Health. (2008). *Commission on social determinants of health final report: Closing the gap in a generation: Health equity through action on the social determinants of health.* Geneva: World Health Organization.

Gordon, R. A. (2000). *Eating disorders: Anatomy of a social epidemic* (2nd ed.). Boston: Blackwell Publishers.

Haines, J., & Neumark-Sztainer, D. (2006). Prevention of obesity and eating disorders: A consideration of shared risk factors. *Health Education Research, 21,* 770-782.

Irving, L. (1999). A bolder model of prevention: Science, practice, and activism. In N. Piran, M. P. Levine, & C. Steiner-Adair (Eds.) (1999). *Preventing eating disorders: A handbook of interventions and special challenges* (pp. 63-83). Philadelphia, PA: Brunner/Mazel.

Leishow, S. J., Best, A., Trochim, W. M., Clark, P. I., Gallagher, R. S., Marcus, S. E., & Matthews, E. (2008). Systems thinking to improve the public's health. *American Journal of Preventive Medicine, 35,* s196-s203.

Levine, M. P., & Maine, M. (2010). Are media an important medium for clinicians? Mass media, eating disorders, and the Boulder model of treatment, prevention, and advocacy. In M. Maine, B. H. McGilley, & D. W. Bunnell

(Eds.), *Treatment of eating disorders: Bridging the research-practice gap* (pp. 53-67). New York: Elsevier.

Levine, M. P., & Piran, N. (2004). The role of body image in the prevention of eating disorders. *Body Image, 1,* 57-70.

Levine, M. P., & Smolak, L. (2006). *The prevention of eating problems and eating disorders: Theory, research, and practice.* Mahwah, NJ: Lawrence Erlbaum Associates.

Maclean, L., Edwards, N., Garrard, M., Sims-Jones, N., Clinton, K., & Ashley, L. (2009). Obesity, stigma, and public health planning. *Health Promotion International, 24,* 88-93.

Maine, M. (2000). *Body wars: Making peace with women's bodies. An activist's guide.* Carlsbad, CA: Gürze Books.

McVey, G., Adair, C., deGroot, J., McLaren, L., Plotnikoff, R., Gray-Donald, K., & Collier, S. (2008). *Obesity and eating disorders: Seeking common ground to promote health.* A national meeting of researchers, practitioners and policymakers. Final Report. November 2007. Retrieved from http://www.ocoped .ca/DNN/PDF/Obesity_eating_disorders_2007.pdf

Muennig, P. (2008). The body politic: The relationship between stigma and obesity-associated disease. *BMC Public Health, 8,* 128.

Neumark-Sztainer, D., Wall, M., Guo, J., Story, M., Haines, J., & Eisenberg, M. (2006). Obesity disordered eating, and eating disorders in a longitudinal study of adolescents: How do dieters fare 5 years later? *Journal of the American Dietetic Association, 106,* 559-568.

Orbach, S. (1978). *Fat is a feminist issue II: A program* to conquer compulsive eating. Berkely, CA: Berkley Books.

Perry, C. L. (1999). *Creating health behavior change: How to develop communitywide programs for youth.* Thousand Oaks, CA: Sage.

Piran, N. (1999). The reduction of preoccupation with body weight and shape in schools: A feminist approach. In N. Piran, M. P. Levine, & C. Steiner-Adair (Eds), *Preventing eating disorders: A handbook of interventions and special challenges* (pp. 194-206). Philadelphia, PA: Brunner/Mazel.

Piran, N. (2001a). Re-inhabiting the body: Girls transform their school environment. In D. L. Tolman & M. Brydon-Miller (Eds.), *From subjects to subjectivities: A handbook of interpretive and participatory methods* (pp. 218-238). New York: New York University Press.

Piran, N. (2001b). Reinhabiting the body. *Feminism and Psychology, 11,* 172-176.

Piran, N. (2010a). A feminist perspective on risk factor research and the prevention of eating disorders. *Eating Disorders, 18,* 183-198.

Piran, N. (2010b). *The developmental theory of embodiment.* (Presented at the International Conference of Eating Disorders, Academy of Eating Disorders, Salzburg, Austria).

Puhl, R. M., & Heuer, C. A. (2010). Obesity stigma: Important considerations for public health. *American Journal of Public Health, 100,* 1019-1028.

Smolak, L., & Murnen, S. K. (2004). A feminist approach to eating problems. In J. K. Thompson (Ed.). *Handbook of eating disorders and obesity* (pp. 590-605). Hoboken, NJ: Wiley and Sons.

Steiner-Adair, C. (1994). The politics of prevention. In P. Fallon, M. A. Katzman, & S. Wooley (Eds.), *Feminist perspectives on eating disorders* (pp. 381-394). New York: Guilford Press.

Striegel-Moore, R. H., & Steiner-Adair, C. (1998). Primary prevention of eating disorders: Further considerations from a feminist perspective. In W. Vandereycken & G. Noordenbos (Eds.), *The prevention of eating disorders* (pp. 1-22). London: Athlone.

Trickett, E. J. (2009). Community psychology: Individuals and interventions in community context. *Annual Review of Psychology, 60,* 195-419.

The Contributors

Gail L. McVey, Ph.D., C.Psych, is a Health Systems Research Scientist and Psychologist in the Community Health Systems Resource Group at the Hospital for Sick Children, Associate Professor in the Dalla Lana School of Public Health at the University of Toronto, and Director of the Ontario Community Outreach Program for Eating Disorders. Her research is focused on the prevention of disordered eating and the promotion of wellness in children and youth. She is currently leading a Canadian National Prevention Knowledge Exchange Group with stakeholders from research, practice, and policy to investigate ways to align prevention efforts across the fields of eating disorders and obesity. Dr. McVey has been honoured for her leadership and advocacy work in the area of eating disorders.

Michael P. Levine, Ph.D., FAED, is Emeritus Professor of Psychology at Kenyon College in Gambier, Ohio, where he taught 33 years. He has authored two books on eating disorders and two prevention curriculum guides, and he has co-edited three books on prevention. Dr. Levine is a Fellow of the Academy for Eating Disorders, which has awarded him their Meehan-Hartley Award for Leadership in Public Awareness and Advocacy and, recently, their Research-Practice Partnership Award.

Niva Piran, Ph.D., C. Psych., FAED, is a Professor at the Ontario Institute for Studies in Education at the University of Toronto. Dr. Piran is co-editor of *A Day Hospital Group Treatment Program for Anorexia Nervosa and Bulimia Nervosa* (with Kaplan) and *Preventing Eating Disorders: A Handbook of Interventions and Special Challenges* (with Levine and Steiner-Adair). She is a Fellow of the Academy for Eating Disorders and the Prevention Editor of the *Eating Disorders* journal. Dr. Piran is internationally recognized for her innovative work on body image development, as well as the prevention and treatment of eating disorders. She is the recipient of mentorship and research awards, and her research is supported by the Social Sciences and Humanities Research Council of Canada.

H. Bruce Ferguson, Ph.D., C.Psych., is the Director of the Community Health Systems Resource Group at the Hospital for Sick Children and a Professor in the Departments of Psychiatry and Psychology and the Dalla Lana School of Public Health at the University of Toronto. Dr. Ferguson works to build networks and improve systems of care and support for children and families. He created the Community Health Systems Resource Group in an effort to advocate for the implementation of evidence-based interventions and standardized outcome measurement in health, mental health, social services, and education, and to promote and facilitate integration and collaboration in service delivery. He has been honoured by many organizations for his leadership in child and youth mental health. His vision is to promote success in children and youth by considering all factors essential to well-being including health, home life, school, community life, and peer relationships.

Carol E. Adair, Ph.D., is Adjunct Associate Professor in the Departments of Psychiatry and Community Health Sciences and the Institute for Public Health at the University of Calgary. Her research is in the fields of psychiatric epidemiology and mental health services research, especially health services outcomes measurement.

Janet deGroot, M.D., FRCP, is Associate Dean, Equity and Professionalism, at the University of Calgary, Faculty of Medicine, and an Associate Professor in the Departments of Psychiatry and Oncology at University of Calgary.

Manuela Ferrari, Ph.D., recently completed her doctoral studies at the Dalla Lana School of Public Health, at the University of Toronto. Her dissertation, entitled Beyond Obesity and Disordered Eating in Youth (BODY), is a qualitative study that sheds light on the different meanings that individuals attribute to the spectrum of weight-related problems. Academically, Dr. Ferrari is interested in understanding the relationship between gender, body size, and weight in relation to prevention and medical practices. At a scholarly level, Dr. Ferrari has produced several important peer-reviewed publications and presented her work at national and international conferences. She was awarded the Enid Walker Graduate Student Award in Women's Health (2008–2012) from the Women's College Hospital Research Institute in Toronto. Dr. Ferrari's contributions to the academic community have earned her the David Hewitt Award and the Gordon Cressy Student Leadership Award.

Joe Kelly, B.Sc., is a Fathering Educator in Emeryville, California. He reports and writes about responsible fathering, girls' issues, and marketing to children. Formerly the fathering educator for The Emily Program in Minnesota, he teaches professionals how to engage and utilize men in families as allies in their work. He is also an eating disorders activist and co-founder of New Moon Girl Media. Kelly's books include *Dads & Daughters: How to Inspire, Support, and Understand Your Daughter* and (with Margo Maine) *The Body Myth: Adult Women and the Pressure to Be Perfect.* His www.The DadMan.com and www.MenInFamilies.com provide resources for fathers, families, and professionals.

Lindsay McLaren, Ph.D., is an Associate Professor and Alberta Innovates — Health Solutions Population Health Investigator in the Department of Community Health Sciences and the Institute for Public Health at the University of Calgary. Her research is focused on population health and social inequalities in health where these apply to a range of health issues, including obesity and body image.

Susan J. Paxton, Ph.D., is Professor in the School of Psychological Science at La Trobe University, Melbourne. She has a particular interest in the development and evaluation of school-based and community prevention for body image and eating problems. Susan was President of the Academy of Eating Disorders in 2009 and a member of the Body Image Advisory Group, which from 2009 to 2011 advised the Australian Federal Minister for Youth on prevention issues.

Leora Pinhas, M.D., FRCP, is a psychiatrist at SickKids Hospital, an Assistant Professor in the Department of Psychiatry at the University of Toronto, and the founding member of the Eating Disorders Association of Canada. Her research interests include the diagnosis and treatment of eating disorders and obesity in children and adolescents. She is the co-editor of the book *Help for Eating Disorders: A Parent's Guide to Symptoms, Causes and Treatments* (2005). She is currently working on her Ph.D. in Epidemiology.

Shelly Russell-Mayhew, Ph.D., is an Associate Professor and Registered Psychologist in Educational Studies in Psychology, Faculty of Education, at the University of Calgary. Her research is focused on the prevention of weight-related disorders and the promotion of healthy body image.

Linda Smolak, Ph.D., is Emerita Professor of Psychology at Kenyon College in Gambier, Ohio, where she has taught for 32 years. Dr. Smolak's research focuses on body image and eating problems in boys and girls. Her work emphasizes developmental contributors to body image and body change strategies. She is also working on research that examines the place of gender role in the development of body image and eating problems.

Benjamin J. Taylor completed his Ph.D. in epidemiology at the Dalla Lana School of Public Health in Toronto. He has published extensively in the area of substance use and health outcomes. He has also consulted to the World Health Organization, the Pan American Health Organization, and various public health agencies through his work at the Centre for Addictions and Mental health

Tanya Teall is completing her Ph.D. in Counselling Psychology at the Ontario Institute for Studies in Education of the University of Toronto. Her clinical training has focused on women's health, primarily in the areas of eating disorders, trauma, and borderline personality disorder. Her research interests, under the supervision of Dr. Piran, have primarily involved a quantitative testing of the Developmental Theory of Embodiment and the construction of the Embodiment Scale for Women.

Index